T0226154

The Prevention
and Management
of Violence

Second Edition

The Prevention and Management of Violence

Guidance for Mental Healthcare Professionals

Second Edition

Edited by

Masum Khwaja
Consultant Psychiatrist, West End Primary Care Network, London

Peter Tyrer
Imperial College, London

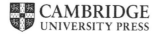
CAMBRIDGE
UNIVERSITY PRESS

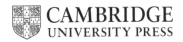

Shaftesbury Road, Cambridge CB2 8EA, United Kingdom

One Liberty Plaza, 20th Floor, New York, NY 10006, USA

477 Williamstown Road, Port Melbourne, VIC 3207, Australia

314–321, 3rd Floor, Plot 3, Splendor Forum, Jasola District Centre, New Delhi – 110025, India

103 Penang Road, #05–06/07, Visioncrest Commercial, Singapore 238467

Cambridge University Press is part of Cambridge University Press & Assessment, a department of the University of Cambridge.

We share the University's mission to contribute to society through the pursuit of education, learning and research at the highest international levels of excellence.

www.cambridge.org
Information on this title: www.cambridge.org/9781911623267

DOI: 10.1017/9781911623274

First published 2013
Second edition 2023

A catalogue record for this publication is available from the British Library.

A Cataloging-in-Publication data record for this book is available from the Library of Congress.

ISBN 978-1-911-62326-7 Paperback

Cambridge University Press & Assessment has no responsibility for the persistence or accuracy of URLs for external or third-party internet websites referred to in this publication and does not guarantee that any content on such websites is, or will remain, accurate or appropriate.

Every effort has been made in preparing this book to provide accurate and up-to-date information that is in accord with accepted standards and practice at the time of publication. Although case histories are drawn from actual cases, every effort has been made to disguise the identities of the individuals involved. Nevertheless, the authors, editors, and publishers can make no warranties that the information contained herein is totally free from error, not least because clinical standards are constantly changing through research and regulation. The authors, editors, and publishers therefore disclaim all liability for direct or consequential damages resulting from the use of material contained in this book. Readers are strongly advised to pay careful attention to information provided by the manufacturer of any drugs or equipment that they plan to use.

Dedicated to the memory of my parents, Abida Mohsin and Anwer Bey Khwaja

Contents

Contributors

Dr Saima Ali, BSc (Hons) MBChB MRCPsych
Specialist Trainee in Forensic Psychiatry, West London NHS Trust, London

Dr Shaazneen Ali
Consultant Psychiatrist and Sleep Specialist, Royal London Hospital for Integrated Medicine, University College London Hospitals NHS Foundation Trust

Dr Alina Bakala
Consultant Psychiatrist in Intellectual Disability, Central and North West London NHS Foundation Trust, Hammersmith & Fulham Learning Disability Service

Dr Shanika Balachandra
Consultant Psychiatrist, Shannon Ward Psychiatric Intensive Care Unit, St Charles Hospital; Deputy Director of Operations, National Association of Psychiatric Intensive Care and Low Secure Units (NAPICU)

Dr Miriam Barrett
Consultant Psychiatrist in Psychotherapy, Cassel Specialist Personality Disorder Service, West London NHS trust, London

Eric Baskind
Visiting Research Fellow, Oxford Brookes University; Chair, SWC Experts Group

Anthony Beschizza
Assistant Director, Mental Health Law, Health and Safety, Emergency Planning and Business Continuity, Central and North West London NHS Foundation Trust

Dr Ingrid Bohnen
Consultant Psychiatrist in Intellectual Disability, Central and North West London NHS Foundation Trust,

Westminster Learning Disability Health Partnership

Dr Juliette Brown
Consultant Psychiatrist, Older Adults: East London NHS Foundation Trust; Honorary Clinical Senior Lecturer in the Centre for Psychiatry, Wolfson Institute of Preventative Medicine, Queen Mary University of London

Dr Elliott Carthy
Specialist Registrar in Forensic Psychiatry, Oxford Health NHS Foundation Trust, Warneford Hospital, Oxford

Dr Maria Clarke
Honorary Consultant Psychiatrist, Central and North West London NHS Foundation Trust and retired Honorary Clinical Senior Lecturer, Imperial College, London

David Cochrane
Head of Forensic Social Work, West London NHS Trust

Hannah Crisford
Clinical Psychologist, Cornwall Partnership NHS Foundation Trust

Kate Crosby
Service User Trainer, Middlesex University, London

Sarah Devereux
Psychotherapist, The Bowlby Centre, London

Dr Dominic Dougall
Clinical Director, Newham Adult Mental Health Directorate, Newham Centre for Mental Health, London

Dr Joanna Dow
Formerly Consultant Forensic Psychiatrist, West London NHS Trust, London

Professor Andrew Forrester
Professor of Forensic Psychiatry, Cardiff University

Dr Heidi Hales
Consultant Adolescent Forensic Psychiatrist and Medical Lead for Community Forensic Services, North West London F-CAMHS

Dr Bradley Hillier
Consultant Forensic Psychiatrist, West London NHS Trust, London

Dr. Laura Humphries
Consultant Psychiatrist, East London NHS Foundation Trust, London

Dr Ryan Kemp
Consultant Psychologist, Director of Therapies, Central & North West London NHS Foundation Trust, London, and Honorary Professor of Clinical Practice Brunel University, London

Tim Kendall
National Clinical Director for Mental Health NHS England; Consultant Psychiatrist for Homeless Mental Health and Medical Director (Research), Sheffield Health and Social Care NHS Foundation Trust; Honorary Professor, University of Sheffield

Dr Masum Khwaja
Consultant Psychiatrist, West End Primary Care Network, Central and North West London NHS Foundation Trust; Chair of the London S12(2) MHA and Approved Clinician Approval Panel and retired Honorary Clinical Senior Lecturer, Imperial College, London

Dr Gabriel Kirtchuk (deceased)
Former Consultant Psychiatrist in Psychotherapy (Forensic) and a Fellow of the British Psychoanalytical Society

Sue Mcdonnell
Former RMN, Service Manager (retired), Kensington & Chelsea Mental Health Service, St Charles MHU, London

Susan McGinnis
Course Coordinator, Certificate in Counselling Children and Young People, Counselling Unit, University of Strathclyde

Dr Mary Moss
Formerly PICU Consultant (retired), Sussex Partnership NHS Foundation Trust

Dr Chan Nyein
Consultant Psychiatrist, Central and North West London NHS Foundation Trust

Dr Rachel O'Beney
Consultant Clinical Psychologist, Operational lead for Westminster Psychology, Westminster Community Mental Health Hub, Central and North West London NHS Foundation Trust, London

Dr Jane Obi-Udeaja, DProf
Physical intervention trainer, Middlesex University, London

Caroline Parker
Lead Pharmacist Community Mental Health Teams, Gloucestershire Health & Care NHS Foundation Trust. Pharmacy Department, Gloucestershire Royal Hospital, Gloucester

Dr Sachin Patel
Consultant Liaison Psychiatrist, Hammersmith & Fulham Liaison Psychiatry Service, West London NHS Trust and Honorary Consultant Psychiatrist at Imperial College Healthcare NHS Trust

Peter Pratt, Bsc Mphil(Dist) FRPharmS FCMHP
National Specialty Advisor, Mental Health Pharmacy, NHS England

Dr Mehtab Ghazi Rahman
Consultant Psychiatrist, Nile Ward
Psychiatric Intensive Care Unit, St Charles
Hospital; Trust-wide Physical Health Lead
in Mental Health Services, Central and
North West London NHS Foundation
Trust, London

Dr Louise Robinson
Consultant and Honorary Senior Lecturer
in Forensic Psychiatry, Lancashire and
South Cumbria NHS Foundation Trust and
University of Manchester

Garry Ryan
Service User Trainer, Middlesex University,
London

Dr Celia Sadie
Honorary Consultant Clinical
Psychologist, Health and Justice Services
Directorate, Central and North West
London NHS Foundation Trust

Dr Joanna Sales
Consultant Child and Adolescent
Psychiatrist, HMYOI Cookham Wood,
Kent

Dr Laura Steckley, PhD
Senior Lecturer, School of Social Work and
Social Policy/CELCIS, University of
Strathclyde

Dr Alexis Theodorou
Specialist Trainee in Forensic Psychiatry
and Medical Psychotherapy, West London
NHS Trust and Tavistock and Portman

NHS Foundation Trust, London and
Honorary Research Fellow, Cardiff
University

Dr Alex Thomson
Consultant Liaison Psychiatrist, Central
and North West London NHS Foundation
Trust, London

Peter Tyrer
Emeritus Professor of Community
Psychiatry, Imperial College, London;
Consultant in Transformation Psychiatry,
Lincolnshire Partnership NHS Foundation
Trust

Emma Valentine
Team Manager, Hammersmith and
Fulham Liaison Psychiatry Service, London

Jonathan Waite
Locum Consultant Liaison Psychiatrist for
Older People: Nottinghamshire Healthcare
NHS Foundation Trust; Honorary Senior
Fellow: Institute of Mental Health,
University of Nottingham

Anusha Wijeratne
Consultant Psychiatrist, Central and North
West London NHS Foundation Trust, The
Kingswood Centre Learning Disabilities
Service, London

Dr Mervyn Yong, MBBS MRCPsych
ST6 in Psychiatry of Intellectual Disability,
Camden and Islington NHS Foundation
Trust, Camden Learning Disability Service,
London

Preface

Since the first edition of this book, also published as the Royal College of Psychiatrists College Report CR177, in 2013, violence has become even more relevant to all mental health professionals in their daily lives.

The illustration on the cover of the first edition is of two chess pieces, a pawn and a queen, on a standard squared board. The metaphor of the chess board and its pieces can be extended greatly in this second edition. As in chess, the effective management and prevention of violence requires concentration; knowledge; pattern recognition; planning; confident, calm decision-making under pressure; and an overall strategy based on a knowledge of the best 'move' in each scenario.

Each potentially violent situation is different; it needs a rapid assessment of the setting and the options available, and no book can ever give a complete account. In the second edition we take the reader through all the options, but we have tried to organise the process systematically into sections so that everything fits neatly. At the same time, we are conscious that many professionals may need advice in only one area (e.g. intellectual disability, safeguarding) and need to consult only one chapter when faced with a problem. We have therefore tried to allow each chapter to stand alone as well as having links to the others.

The first five chapters are relevant to every reader. Guidelines to manage violence are still haphazard and contradictory, and Eric Baskind (Chapter 1) makes a sound case for a common approach across all settings. The legislation of mental illness (Chapter 2), always changing but never seemingly fit for purpose, then as in chess, sets the rules of engagement. Protecting vulnerable adults and children exposed to violence (Chapter 3) is an essential part of clinical practice and the safeguarding chapter has been significantly developed from the first edition version to reflect this. The additional expectations of NHS services in dealing with violence (Chapter 4) are developed further in the advice from the National Institute for Health and Care Excellence (better known as NICE) and, like opening strategies in chess, have particular value in managing the early stages of a likely violent incident. After an incident of violence there should be a post-incident review (Chapter 5), and here, the equivalent of engine analysis after a game of chess, teams may often fail to prevent repeat violent episodes if they do not pick up on previous mistakes.

The pharmacological and psychological treatments are comprehensively covered in Chapters 6 and 7; we have most evidence of efficacy for the former, but it is also the most contentious. The final chapter in this section (Chapter 8) provides a useful summary of how to prevent and manage violence in inpatient settings.

Chapters 9 to 12 cover the management of violence in different settings and, as statistics show that the incidence of violence is increasing everywhere and management is not always coherent, it is clear that Baskind's wish for a common guideline is a cogent one. Violence in prisons is a serious concern, made worse by Penrose's Law – as the number of psychiatric inpatients declines, the number of prisoners increases [1] – which is probably even more true today; Robinson and Forrester (Chapter 12) make a strong case for urgent reform. It is paradoxical that some lessons can be learnt from the COVID-19 pandemic as violence has unexpectedly been reduced in these settings as a consequence of changes forced on prisons by the virus.

To illustrate the comprehensive cover of the subject, Section 4 has chapters on the management of violence in different groups and opens with discussions on violence in children (Chapter 13) and in older adults (Chapter 14). The management of violence in those with intellectual disability is one of the biggest challenges in psychiatry and is addressed in Chapter 15. The final chapter in this section explores mental health inequality in the Black, Asian and minority ethnic communities (Chapter 16)and explains why assessing the impact of discrimination, using our chess metaphor, is as complicated as evaluating the strategic value of a black or white piece in a game of chess when there are material imbalances between the players.

Section 5 of the book covers the criminal and youth justice liaison and diversion systems (Chapter 17) and has extended chapters, compared to the first edition, on information-sharing and on the victims of violence (Chapters 18 and 19). In the past, victims of violence were often forgotten about. Some became perpetrators of violence too, and in trying to help both we can be stymied, rather like the position of stalemate in chess that prevents either from winning. Increasingly, we are recognising the needs of victims with better understanding and support; the latter rounded chapters of the final section of the book, showing the value of consulting/learning from service users including in the training of staff, present an optimistic way forward (Chapters 20 and 21).

By the end of the book we hope the reader will have proceeded like Alice in *Through the Looking Glass*: from being a pawn in the second row at the beginning of a game of chess to a superior position further down the board of violence prevention. An exceptionally diligent student may have even come to the end of the board and become a queen. This may appear to be an extravagant joke, but it is not. We all know people who have amazing skills in defusing violence; learning from them and this book should make us all better practitioners in this key part of psychiatry.

References

1. Penrose, L. S. Mental disease and crime: outline of a comparative study of European statistics. *British Journal of Medical Psychology* 1939; 18:1–15.

Abbreviations

A&E	Accident and Emergency
AA	appropriate adult
AAT	animal-assisted therapy
ABD	acute behavioural disturbance
ACR	age of criminal responsibility
ACT	Assertive Community Treatment
ADHD	Attention-Deficit/Hyperactivity Disorder
AMCP	approved mental capacity professionals
AMHE	advancing mental health equality
AMHP	approved mental health professional
ART	aggression replacement therapy
ASD	Autism Spectrum Disorder
ATR	alcohol treatment requirement
BAME	Black, Asian and minority ethnic
BAP	The British Association for Psychopharmacology
BAWSO	Black Association of Women Step Out
BBC	British Broadcasting Corporation
BIA	best interest assessors
BILD	British Institute of Learning Disabilities
BLM	Black Lives Matter
BMJ	British Medical Journal
BNF	British National Formulary
BPSD	behavioural and psychiatric symptoms of dementia
BRAVE	Better Reduction through Assessment of Violence and Evaluation
CAMHS	child and adolescent mental health services
CBT	cognitive behavioural therapy
CCGs	clinical commissioning groups
CCQI	College Centre for Quality Improvement
CDR	conditional discharge report
CEDAR	Children Experiencing Domestic Abuse Recovery
CFT	community forensic team
CHAT	comprehensive health assessment tool
CICA	Criminal Injuries Compensation Authority
CJS	criminal justice system
CMHT	community mental health team
CNWL NHS FT	Central and North West London NHS Foundation Trust
COVID-19	Coronavirus disease 2019
CPA	Care Programme Approach
CPS	Crown Prosecution Service
CPT	European Committee for the Prevention of Torture and Inhuman or Degrading Treatment or Punishment
CQC	Care Quality Commission

CROMs	clinician rated outcome measures
CSIP model	challenge support and intervention plan
CSPF	clinical secure practice forum
CSPs	community safety partnerships
CSRA	cell-sharing risk assessment
CTO	community treatment order
CYP	child or young person
DABS	directory and book services
DBT	dialectical behaviour therapy
DoH	Department of Health
DoLS	deprivation of liberty safeguards
DRR	drug rehabilitation requirement
DVCA	Domestic Violence, Crime and Victims Act
E&W	England and Wales
ECG	electrocardiogram
ECHR	European Court of Human Rights
ECT	electroconvulsive therapy
ED	emergency department
EPS	extrapyramidal side effects
ExD	excited delirium
FACT	flexible assertive community treatment
FAIV	framework for assessment and intervention
F-CAMHS	forensic child and adolescent mental health services
FFT	functional family therapy
FME	forensic medical examiner
GDPR	general data protection regulations
GMC	General Medical Council
GP	general practitioner
GSA	general services association
HBPoS	health-based place of safety
HCR-20	historical, clinical, risk management
HMIP	His Majesty's Inspectorate of Prisons
HMPPS	His Majesty's Prison and Probation Service
HoNOS	health of the nation outcome scales
HSCIC	Health and Social Care Information Centre
HSE	Health and Safety Executive
IAPT	improving access to psychological therapies
ICS	integrated care systems
ID	intellectual disability
IM	intramuscular
IPP	imprisonment for public protection
IRC	immigration removal centre
IRIS	identification and referral to improve safety
IV	intravenous
IVDA	Independent Domestic Violence Advisors
JWA	Jewish Women's Aid
KPIs	key performance indicators

L&D	liaison and diversion
LARA–VP	Linking Abuse and Recovery through Advocacy (for Victims and Perpetrators)
LD	learning disability
LGBTQ+	Lesbian, gay, bisexual, transgender, queer or questioning and other identities
LPS	liberty protection safeguard scheme
LPT	Leicestershire Partnership NHS Trust
MAC-UK	Music and Change – United Kingdom
MAPPA	multi-agency public protection arrangements
MARAC	Multi-Agency Risk Assessment Conference
MASH	multi-agency safeguarding hub
MBT	mentalisation-based therapy
MCA	Mental Capacity Act
MDFT	multi-dimensional family therapy
MDOs	mentally disordered offenders
MDT	Multidisciplinary team
MHA 1983	Mental Health Act 1983
MHCS	mental health casework section
MHRA	Medicines and Healthcare Products Regulatory Agency
MHT	mental health tribunals
MHTR	mental health treatment requirement
MoJ	Ministry of Justice
MOPAC	Mayor's Office of Policing and Crime
MoU	memorandum of understanding
MPGP	Maudsley Prescribing Guidelines in Psychiatry
MST	multisystemic therapy
NAPAC	National Association for People Abused in Childhood
NAPICU	National Association of Psychiatric Intensive Care and Low Secure Units
NatSCEV	National Survey of Children's Exposure to Violence
NCCMH	National Collaborating Centre for Mental Health
NFA	no further action
NGRI	not guilty by reason of insanity
NHS	National Health Service
NHSE	NHS England
NICE	National Institute for Health and Care Excellence
NMC	Nursing and Midwifery Council
NOG	national oversight group
NPS	novel psychoactive substances
NPSU	novel psychoactive substances users
NRM	national referral mechanism
NSPCC	National Society for the Prevention of Cruelty to Children
NVR	non-violent resistance
OASys	offender assessment system
OCF	organisational competence framework
OM	offender manager

OPD	offender personality disorder
PACE	Police and Criminal Evidence Act 1984
PALS	Patient advice and liaison service
PCCs	Police and Crime Commissioners
PCL-R	Hare Psychopathy Checklist – Revised
PCN	primary care network
PCREF	patient and carers race equalities framework
PICU	psychiatric intensive care
PMVA	prevention and management of violence and aggression
PO	oral route
PPG	penile plethysmograph(y)
PRN	pro re nata (when required)
PROMs	patient-related outcome measures
PR	physical restraint
PRU	pupil referral network
PS	probation service
PTSD	post-traumatic stress disorder
QI	quality improvement
QIP	quality improvement projects
QNFMHS	Quality Network for Forensic Mental Health Services
RAID	Reinforce Appropriate, Implode Disruptive
RAR	rehabilitation activity requirement
RC	responsible clinician
RCN	Royal College of Nursing
RCPsych	Royal College of Psychiatrists
RIDDOR	Reporting of Injuries, Diseases and Dangerous Occurrences Regulations 2013
RJC	Restorative Justice Council
RMN	registered mental health nurse
RRN	restraint reduction network
RT	Rapid tranquillisation
RUI	released under investigation
SARCs	sexual assault referral centres
SCFT	specialist community forensic team
SCIE	Social Care Institute for Excellence
SCM	structured clinical management
SDVC	specialist domestic violence courts
SIGN	Scottish Intercollegiate Guidelines Network
SMI	severe mental illness
SOAD	second opinion appointed doctor
SPOC	nominated single point of contact
SSC	sexual safety collaborative
STAMP	supporting treatment and appropriate medication in paediatrics
STC	secure training centre
STOMP	stopping over-medication of people with an intellectual disability, autism or both
SWC	safety without compromise

TREC	Tranquilização RápidaEnsaio Clínico (Rapid Tranquillisation Clinical Trial)
TULIPS	Talk, Understand, Listen for In-Patient Settings
UN	United Nations
UNCRC	United Nations Convention on the Rights of the Child
VCS	Victim Contact Scheme
VLO	victim liaison officer
VLP	victim liaison protocol
VP	vulnerable prisoners
WEMSS	women's enhanced medium secure service
WHA	World Health Assembly
WHO	World Health Organisation
YJLD	Youth Justice Liaison and Diversion
YOI	young offenders' institution
YOS	youth offending service
YOT	youth offending team

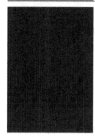

Section Introductions

Section 1: General Advice and Recommendations

This section sets the tone for the rest of this book. The management of the threat of violence is a highly individual matter that cannot be decided unilaterally by any official guidance. But all management requires a framework within which practitioners have to work, only going outside it under exceptional circumstances. In Chapter 1, Eric Baskind makes a bold attempt to bring all together with the suggestion of a common set of guidelines, as violence can show itself, often Medusa-like in its sudden venom, in every possible setting. So, it is wise to have a common policy of management. But we are not there yet, and Chapter 2 tells us exactly where we are at present in terms of legislation, a subject that changes often and which depends on the locality. This is an excellent aide-memoire to those who organise management programmes and need to ensure that they are both legal and justified.

Chapter 3 explores the hinterland of violence, the territory where the effects of violence or its threat can affect others of all ages. Safeguarding is an essential element here; we may not be able to prevent all violence but good safeguarding can nullify its effects.

Chapter 4 describes the advice given by the National Institute for Health and Clinical Excellence (NICE), which requires all services to follow in England and Wales but with some modifications in Scotland and Northern Ireland. It also includes a section on risk and its management, one of the most difficult subjects in the study of violence, as so much of risk is dependent on individual circumstances that cannot be anticipated. Standard assessments of risk are suspect and we need more dynamic assessments that do not just rely on often distant past behaviour.

The last part of this section (Chapter 5) describes what should take place in a service after a significant incident of violence. Post-incident review of a violent episode is an essential part of management, not a luxury to be taken on at some distant point in the future when time permits, as almost invariably such reviews show what might have been done differently to either prevent or minimise the violent episode. Lessons are always learnt from a good post-incident review; it can be a powerful brake on repetition.

The Need for a Common Set of Guidelines

Eric Baskind

Violence and aggression never present themselves in a vacuum, yet this is typically the way policymakers approach the subject, its prevention and its management. Although guidelines exist in different sectors, apart from a few common messages, too often little or no consideration is given to many of the wider issues in play, particularly the use of restraint whenever it becomes necessary.

Numerous commentators have described the harm that can result from restraint. It has been described as inherently dangerous [1] and, even if used appropriately, can result in physiological and/or physical harm [2]. Restraint can be *'humiliating, terrifying and even life-threatening'* [3; emphasis added]. Accordingly, with the exception of acting in self-defence, the use of physical interventions should be based on a careful assessment that it will cause less harm than not intervening.

Because the risk of serious harm is greater the longer the restraint is applied, it is generally accepted that the safest way of bringing a violent person under control is rapid initial restraint, carried out by those who have had proper training [4, 5]. Any suggestion that such an approach to gaining control is excessive is misconceived because the use of forceful restraint is only needed in cases of significant violence: minor incidents should not need any forceful restraint and, in most cases, require no physical intervention at all. When considering the question of safety, it is important to consider the safety of all parties: an intervention that reduces risk for patients but places staff and others at risk is undesirable and detrimental to the overall safety and efficient management of the service.

In comparison to other settings, the use of restrictive interventions in healthcare services is highly regulated, and rightly so. For example, in the United Kingdom, the National Institute of Health and Care Excellence (NICE) Guideline NG10, 'Violence and aggression: Short-term management in mental health, health and community settings', aims 'to safeguard both staff and people who use services by helping to prevent violent situations and providing guidance to manage them safely when they occur'. Since April 2021, certification of training services has been a requirement for certain NHS-commissioned services, and the Care Quality Commission (CQC) will expect regulated services to use certified training [6].

The call for the regulating and accrediting of the use of physical interventions is not new and in recent years has become more vocal. At the 2013 Royal College of Nursing (RCN) Annual Congress, the motion 'That this meeting of RCN Congress asks Council to lobby UK governments to review, accredit and then regulate national guidelines of approved models of physical restraint' was passed by 99.8% of delegates.

For any common guidelines to be beneficial they need to be universally adopted, and this requires the broad support of those who will be affected by them, including staff and the users of the services. They also need to take account of the best available evidence. There are many examples where the evidence has not been followed, leading to confusion and uncertainty. A good example of this confusion concerns the so-called banning of prone restraint and pain-compliance interventions, as well as the curious antipathy towards mechanical restraining devices, even in circumstances where these kinds of intervention might be the safest and least restrictive methods, taking into account all the circumstances of an incident.

The Winterbourne View scandal [7] brought the question of prone restraint into public focus. Despite Winterbourne being principally about the abuse of its vulnerable residents rather than restraint per se, the subsequent serious case review made the following recommendation in relation to restraint positions: 'The Department of Health, Department for Education and the Care Quality Commission should consider banning the t-supine restraint of adults with learning disabilities and autism in hospitals and assessment and treatment units' [7, p. 135]. T-supine restraint is a face-up position and is defined in the report as 'restraint that results in people being placed on the ground with staff using their body weight to subdue them' [7, p. xi].

Just how a recommendation to *consider* banning a kind of supine restraint led to an attempt to ban prone restraint remains debatable, yet provides further evidence of the confusion amongst policymakers. Yet further confusion can be seen in the backtracking of the policy to ban positions of prone restraint in subsequent guidelines, policies and announcements, with the Department of Health stating that what people considered to be a ban was no more than guidance. Widespread (but by no means universal) concern was expressed by practitioners as to this so-called ban, and it was pointed out that in many cases, especially those involving extreme levels of violence, trying to restrain the subject in a position other than prone is often unsafe, unpredictable and, in many cases, impossible.

To some extent, the United Kingdom's NHS Protect (now disbanded) clarified the position on prone restraint positions following a consultation with the Department of Health and the Health and Safety Executive. It concluded that it was 'not acceptable for restrictive interventions, such as face-down restraint, to have become normalised' but there 'may be exceptional circumstances where prone restraint will happen'. It acknowledged that 'on rare occasions, face-down restraint may be the safest option for staff and service users, with few, if any, viable alternatives'. It concluded by pointing out that 'if Boards decide that they need staff to be trained in prone restraints it is vital that they are trained in the risks and appropriate techniques' [8].

These clarifications met with the approval of many practitioners, but those against the use of prone restraints were unmoved in their views that they should be banned, with some forbidding their use in their own services. Regrettably, this has led to the use of prone restraint being unreported in some services.

However, just one month later, NICE Guideline NG10 [9] declared a preference for supine positions over prone positions (para. 6.5.1). NICE NG10 recommended that for manual restraint, staff should avoid taking the service user to the floor, but if this becomes necessary they should use the supine position where possible; if the prone position is deemed necessary, it should be used for as short a time as possible (paras. 6.6.3.8 and 8.4.5.2).

Furthermore, the Welsh Assembly Government clarified their position on the use of prone restraints by advising practitioners that they should 'continue to use their professional judgement to determine whether use of a particular restraint technique is an appropriate response to a given situation' [10].

Smallridge and Williamson [11] carried out a comprehensive review of restraint in juvenile secure settings. They concluded that

> Some, but not all, prone restraint positions have a significant effect on breathing. It is clear that recommendations given previously, either to consider all prone restraint as dangerous or to consider prone restraint as presenting no additional risk, are not supported by empirical results ... We are aware that the secure estate is looking to us for guidance on prone restraint. But there are no simple answers. We are wary of over-simplification over prone restraint and are cautious on the issue. Where a young person is held face down with pressure only on the limbs the evidence is that there is likely to be only a small effect on lung function, and in these cases prone may be quite safe for most young people, for most of the time. However, more 'forced' prone restraint, when body weight is applied to the back or hips may be unsafe for almost everyone. In the light of the competing evidence we feel that we cannot make any recommendation to ban prone restraint, but we consider it prudent that when prone restraint is used there should be a re-assessment of the risks after control has been obtained in the initial restraint. There should be procedures in place to ensure that a senior member of staff responds to the incident, assesses the situation, evaluates the competing risks and implements an alternative to prone if safety demands. (paras. 6.34 and 6.35)

Another example where the evidence has not been followed concerns the issue commonly referred to as 'prolonged restraint'. The longer a person is held in restraint, especially on the ground, the greater the risk of harm, including the risk of death. A question that is often asked is whether there is a maximum period of time for which it is considered safe to maintain restraint. Since it is known that death can occur extremely quickly this question must be answered in the negative. Despite this, several attempts have been made to prescribe such a time limit, the latest being NICE Guideline NG10 [9] which advises practitioners that manual restraint should not routinely be used for more than ten minutes (para. 6.6.3.13). This guidance was provided despite the earlier Bennett Inquiry recommendation that a person should not be restrained in a prone position for more than three minutes [4] being rejected by the profession as misleading and unworkable.

The confusion around these issues is manifest. It is also damaging, for the reason given at the beginning of this chapter: namely, that violence and aggression never present themselves in a vacuum. The reluctance of some staff to intervene in an incident is understandable when there is so much confusion about how they should intervene, and with the real prospect of sanctions if their response fails to follow policy, yet at the same time suspecting that adhering to policy could place themselves and patients at risk. With that in mind, it might be thought that a policymaker seeking to ban a particular intervention would have alternatives in mind, but policymakers have consistently stated that alternative interventions are not matters for them. This leaves a wholly unacceptable vacuum which is regrettably all too often filled by the police, who work to an entirely different set of standards to those that operate within healthcare settings. Not only are police officers not constrained by the prohibitions referred to earlier, they are also trained in techniques that healthcare staff would not wish to see used on patients. The answer must be to provide those within healthcare settings with appropriate training to increase the organisation's capacity and capability to deal with potentially violent situations without recourse to external agencies.

Effective training will enable staff to be more self-sufficient so as to minimise requests for police attendance [12]. This was the approach taken in the memorandum of understanding (MoU) made between a number of parties, including the RCN, the Royal College of Psychiatrists and the College of Policing [12]. The aim of the MoU was to provide clarity on the role of the police service in responding to incidents, with the intention of outlining when and how the responsibilities of the police service fit in to the established roles and responsibilities of care providers.

Much of the debate about common standards concentrates on the type of individual interventions used by different organisations, which are often influenced by trainer choice. The choice of intervention ought to be secondary to, and informed by, principles and guidelines. Before considering these principles, it is important to emphasise that in all cases there needs to be a shift in focus from the reactive and limited approaches seen in restraint to more holistic approaches emphasising human rights, the better meeting of specific needs, prevention, non-escalation, de-escalation, reflective practice and, where appropriate, recovery. This shift in focus is crucial if we are to prevent over-reliance or dependence on restraint so as to give proper meaning to last-resort principles, thereby helping prevent the organisation becoming 'dysfunctional and ultimately toxic' to those who work in it and those it seeks to support [13, p. 28]. The practice of providing training in restraint, as an isolated set of skills, is outdated and should not be used. Restraint training should be seen as part of the overall practice of patient and staff safety, wherein a range of skills aimed at minimising its use should be emphasised. Similar principles should apply to all forms of restrictive practice.

So, what would a common set of guidelines look like? The essential ingredients should include the following principles:

- A human rights-based approach which emphasises the need to minimise the use of all restrictive interventions and ensures those that are absolutely necessary are rights respecting. Although the Human Rights Act 1998 applies only to public authorities, its principles ought to be adopted in other settings.
- With regard to children, reference should be made to the United Nations Convention on the Rights of the Child, which ensures that all children have the right to be heard and protected from harm. Reference should be made to Article 3 (the best interests of the child shall be a primary consideration), Article 16 (no arbitrary or unlawful interference with the child's privacy, etc.) and Article 19 (protection from all forms of physical or mental violence, injury or abuse, neglect or negligent treatment, maltreatment or exploitation).
- For people with disabilities, reference should be made to the United Nations Convention on the Rights of Persons with Disabilities and, in particular, to Article 10 (right to life), Article 12 (equal recognition before the law), Article 14 (liberty and security of person), Article 15 (freedom from torture or cruel, inhuman or degrading treatment or punishment) and Article 16 (freedom from exploitation, violence and abuse).
- Compliance with the legislative framework governing restrictive interventions. This requires a thorough understanding of both primary and secondary legislation pertaining to the country and specific setting. We will only consider the legislation pertaining to England and Wales, although a significant part also applies elsewhere in the United Kingdom and the legislation in other countries is often drafted in similar terms. The principal pieces of legislation for all settings include the Human Rights Acts 1998, Health & Safety at Work etc. Act 1974, Management of Health and Safety at Work Regulations 1999, Manual Handling Operations Regulations 1992, Equality Act 2010, Criminal Law

Act 1967 (section 3(1)) and Criminal Justice and Immigration Act 2008 (especially sections 76 and 119–22). In the healthcare settings, the principal legislation includes the Mental Health Units (Use of Force) Act 2018, Mental Health Act 1983 (as amended, most recently by the Mental Health Act 2007), Mental Capacity Act 2005, Mental Capacity (Amendment) Act 2019 (including the Liberty Protection Safeguards (LPS), which replaces the Deprivation of Liberty Safeguards (DoLS)) and the Care Act 2014. The relevant sections from the legislative framework should be incorporated into policy and training.

- A statement about compliance with relevant guidelines, setting out which guidelines are relevant. Where guidelines cannot be complied with, the reasons must be clearly documented.
- A statement setting out the organisation's position in respect of the tension between the rights of the patient and those of staff insofar as the use of restrictive interventions is concerned.
- Where it applies, conformity to the Restraint Reduction Network (RRN) Training Standards: 'These standards will be mandatory for all training with a restrictive intervention component that is delivered to NHS-commissioned services for people with mental health conditions, learning disabilities, autistic people and people living with dementia in England. Implementation will be via commissioning requirements and inspection frameworks from April 2021' [6].

The RRN training standards [6] are divided into four sections. Section 1 deals with the process that needs to be completed before a training curriculum is developed. Section 2 covers what needs to be included in the curriculum. Section 3 covers the post-delivery processes. Section 4 relates to trainer standards. We will refer to the relevant RRN standards as they apply.

Before a Training Curriculum is Developed

Before developing a training curriculum, it is necessary to carry out a suitable and sufficient assessment of the risks. The curriculum must be based on a training needs analysis (RRN 1.1). Training is typically provided either by in-house trainers or by an external training provider. In-house trainers should already have detailed knowledge of the service or services for which the training is being provided, including the population being supported and the needs and characteristics of the staff providing such support. External training providers will need to understand as much about the population and staff as their in-house counterparts before developing any package of training. This helps to ensure that all training is appropriate, proportionate and fit for the specific needs of the population, named individuals and staff, taking account of any specific needs that were identified during the initial fact-finding process. This process should be reviewed on a regular basis and updated where changes are identified with the population, specific individuals or staff, or where specific risks have been acknowledged.

Commissioning organisations should check with prospective training providers that they have appropriate professional indemnity and public liability insurance cover (RRN 4.5) and that this insurance is maintained throughout the period of the contract.

What Needs to be Included in the Curriculum

Physical intervention techniques should be considered as part of the overall process in the prevention and management of violence and aggression (PMVA) rather than being taught in isolation. This helps ensure that these techniques are not seen as the only, or even the main, response to PMVA. In practice, physical intervention techniques ought to be a small part of the overall approach to PMVA, albeit an important one.

In terms of the training provided to staff, the emphasis should be on primary prevention skills, consisting largely of skills aimed at predicting and preventing violence and aggression and proactive de-escalation strategies. Where such primary prevention skills are unsuccessful, secondary intervention skills may be deployed. These consist mainly of supportive holds aimed at preventing any escalation in the incident. To achieve this, the secondary intervention skills should include active de-escalation responses. Only where the incident cannot safely be managed at the primary or secondary level should reactive responses be considered. These consist of physical intervention techniques aimed at bringing the incident under control as safely as possible.

All physical intervention techniques need to be risk assessed by a competent person before being considered for inclusion in any training package (RRN 1.3). This assessment should consider the risks associated with each technique with respect to its biomechanical properties, its physical and psychological risks, and its suitability both for the general population and for any specific individuals that the service supports, as well as for the staff who might need to use the skills. A legal review of the proposed training package should also be carried out to ensure compliance with all relevant legislation and guidance. Trainers should be provided with copies of all pertinent risk assessments prior to the training taking place. Because physical intervention is a manual handling activity, this review should ensure compliance with the relevant manual handling regulations.

A process for the periodic review of each physical intervention technique should be included, the timing of which should be determined during the initial review. Such periodic review ought to be undertaken at least every two years (RRN 1.3.3), or immediately in the case that any variation to a specific technique is to be considered or where a reassessment or incident reasonably calls into question its safety or efficacy.

The choice of techniques to be included in the curriculum will, to a large extent, be dependent on a number of variables, including the population and any specific individuals that the service supports as well as the staff who might need to utilise the skills. This will require regular monitoring to ensure that the techniques selected remain appropriate. Pain-compliance techniques (i.e. techniques that deliberately use a painful stimulus to control or direct a person's actions, typically used to break the cycle of harmful, violent or resistant behaviour and achieve compliance) remain the subject of huge controversy and debate. The RRN training standards 'do not support the use of pain to gain compliance. Training providers must not include the teaching of any restrictive intervention that uses pain to force an individual to comply' (RRN 1.3.7, Appendix 21A). Notwithstanding that Appendix 21A confirms that 'the cross sector RRN steering group does not endorse the use of pain-based techniques', Appendix 21B acknowledges the argument that pain-compliance techniques may be needed 'for escape or rescue purposes' and that 'where there is an immediate risk to life, the NICE guidelines (NG10) refer to the use of techniques which may cause pain-based stimulus to mitigate the risk to life'. Although the expression 'immediate risk to life' is open to wide interpretation, the proper use of pain-compliance techniques should only be considered as an exceptional intervention.

A recent review [14] of international evidence and practice on non-pain-inducing techniques which was commissioned principally to identify, review and assess alternatives to pain-compliance techniques across the secure juvenile estate concluded that 'it was . . .

not possible, based on the evidence available, to identify a safe, more effective system of restraint readily available to specifically manage volatile and serious situations within the youth secure estate in England and Wales'.

Whichever techniques are chosen for inclusion, it is important that training is provided within the context of an explicit commitment to the reduction of all restrictive practices (RRN 1.4) and that the views of appropriate people who have experienced restrictive practices should help inform the content of training (RRN 1.5). The content of the training should be person centred and rights based (RRN 2.1), both in respect of the people being trained and those upon whom the techniques may be used.

Once the initial training has been delivered, staff should undergo refresher training at least annually (RRN 1.6), with the full programme attended every fourth year (RRN 1.6.1). This means that the full training programme, as agreed with the commissioning organisation, will be delivered in full in year one, with refresher training in years two and three and the full programme repeated in year four. This is a curious requirement and does not reflect how training is, or should be, delivered. Accordingly, it is hoped that this requirement will be removed from the RRN standards. In any event, the frequency of refresher training may need to be increased if indicated by risk assessment, staff or organisational circumstances.

Neither the RRN standards nor the associated British Institute of Learning Disabilities (BILD) Association of Certified Training (ACT) certification scheme lay down a syllabus or specify which techniques should be included. Instead, the standards describe the principles which need to be followed when compiling the training syllabus. Questions as to which physical techniques or systems ought to be taught are complex and are often used by training providers seeking to demonstrate the superiority of their own methods. It is hoped that future editions of the standards, or alternative standards, will look more closely at the specific techniques as it is often the use of inappropriate techniques, or appropriate techniques applied inappropriately, that cause the most harm. The Safety Without Compromise (SWC) Experts Group has developed a guidance and approval-rating system for physical techniques which can be used alongside the RRN standards or as a standalone system [15].

Before considering which physical techniques to include, it is important to consider how they will fit in with an organisation's overall violence and restraint reduction plans. A good example of this can be seen in Figure 1.1, which illustrates the 'hierarchy of responses' approach used by the West London NHS Trust and incorporated into the training manual used by the United Kingdom's four high-security hospitals (and which, at the time of writing, is the only such training manual to be endorsed by NICE), as well as by a number of other organisations. (The author was the Independent Expert Advisor to the High Secure Services Violence Reduction Manual Steering Group and wrote significant parts of the manual.) The 'hierarchy of responses' approach illustrates how the risks associated with a strategy increase as staff move up the hierarchy from primary through secondary and then to tertiary/escape and rescue interventions. Staff should aim, as far as possible, to keep strategies in the primary proactive prevention section and only move to secondary interventions when necessary.

Primary responses are non-physical and include, as part of a proactive de-escalation process, a range of prediction and prevention strategies aimed at managing the incident without recourse to any hands-on intervention. Secondary interventions include supportive holds as part of the active de-escalation process. By contrast, tertiary/escape and rescue responses should be considered as medical/psychiatric or environmental/situational

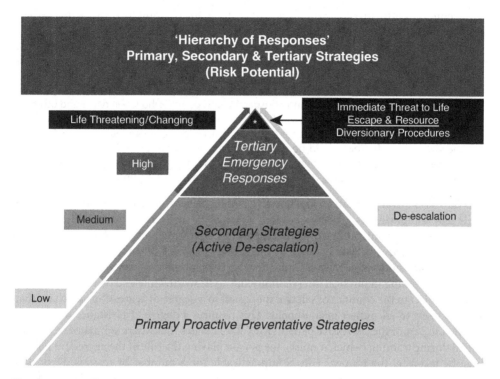

Figure 1.1 Hierarchy of responses

emergencies and are therefore exceptional interventions. Their use must be necessary, reasonable and proportionate to the risks presented by the patient or incident, and they must only be used by staff who have been adequately trained in their use. A tertiary/escape and rescue response is the most restrictive of interventions and is designed to manage significant increases in risk in a patient's violence and aggression to themselves or others. Tertiary responses may include, where appropriate, placing or holding the subject on the ground, in the most appropriate and safe position, and/or using one of the approved emergency distraction techniques. Such techniques may be justified when the patient cannot safely or reasonably be managed with less restrictive techniques, or to prevent the dangers associated with prolonged restraint in any position, and then only for the shortest possible time and with appropriate monitoring to help ensure the patient's safety.

The diagram also provides staff and patients with a visual tool to work collaboratively and design person-centred individualised support plans to manage differing levels of risk (RRN 2.6.1). Plans can be agreed at each stage of the triangle to provide advanced directions and expressed wishes to better predict and prevent behavioural disturbances that can often lead to acts of serious self-harm and interpersonal violence.

The black triangle at the tip of the diagram covers a range of emergency interventions, such as wrist flexion and so-called 'distraction' techniques. These techniques are intended to cause pain and should be considered as truly exceptional interventions. They are referred to in the RRN standards under Appendix 21B: 'The use of pain for escape or rescue purposes'. The double-headed arrow on the right of the triangle emphasises the importance of de-escalation throughout the entire process, with the aim of bringing the restraint to an end at the earliest possible time.

The duty of candour is of particular importance to healthcare professionals and it is unsurprising that RRN 2.2 requires training content to cover this in all settings. The duty of candour is also a CQC requirement; Regulation 20 explains that its aim is

> to ensure that providers are open and transparent with people who use services and other 'relevant persons' (people acting lawfully on their behalf) in relation to care and treatment ... Providers must promote a culture that encourages candour, openness and honesty at all levels. This should be an integral part of a culture of safety that supports organisational and personal learning. There should also be a commitment to being open and transparent at board level, or its equivalent such as a governing body.

This duty also includes a duty of 'openness', enabling concerns and complaints to be raised freely and without fear, with any questions asked to be answered, and including specific reference to the commissioning organisation's whistle-blowing policy and procedures. This is to be welcomed not least because of the serious problem of under-reporting uses of restrictive interventions at both the individual and organisational levels.

For any training in physical intervention skills to be worthwhile and beneficial to staff it should, subject to the confines of safety, expose staff to a degree of aggression and chaos that they are likely to encounter operationally. This requires a degree of resistance from those playing the part of the aggressive patient. RRN 2.8.11 states that where simulated resistance is used during training (which it must), the person playing the role of the aggressive patient must be taken by the trainer. This is impracticable for a number of reasons. First, it is beneficial for staff to have the technique applied on them so they can appreciate the same from the patient's perspective. Second, staff need to practise the techniques on people of different sizes, weights, etc. Third, staff need to practise the techniques a number of times before they are familiar with them and are able to perform them under stress. Restricting this training so that staff only practise the techniques on the trainers would tie up the trainers, preventing them from carrying out their other duties, including teaching other skills and supervision/assessment. Fourth, with certain types of intervention, practising them only on the trainers would give rise to foreseeable risk of injury to the trainers by having the same technique repeated on them by every member of the class. The normal method of practising these techniques, whereby the trainers demonstrate the skills and then supervise the trainees whilst they practise them, works perfectly well and should not be abandoned. It may be appropriate for trainers to play the role of the aggressive patient in scenarios that incorporate higher levels of aggression.

Any use of mechanical restraint needs to be approved at board level (RRN 2.8.A.1) and only considered for use 'in exceptional circumstances in specific settings and under specific circumstances' (RRN 2.8.A.2). Moreover, the use of mechanical restraint should represent the least restrictive option for the individual upon whom it is to be used, and it needs to be shown why alternatives would not be appropriate [15]. In no circumstances should mechanical restraint be used for the convenience of staff.

The training should make it clear that there is no such thing as a safe physical intervention as they all carry risks of physical, psychological or emotional harm (RRN 2.9.1). Accordingly, the training should include all known risk factors associated with each technique, with instructions on how to perform each manoeuvre as safely as possible, setting out the factors that might contribute to or elevate the risk. Furthermore, the training should include instruction in emergency procedures in the event of a medical emergency arising during the intervention (RRN 2.10). These emergency procedures should extend to the period following the intervention as this period is also known to carry risks to the patient. The main risks associated with physical intervention include positional asphyxia; aggravation of acute behavioural disturbance, including excited delirium; and limb deformity/fractures. These risks should be clearly explained, setting out their warning signs (RRN 2.10.2) and the appropriate response from staff should they occur. Most importantly, staff must be told that these conditions are medical emergencies, and the well-being of the patient must take priority over the continuance of the intervention. Careful monitoring of the patient's airway, breathing and circulation during the intervention is crucial, as is the appropriate monitoring of any known existing medical conditions or injuries (RRN 2.10.2). The abovementioned list of conditions is not exhaustive, and staff must ensure the overall well-being of the patient.

The training curriculum should also include reference to the necessity for post-incident reviews [16, RRN 2.13], emphasised in other chapters in this book. Two discrete components of post-incident review are important for the present purposes: post-incident support covering both the physical and emotional well-being of those involved in the intervention, and a review covering post-incident reflection and learning [17]. Both of these components should be covered in the curriculum.

Post-Delivery Processes

All training providers and in-house training departments should routinely review their training to ensure quality, effectiveness and continued fitness for purpose, covering both the theoretical and the practical elements of the curriculum (RRN 3.1).

Training providers and in-house training departments should complete and maintain records for each course delivered (RRN 3.2.1). These records should include the date and duration of the course, the names and status of the trainers and the names of the participants. The records should also include details of the techniques taught and, against each participant's name, whether they have been assessed as competent or whether further training is needed, together with specific details of any such further training. A graded system of assessment (rather than merely recording pass or fail) can be hugely beneficial. The date when refresher training is due should also be recorded against each participant's name. A record confirming each participant's fitness to participate in the training and details of any injuries sustained during the training should also be kept.

To help ensure the training meets the requirements of the organisation and its staff, all participants should be encouraged to complete a post-delivery evaluation questionnaire (RRN 3.4.1) and the responses used to improve the quality of the training and its effectiveness.

Trainer Standards

Physical intervention trainers have three important tasks, and these should be explained in the organisation's policy documents. These tasks are the same whether the organisation uses in-house trainers or engages an external training provider to facilitate the training: first, to deliver high-quality and safe training according to the agreed curriculum; second, to ensure that staff understand the need to minimise the use of all restrictive interventions; and third, to challenge any unhelpful attitudes from staff or elsewhere within the organisation.

Trainers have an important role in influencing staff attitudes, and employers need to ensure that this role is exercised properly and effectively. To help achieve this, those providing training should have in place good-quality assurance systems which, amongst other things, should monitor the competence of trainers (RRN 4.1). All trainers must hold, or be working towards, relevant qualifications and be able to demonstrate competence to deliver the training (RRN 4.2). In addition, all trainers should hold current first-aid certification, including immediate life support (RRN 4.2.2). The RRN also requires trainers to 'be able to evidence that they have the qualifications, experience and competence in supporting people in the sector in which they are delivering training' (RRN 4.3). This requires trainers to have 'a professional qualification (with current, up-to-date registration) or have completed a programme of relevant vocational training, having received a qualification within health, education or social care'. Evidence of this professional competence may include relevant vocational qualifications, social work qualifications, teaching or education-based qualifications, nursing qualification with current registration or other health professional qualifications (RRN 4.3.1). Furthermore, 'all trainers must have been continuously employed in a support or care role within social care, education or a health care environment for a period of not less than two years' (RRN 4.3.2). Whilst experience of relevant healthcare settings is clearly beneficial, these requirements will mean that many training providers and trainers will become ineligible to provide training to these sectors, including some exceptional trainers with considerable knowledge and expertise. It remains to be seen what resource implications this might have.

Not only should the curriculum be based on a training needs analysis (RRN 1.1) but the delivery of training must be informed by training needs analyses, with which trainers need to be familiar (RRN 4.4).

A number of factors have been identified that should be considered for a 'charter' for PMVA trainers [18]. These factors are split into three sections: (a) the role of the trainer as a professional, (b) the content of the training and (c) the provision of the training. With regard to the role of the trainer as a professional, trainers should not provide training outside their scope of competence, they should embrace continuing professional development, and they should act in a professional and ethical manner at all times. The training should be safe, evidence-based and meet best-practice standards. Training should be designed following a needs analysis, be fit for the specific purpose of the organisation rather than delivered on a one-size-fits-all basis, conform to relevant legal and ethical guidance, and emphasise the importance of prevention and minimisation of restrictive practices. The training should be delivered in such a way that it is integrated into a broader organisational agenda and carried out in a way that respects the safety, dignity and diversity of those participating.

Conclusion

The aim of any good guidance seeking to influence practices in the prevention and management of violence and aggression should be to minimise the need for any kind of restrictive intervention but, where necessary, to apply techniques as safely as possible within the relevant legislative framework.

Some staff working in healthcare settings are required to receive training to increase the organisation's capacity and capability to deal with potentially violent situations without recourse to external agencies (such as the police) who operate to an entirely different set of standards to those that operate within healthcare settings, and who use techniques that healthcare staff would not wish to see used in their settings.

We are only now looking at the introduction of the RRN training standards and it seems that, despite the need for a set of common guidelines in all settings, success is still a long way away.

References

1. Knox, D. K. and Holloman, G. H. Jr. Use and avoidance of seclusion and restraint: Consensus Statement of the American Association for Emergency Psychiatry Project BETA Seclusion and Restraint Workgroup. *Western Journal of Emergency Medicine* 2012 13(1):35–40. https://doi.org/10.5811/westjem.2011.9.6867. PMID: 22461919; PMCID: PMC3298214.

2. Sequeira, H. and Halstead, S. 'Is it meant to hurt, is it?' Management of violence in women with developmental disabilities. *Violence Against Women* 2001 7 (4):462–476. https://doi.org/10.1177/10778010122182550.

3. Campbell, D. Figures reveal alarming rise in injuries at mental health units. *The Guardian*. 2018. https://bit.ly/2kYBkc8 [Accessed 24.4.2022].

4. Norfolk, Suffolk and Cambridgeshire Strategic Health Authority. Independent Inquiry into the death of David (Rocky) Bennett. [online] 2003. http://image.guardian.co.uk/sys-files/Society/documents/2004/02/12/Bennett.pdf [Accessed 24.4.2022].

5. College of Policing. Detention and custody: Control, restraint and searches. [online] 2018. www.app.college.police.uk/app-content/detention-and-custody-2/control-restraint-and-searches/?highlight=restraint?s=+restraint [Accessed 24.4.2022].

6. BILD Association of Certified Training. Website [online] 2019. www.bild.org.uk/bild-act/ [Accessed 24.4.2022].

7. South Gloucestershire Safeguarding Adults Board. Winterbourne View Hospital: A serious case review. [online] 2012. www.basw.co.uk/system/files/resources/basw_85617-10_0.pdf [Accessed 24.4.2022].

8. NHS Protect, March 2015. Team Teach News: Is prone restraint banned? [online] 2016. www.teamteach.co.uk/is-prone-restraint-banned/ [Accessed 24.4.2022].

9. National Institute of Clinical Excellence. Violence and aggression: Short-term management in mental health, health and community settings. NICE guideline NG10 28 May 2015. www.nice.org.uk/guidance/ng10/resources/violence-and-aggression-shortterm-management-in-mental-health-health-and-community-settings-pdf-1837264712389 [Accessed 26.8.2021].

10. Welsh Assembly Government. Reducing restrictive practices framework. 20 January 2009. https://gov.wales/sites/default/files/publications/2021-07/reducing-restrictive-practices-framework.pdf.

11. Smallridge, P. and Williamson, A. Independent review of restraint in juvenile secure settings. London: HMSO. [online] 2008. www.positivehandling.co.uk/wp-content/uploads/2015/07/restraint-review.pdf [Accessed 24.4.2022].

12. College of Policing. Memorandum of understanding: The police use of restraint in mental health & learning disability settings. [online] 2017. https://rcem.ac.uk/wp-content/uploads/2021/11/Police_Use_of_Restraint_in_Mental_Health_and_LD_Settings.pdf [Accessed 24.4.2022].

13. Paterson, B. How corrupted cultures lead to abuse of restraint interventions. *Learning Disability Practice* 2011 14 (7):24–28.

14. Youth Justice Board for England and Wales. Research and analysis: Review of non-pain inducing techniques and systems of restraint. www.gov.uk/government/publications/review-of-non-pain-inducing-techniques-and-systems-of-restraint [Accessed 24.4.2022].

15. SWC Experts. Group guidance and approval-rating system for physical techniques. www.swcexperts.com [Accessed 24.4.2022].

16. Care Quality Commission. Brief guide: Restraint (physical and mechanical). [online] 2016. www.cqc.org.uk/sites/default/files/20180322_900803_briefguide-restraint_physical_mechanical_v1.pdf [Accessed 24.4.2022].

17. National Institute for Health and Care Excellence (NICE). Violent and aggressive

behaviours in people with mental health problems. Quality Standard QS154. [online] 2017. www.nice.org.uk/guidance/qs154 [Accessed 24.4.2022].

18. Baker, P. Attending to debriefing as post-incident support of care staff in intellectual disability challenging behaviour services: An exploratory study. *International Journal of Positive Behavioural Support* 2017 7(1):38–44.

19. Paterson, B., McKenna, K., and Bowie, V., A charter for trainers in the prevention and management of workplace violence in mental health settings. *Journal of Mental Health Training, Education and Practice* 2014 9(2):101–8.

Chapter

Legislation Relevant to the Management of Violence by Persons With Mental Disorders

Anthony Beschizza, Dominic Dougall and Masum Khwaja

Introduction

This chapter provides an overview of the legislative frameworks that are relevant to the management of violence by persons with mental disorders in the United Kingdom. Three jurisdictions apply (England and Wales, Scotland, and Northern Ireland), but individual frameworks and their variants are not discussed in detail. Instead, any substantial differences relevant to the management of violence are highlighted. Professionals should refer to the respective frameworks for detailed guidance.

The legislative and ethical framework and guidance regarding children and adolescents is discussed in Chapter 13.

Management of violence refers not only to acute episodes but also to the prevention or reduction of the risk of future violence. The core principles guiding routine medical practice of 'consent' and 'do no harm' remain relevant. Legislation provides a framework when coercion may be necessary to manage an acute violent act, to manage the immediate risk of further violence or to manage longer-term risk of violence.

Three strands of legislation are relevant to this report: The Human Rights Act 1998, mental health acts and mental capacity acts. The Human Rights Act applies to all three jurisdictions. The Mental Capacity Act 2005 and the Mental Health Act 1983 apply to England and Wales. Scotland is covered by the Mental Health (Care and Treatment) (Scotland) Act 2003 and the Adults with Incapacity (Scotland) Act 2000. Mental health legislation in Northern Ireland comprises the Mental Health (Amendment) (Northern Ireland) Order 2004 and the Mental Capacity Act (Northern Ireland) 2016.

Human Rights Act 1998

Compliance with the Human Rights Act is required when a function is of a public nature. The Act requires public authorities to act in accordance with the European Convention on Human Rights and the European Court of Human Rights (ECHR) which came into force in 1953. The Act would, for example, apply to the NHS and local authorities. It recognises certain rights and freedoms, with the ECHR hearing alleged breaches. The Act serves to allow UK citizens to seek redress in the United Kingdom regarding possible contraventions without having to apply immediately to the ECHR.

The Human Rights Act includes the notion of proportionality, which is highly relevant in the management of violence. It recognises that on occasions it may be necessary to restrict someone's rights, but any restriction must be kept to the minimum necessary to achieve the required objective.

Articles 2, 3, 5 and 8 are most relevant to this report and are described in more detail. Article 6 relates to the provision of the Mental Health Act, but less so to violence; however, it does state that everyone has the 'right to a fair trial' in relation to both civil rights and criminal charges. The tribunal or court should be independent and impartial. The remaining articles are less relevant.

Article 2: Right to life – Article 2 states that 'Everyone's right to life shall be protected by law' and

> Deprivation of life shall not be regarded as inflicted in contravention of this article when it results from the use of force which is no more than absolutely necessary:
>
> (a) In defence of any person from unlawful violence
> (b) In order to effect a lawful arrest or to prevent the escape of a person lawfully detained
> (c) In action lawfully taken for the purpose of quelling a riot or insurrection.

It has been held that Article 2 implies 'in certain well-defined circumstances a positive obligation on the authorities to take preventive operational measures to protect an individual whose life is at risk from the criminal acts of another individual' (*Osman* v. *United Kingdom* [2000]) [1].

The work of public authorities may be affected by Article 2 in a variety of ways. A public authority with knowledge of the 'existence of a real and immediate risk to someone's life from the criminal acts of another individual' should act to protect that person. A public authority should ensure those in its care are safe. If 'planning an operation which may result in a risk to life', then 'the minimum necessary force' must be used. If working with 'persons known to be dangerous', then steps should be taken to maintain public safety [2].

Article 3: Prohibition of torture – Article 3 states that 'no one shall be subjected to torture or to inhuman or degrading treatment or punishment'. Measures need to be taken to ensure this does not occur in psychiatric hospitals where individuals are potentially more vulnerable. The exact scope of this article has been regularly considered by the ECHR, which has found that 'compulsory treatment is capable of being inhuman treatment (or in extreme cases even torture) contrary to Article 3, if its effect on the person concerned reaches a sufficient level of severity', but that 'a measure which is convincingly shown to be of therapeutic necessity from the point of view of established principles of medicine cannot in principle be regarded as inhuman and degrading' (*Herczegfalvy* v. *Austria* [1993]) [3].

Article 5: Right to liberty and security – Article 5 states that everyone has the right not to be 'arrested or detained' apart from exceptions such as 'the lawful detention of a person after conviction by a competent court' and 'persons of unsound mind'. Lawful detention in relation to persons of unsound mind would more likely be under the auspices of the Mental Health Act, although circumstances may occur where detention under the Mental Capacity Act or, in limited circumstances, under common law 'best interests' is necessary.

Article 8: Right to respect for private and family life – Although everyone has the right to private and family life and private correspondence (letters, telephone calls, emails, etc.), certain restrictions exist. Relevant exclusions include public safety, prevention of crime, protection of health or morals and the protection of the rights and freedoms of others. Compulsory administration of treatment would infringe Article 8 unless it is covered by law, such as the Mental Health Act. Such treatment would need to be proportionate and legitimate, such as reducing the risk associated with a person's mental disorder and improving their health.

Mental Capacity Act 2005

England and Wales – The Mental Capacity Act 2005 provides a statutory framework for professionals and others who care for people with impaired capacity. Any action resulting from the use of the Act must be assessed as being in the person's best interests (*Herczegfalvy v. Austria* [1993]) [3]. Consideration must also be given as to whether the decision can be deferred until the person regains capacity. It is important to recognise when the Act may be indicated or when the Mental Health Act is more appropriate: a patient with a mental disorder who lacks capacity to consent to treatment in a psychiatric hospital is liable to be detained under the Mental Health Act rather than receive treatment under the Mental Capacity Act.

The Mental Capacity Act and an evaluation of 'best interests' are both relevant when considering the legality of administering rapid tranquillisation to a patient who is refusing treatment or lacks capacity to consent to treatment. Subject to the Mental Health Units (Use of Force) Act 2018, sections 5 and 6 of the Mental Capacity Act provide a defence against liability in relation to acts such as restraining mentally incapacitated adults using reasonable force or giving them medication without consent which is necessary in their best interests. Where treatment or restraint is necessary not because it is in the patient's best interests but for the protection of others, defence would come from the common law doctrine of necessity.

The procedure for determining the best interests of a person with impaired capacity is laid down in section 4 of the Mental Capacity Act. This takes into account any valid advanced decisions and statements, the patient's past and present feelings, beliefs and values likely to influence their decision, and any other factors which they would be likely to consider if able to do so. If practicable and appropriate, the views of anyone named by the patient, such as a carer or person interested in their welfare, must also be consulted

In relation to the management of violence, the Mental Capacity Act Code of Practice attempts to make clear the nature of restraint that is acceptable. Section 6 of the Act provides authority to restrain a person who lacks capacity. Restraint is defined as: 1. 'the use, or the threat of the use of force against a person who resists the action', and 2. 'restricts a person's liberty of movement, whether or not the person resists'. Two conditions are applied to the use of restraint: 1. 'to reasonably believe that it is necessary to prevent harm to a person', and 2. 'that it is a proportionate response to the likelihood of the person suffering harm and the seriousness of that harm'. In addition, the Code of Practice describes circumstances where the Mental Capacity Act may be relevant in the prevention of violence: 'a person may also be at risk of harm if they behave in a way that encourages others to assault or exploit them (for example, by behaving in a dangerously provocative way)' [4].

Restraining a person who is likely to cause harm but is not at risk of suffering harm themselves appears not to be covered by the Mental Capacity Act. Any such action would have to be justified in terms of the professional's duty of care to the person at risk of suffering harm and may need to be managed under common law.

If restraint is used frequently, this may amount to a deprivation of liberty. This is not covered by Section 6, and if a patient in a hospital or a resident in a care home is at risk of deprivation of liberty, authorisation should be sought. This is currently carried out by

Deprivation of Liberty Safeguards (DoLS) from the appropriate supervisory body, but this will be replaced by a new scheme, the Liberty Protection Safeguard Scheme (LPS), which was due to come into force in April 2022. On 16 December 2021, the Department of Health and Social Care announced that this implementation date could not be met, given the impact of the pandemic. A new implementation date has not been set. The key changes that will be introduced by the LPS are:

- Three assessments will form the basis of the authorisation of the LPS: mental capacity assessment, medical assessment, necessary and proportionate assessment.
- Greater involvement for families: there will be an explicit duty to consult those caring for the person.
- Best interest assessors (BIA) to be replaced with approved mental capacity professionals (AMCP). This will mean that LPS will become everybody's business and assessments will form part of routine care-planning considerations.
- LPS scheme extending to 16- and 17-year-olds.
- LPS scheme will extend to domestic settings, residential schools, day services and commuting from one place to another without the need for a court order.
- Clinical commissioning groups (CCGs)/integrated care systems (ICS), NHS trusts and local authorities as responsible bodies. The LPS creates a new role for CCGs/ICS and NHS trusts in authorising arrangements.

It should be noted that both DoLS (and the LPS in the future) cannot normally be used for a patient in hospital if the necessary care or treatment consists in whole or in part of the medical treatment for a mental disorder. The interface between the Mental Capacity Act and the Mental Health Act continues to cause confusion, with a lack of 'clarity and consistency' both in practice and in research [5].

Under the provisions of 'advance decisions to refuse treatment' (Sections 24–26), it is possible to make an advance decision to refuse any specified medical treatment; this might include medication for the management of potential violence [6]. Medication given under Part IV of the Mental Health Act is not covered by these provisions.

Scotland

Adults with Incapacity (Scotland) Act 2000 – This is broadly similar to the Mental Capacity Act. Guidance specific to violence is found in Section 47[7]. This states that the use of force or detention is not authorised unless it is immediately necessary. The use of force or detention should only be maintained for as long as is necessary and should be consistent with a decision that may be made by a competent court. The Act should not be used to treat a patient for a mental disorder in hospital against their will.

Northern Ireland

The Mental Capacity Act (Northern Ireland) 2016 was enacted by the Assembly in May 2016. The first Phase of the Act came into operation in two stages: research provisions commenced on 1 October 2019, and provisions in relation to deprivation of liberty, offences, and money and valuables in residential care and nursing homes commenced on 2 December 2019. The Act provides a statutory framework for people who lack capacity to make a decision for themselves and for those who have capacity now but wish to prepare for a time in the future when they lack capacity. Restraint and detention amounting to a deprivation of liberty are closely interlinked as they relate to compulsory limitations to a person's liberty. Restraint is not covered by the first phase commencement of the Act. However, restraint that is ongoing, planned or regular will most likely be regarded as deprivation of liberty [7].

Mental Health Act 1983

England and Wales – The potential for a mental health service user to imminently be responsible for acts of violence is frequently the reason for seeking detention under the Mental Health Act. It is recognised that where a patient has been detained under the Mental Health Act, there is an implied right for staff to exercise a degree of control over the activities of patient [8].

The Act requires appropriate medical treatment to be available to a patient in order to meet the criteria for section 3 detention or a community treatment order (CTO) as defined by Section 145 [1] and Chapter 23 of the Code of Practice. The Code of Practice states that medical treatment also includes interventions other than medication. This may consist of nursing treatment only, which could include restraint [6].

In the statute, specific reference to violence is made in two places in relation to emergency treatment. Section 62 authorises treatment which is immediately necessary and of minimum interference to prevent a 'patient from behaving violently or being a danger to himself or to others'. In Section 64C there is provision for treatment which would normally require either consent from the patient or authorisation from a second opinion appointed doctor (SOAD) in certain circumstances where the treatment 'is immediately necessary, represents the minimum interference necessary to prevent the patient from behaving violently or being a danger to himself or to others and is not irreversible or hazardous'.

The Code of Practice contains extensive guidance on responses to violence, principally in Chapter 26: 'Safe and therapeutic responses to behavioural disturbance'. Recommendations include suitable assessment for potential risk of violence, identification of warning signs, de-escalation, control and restraint, and seclusion policies [6].

Community treatment orders – CTOs have been in place for some years in the USA, Canada, Australia and New Zealand. They were introduced in Scotland in October 2005, and in England and Wales in November 2008. Under a CTO, patients who have been detained in hospital for treatment under Section 3 and unrestricted Part III (forensic) patients will, on discharge, become subject to a CTO, requiring them to comply with certain conditions. Patients have to be considered for a CTO if they are receiving more than seven days of home leave under Section 17, and if a CTO is not implemented then the responsible clinician must document the reason for not doing so. Equally responsible clinicians must not discharge patients onto a CTO prematurely before there is good evidence, including trials of section 17 leave, that demonstrates that the patient is sufficiently stable, and that the use of a CTO is appropriate and workable. A CTO can only be imposed on a patient directly following a period of compulsory detention in hospital. Patients with mental disorders who do not continue with their treatment (in particular, their medication) when they are discharged from hospital may, if their mental health deteriorates, become a danger either to themselves or to other people, and may eventually have to be compulsorily readmitted to hospital. The aim of a CTO is to maintain stability and reduce the risk of relapse through the use of conditions that ensure the patient receives the necessary treatment. Supervised community treatment allows for recall to a designated hospital. This may allow risks associated with relapse, such as violence, to be more effectively managed and reduced through earlier readmission. Ideally, the conditions of the CTO will have prevented a relapse in the first case. Recall to an outpatient facility, as well as to a designated hospital, is legally permitted, but other than to consider renewal of a CTO under Section 20 or to allow an assessment by a SOAD, recall to an outpatient facility is usually an impracticable approach as the patient may require inpatient care, and transporting the patient safely from an outpatient to an inpatient facility may prove problematic. The use of a CTO is further described in Chapter 29 of the Code of Practice [6].

Before the advent of the CTO, the Mental Health Act included various powers to manage patients by compulsion in the community and these included guardianship (Sections 7 and 37), supervised aftercare (Section 25) and leave of absence (Section 17). Of these, guardianship remains relevant (although longer term Section 17 leave is still indicated in some cases the majority of Section 17 leave is now mostly short-term leave) and enables patients to receive care in the community where it cannot be provided by the use of compulsory powers. The powers of a guardian (who may be a local authority or a named private individual) may include requiring a person to live at a specified address, attend for treatment at a specified place and allow health professionals access to their home. However, unless the patient consents, treatment cannot be imposed. Further, the guardian does not have powers to use force to make a patient attend for treatment or to enter their home.

Are CTOs Effective?

The benefits of CTOs have long been questioned and evidence for their effectiveness is small [9].

Three randomised controlled trials [10–12] have failed to show any benefits of CTOs in reducing the primary outcome measure of readmission to hospital, reduction in clinical symptoms or use of services. CTOs also fail to show improvement in secondary outcome measures such as quality of life, substance abuse, employment and satisfaction with services.

Meta-analyses have failed to support benefits of CTOs in terms of readmission, social functioning or symptomatology [13, 14]. Burns et al.'s follow-up of their OCTET study [15] found no evidence that CTOs improved readmission outcomes or reduced likelihood of disengagement from services in patients with psychosis over 36 months. Readers should note that the OCTET trial has been criticised by some, including David Curtis [16] who robustly states that 'OCTET does not demonstrate a lack of effectiveness for community treatment orders' arguing that 'the patients studied were not those who might have benefited from a CTO and that the psychiatrists involved were unlikely to have used the provisions of a CTO assertively'.

Are CTOs effective in reducing risk of violence to others or of homicide? The answer appears to be 'yes' when compared to no action, but 'probably not' when compared with good community mental health care. The difficulty in predicting a risk incident is acknowledged and there is no reliable way of calculating exactly how many homicides might be prevented by a CTO. It has also been suggested that thousands of people may have to be placed under compulsion in the community to prevent one homicide [17, 18]. There has been no discernible reduction in the overall rates of homicides by people with a mental illness in Canada, Australia or New Zealand as a result of CTOs having been in place for some years. In England, independent inquiries into cases of homicide committed by those who have been in contact with the psychiatric service, mandatory since 1994, have commonly cited non-adherence to medication as one factor leading to the incident [19]. In such cases it is possible that, had the individual been under a CTO, they may have adhered to their treatment regime, potentially averting a homicide, but in the absence of other evidence this remains speculative.

Despite a lack of evidence of their effectiveness, CTOs continue to be used. They are perceived as useful in clinical practice and they remain a less restrictive alternative to compulsory admission to hospital. In justifying the use of CTOs, supporters also point towards the limitations of randomised [20, 21] and non-randomised controlled studies [22].in evaluating CTOs and, in particular, the inability of randomised trials to recruit representative patients [23].

Continued 'targeted' use of CTOs is supported by the government's independent review of the Mental Health Act [24], the summary report of which states: 'During the course of the Review we have become convinced that there are some service users for whom, despite our doubts, the CTO does play a constructive role. For these reasons we do not propose their abolition at this stage' (p. 28).

The report acknowledges that CTOs are 'significantly overused' and that the authors would like to see a 'dramatic reduction' in their use, hence a recommendation that the criteria for CTOs should be tightened and that it should be made particularly difficult to extend a CTO beyond two years without a compelling reason.

Whilst the debate continues and CTOs remain available, clinicians must ensure that they are only considered for use with patients for whom they were originally intended – namely, those with severe mental illnesses, an established history of non-adherence with medication and disengagement from services, and for whom the use of a CTO is proportionate to the risks associated with the patient's history and presentation. It is also important to regularly review whether a CTO is indicated, and CTOs should only be continued if use has demonstrated benefit.

Additionally, when considering conditions of a CTO, clinicians must also consider representations from victims who may be involved with or connected to the patient. The responsible clinician must inform the hospital managers if the patient comes within the scope of the Domestic Violence, Crime and Victims Act 2004. Information-sharing with victims is discussed in Chapter 18.

Consent to Treatment and Community Treatment Orders

Consent to treatment regarding CTOs is discussed in Chapter 6.

Restriction Orders

Restriction orders (such as Section 41) may be imposed by a Crown Court alongside a hospital order (e.g. Section 37) if the court thinks it necessary for protecting the public from harm. Restriction orders can last indefinitely and require consent from the Secretary of State for Justice to approve aspects of management such as discharge from hospital and the approval of community placement. Although the order can be indefinite, it may be lifted by the Secretary of State when the order is no longer considered necessary for the protection of others.

Review of the Mental Health Act

In October 2017, the government announced an independent review of the Mental Health Act 1983. The review was tasked with making recommendations for improvements 'in relation to rising detention rates, racial disparities in detention, and concerns that the act is out of step with a modern mental health system'. The review team were asked to look at both legislation and practice.

On 1st May 2018, an interim report was published which summarised the work to date and outlined emerging priority areas. The review's final report was published on 6 December 2018 and makes a total of 154 recommendations. The review proposes the following principles:

- Choice and autonomy: Ensuring service users' views and choices are respected
- Least restriction: Ensuring the act's powers are used in the least restrictive way
- Therapeutic benefit: Ensuring patients are supported to get better so they can be discharged from the act
- The person as an individual: Ensuring patients are viewed and treated as rounded individuals

These four principles form the basis for the 154 recommendations set out by the review. The following section summarises those proposed actions.

Of the 154 recommendations, there is frequent reference to the criminal justice system. A large number of recommendations are made by the review relevant to the provision of care of service users in the criminal justice system, and in part relate to the powers of magistrates' courts and tribunals. Further, it is recommended that prison should never be used as 'a place of safety' for individuals who meet the criteria for detention under the Mental Health Act. In addition, it is recommended that a new statutory, independent role should be created to manage transfers from prisons and immigration removal centres. The time from referral for a first assessment to transfer should have a statutory time limit of 28 days [24].

Scotland

Mental Health [Care and Treatment] (Scotland) Act 2003 – The key differences between this Act and the Mental Health Act have been described elsewhere [25]. These relate to capacity, compulsion for more than 28 days and responsibilities of practitioners, of which capacity is most relevant to this report. Scottish legislation does not allow compulsion when a person retains capacity, whereas the Mental Health Act will allow compulsion when there is risk to the safety of others (as well as risks to self and health), even when capacity is retained.

Northern Ireland

Mental Health (Amendment) (Northern Ireland) Order 2004 – Legislation in Northern Ireland does not provide for the use of CTOs; it is otherwise not substantially different to the Mental Health Act.

Indeterminate sentences for public protection – The sentence of Imprisonment for Public Protection (IPP) was created by the Criminal Justice Act 2003 and implemented in April 2005. Similar arrangements were legislated for in Northern Ireland by the Criminal Justice (Northern Ireland) Order 2008. The legislation is not specific to mental health patients, but it may be applied to offenders with a mental health disorder. It is issued to those offenders who are seen by the courts as dangerous but who do not require a life sentence. Similar to a life sentence, prisoners are given a tariff or minimum term which they must serve before being considered for release. After release they are subject to recall if they breach the terms of their licence.

In England and Wales, IPP sentences were abolished in 2012. Those who remain jailed under them can only be freed by a parole board, and at the time of writing there are still more than 1,700 people in prison today serving an IPP sentence without a release date [26].

In Northern Ireland, public protection sentences, such as an indeterminate or an extended custodial sentence, remain sentencing options for adult offenders [27].

Conclusion

Legislation provides a framework when coercion may be necessary to manage violence or the risk of violence. Health professionals should be familiar with the Human Rights Act 1998, mental health and mental capacity acts, and with legal frameworks pertinent to whichever country in the United Kingdom they are working in.

The Mental Health Act Code of Practice offers guidance on when to use the mental health or mental capacity acts and when to use DoLS. Although no definitive date has been given by the government, DoLS are likely to be replaced by Liberty Protection Safeguards (LPS) either later this year or next year.

CTOs should only be considered for patients for whom they were originally intended, namely those with severe mental illnesses or established history of non-adherence with medication and disengagement from services, and for whom the use of a CTO is proportionate to the risks associated with the patient's history and presentation.

References

1. European Court of Human Rights. *Osman* v. *United Kingdom* [2000] 29 ECHR 245 https://hudoc.echr.coe.int/eng#{%22dmdoc number%22:[%22696134%22],%22itemid%22 :[%22001-58257%22]} [Accessed 25.4.2022].

2. Equality and Human Rights Commission. Human rights: Human lives. A guide to the Human Rights Act for public authorities. 2014. www.equalityhumanrights.com/en/p ublication-download/human-rights-human -lives-guide-human-rights-act-public-authorities [Accessed 25.4.2022].

3. European Court of Human Rights. *Herczegfalvy* v. *Austria*, 24 September 1992 (A/244) (1993) 15 EHRR 437 1993.

4. Office of the Public Guardian. Mental Capacity Act Code of Practice: Giving guidance for decisions made under the Mental Capacity Act 2005. Published 2013. Updated 2020. www.gov.uk/government/pu blications/mental-capacity-act-code-of-practice#history [Accessed 25.4.2022].

5. Gilburt, H. A tale of two Acts: The Mental Health Act, the Mental Capacity Act, and their interface. The Kings Fund 2021. www .kingsfund.org.uk/blog/2021/02/tale-two-acts-mental-health-act-and-mental-capacity -act [Accessed 25.4.2022].

6. Department of Health and Social Care. Statutory guidance. Code of Practice: Mental Health Act 1983. Published 15 January 2015. Updated 31 October 2017. www.gov.uk/government/publications/cod e-of-practice-mental-health-act-1983 [Accessed 25.4.2022].

7. Department of Health, NI. Mental Capacity Act (Northern Ireland) 2016 – Deprivation of Liberty Safeguards: Code of Practice, November 2019. www.health-ni.gov.uk/pub lications/mcani-2016-deprivation-liberty-safeguards-code-practice-november-2019 [Accessed 25.4.2022].

8. *Pountney* v. *Griffiths*; *Regina* v. *Bracknell Justices*, Ex parte Griffiths HL 1976 [1976] AC 314.

9. Moncrieff, J. and Smyth, M. Community treatment orders – a bridge too far? *Psychiatric Bulletin* 1999 23:644–6.

10. Steadman, H. J., Gounis, K., Dennis, D. et al. Assessing the New York City involuntary outpatient commitment pilot program. *Psychiatric Services*. 2001 52 (3):330–6. https://doi.org/10.1176/appi.ps.52.3.330. PMID: 11239100.

11. Burns, T., Rugkåsa, J., Molodynski, A. et al. Community treatment orders for patients with psychosis (OCTET): A randomised controlled trial. *The Lancet* 2013 May 11;381(9878):1627–33. https://doi.org/10.1016/S0140-6736(13)60107-5. Epub 2013 Mar 26. PMID: 23537605.

12. Swartz, M. S., Swanson, J. W., Wagner, H. R. et al. Can involuntary outpatient commitment reduce hospital recidivism? Findings from a randomized trial with severely mentally ill individuals. *American Journal of Psychiatry* 1999 Dec;156(12):1968–75. https://doi.org/10.1176/ajp.156.12.1968. PMID: 10588412.

13. Kisely, S. and Hall, K. An updated meta-analysis of randomized controlled evidence for the effectiveness of community treatment orders. *Canadian Journal of Psychiatry* 2014 Oct;59(10):561–4. https://doi.org/0.1177/070674371405901010. Erratum in: *Canadian Journal of Psychiatry* 2017 May;62(5):357. PMID: 25565690; PMCID: PMC4197791.

14. Barnett, P., Matthews, H., Lloyd-Evans, B. et al. Compulsory community treatment to reduce readmission to hospital and increase engagement with community care in people with mental illness: A systematic review and meta-analysis. *Lancet Psychiatry* 2018 Dec;5 (12):1013–22. https://doi.org/10.1016/S2215-0366(18)30382-1. Epub 2018 Nov 1. PMID: 30391280; PMCID: PMC6251967.

15. Burns, T., Yeeles, K., Koshiaris, C. et al. Effect of increased compulsion on readmission to hospital or disengagement from community services for patients with psychosis: Follow-up of a cohort from the OCTET trial. *Lancet Psychiatry* 2015 Oct;2(10):881–90. https://doi.org/10.1016/S2215-0366(15)00231-X. Epub 2015 Sep 8. PMID: 26362496.

16. Curtis, D. OCTET does not demonstrate a lack of effectiveness for community treatment orders. *The Psychiatric Bulletin* 2014;38(1):36–9.

17. Crawford, M. Homicide is impossible to predict. *Psychiatric Bulletin* 2000 24(4):152.

18. Szmukler, G. (2000) Homicide inquiries. What sense do they make? *Psychiatric Bulletin* 2000 24:6–10.

19. University of Manchester. Five year report of the national confidential inquiry into suicide and homicide by people with mental illness. https://documents.manchester.ac.uk/display.aspx?DocID=37602 [Accessed 25.4.2022].

20. Mustafa, F. A. Notes on the use of randomised controlled trials to evaluate complex interventions: Community treatment orders as an illustrative case. *Journal of Evaluation in Clinical Practice* 2017; 23:185–92.

21. Segal, S. P. Assessment of outpatient commitment in randomised trials. *Lancet Psychiatry* 2017; 4:e26–28.

22. Mustafa F. A. Naturalistic studies evaluating 'real world' OPC patients are welcome. *BJPsych Bulletin* 2015; 39:101.

23. Mustafa, F. Compulsory community treatment: beyond randomised controlled trials. *Lancet Psychiatry* 2018; 5. 10.1016/S2215-0366(18)30420-6.

24. HM Government. Modernising the Mental Health Act: Increasing choice, reducing compulsion. Final report of the Independent Review of the Mental Health Act 1983, (December 2018) [online pdf]. www.gov.uk/government/publications/modernising-the-mental-health-act-final-report-from-the-independent-review [Accessed 25.4.2022]

25. Zigmond, T. Changing mental health legislation in the UK. *Advances in Psychiatric Treatment* 2008 14:81–3.

26. UK Parliament. Justice Committee launches inquiry into IPP sentences. 2021 [online]. https://committees.parliament.uk/committee/102/justice-committee/news/157647/justice-committee-launches-inquiry-into-ipp-sentences/ [Accessed 22.4.2022].

27. NI Direct Government Services. Indeterminate custodial sentence. [online] www.nidirect.gov.uk/articles/indeterminate-custodial-sentence [Accessed 22.4.2022].

Protection and Safeguarding of Vulnerable Adults and Children Exposed to Violence

Alex Thomson, Chan Nyein and Maria Clarke

Introduction

In popular culture, the widespread prejudice that people with mental disorders are prone to violence persists [1]. Although some mental disorders (such as harmful alcohol and drug use and dissocial personality disorders) are associated with higher rates of perpetrating violence, the other side of the coin is that people with mental disorders are much more likely to be victims of violence than others. The odds of a person with a mental disorder being subject to physical, sexual or domestic violence are almost four times higher than for an adult without disabilities [2]. Studies in the United Kingdom have found that people with a severe mental disorder were the victims of violent crime, physical and sexual violence and domestic violence at higher rates than others [3, 4]. The reasons for this are complex but many factors are common to both mental disorders and violence, including marginalisation or poverty, exclusion from education or employment and increased contact with institutions and statutory services. People in institutional care are often trained or encouraged to behave passively, and assertive behaviour is generally discouraged or framed as challenging. People with a mental disorder may be more likely to be the targets of violence, and they often experience a differential response in criminal justice, safeguarding and protection agencies when violence is disclosed. Violence also has an impact on mental health, and may lead to depression, anxiety, post-traumatic stress disorder, harmful alcohol and drug use, self-harm, suicide and emotional or behavioural problems in children [5].

Given the impact of violence on health and the high prevalence of victimisation of people with mental disorders, actions to create conditions where violence can be prevented, to protect people from violence and to train practitioners in talking to patients about experiences of violence and defusing violent situations must all be core parts of clinical practice.

Safeguarding

Safeguarding means protecting a person's right to live in safety, free from abuse and neglect. It includes providing additional measures for those least able to protect themselves from harm or abuse. Child protection additionally involves protection from maltreatment, preventing impairment of health or development, supporting the provision of safe and effective care, and enabling all children to have the best outcomes [6]. Activity is on a continuum from prevention to protection.

The Children Act 1989 gave every child the right to protection from abuse. The act established the key principles which govern the way decisions concerning the welfare and safety of children are made, including the 'Paramountcy Principle': the principle that the child's best interest and welfare is the first and paramount consideration. The Children Act 2004 established the formation of multi-agency local safeguarding children boards. These consist of representatives from local partner agencies, such as housing, health, police and probation services. The boards are charged with coordinating the functions of all partner agencies in relation to safeguarding children.

'Working Together to Safeguard Children' offers statutory guidance on inter-agency working to safeguard and promote the welfare of children and young people in accordance with the Children Act 1989 and the Children Act 2004 [6]. The Care Act 2014 replaced the 'No Secrets' adult safeguarding guidance with statutory guidance for England and Wales [7, 8]. The act makes provision in respect of care and support for adults, and support for adult carers. It sets out empowerment, prevention, proportionality, protection, partnership and accountability as the fundamental principles that should underpin approaches to safeguarding and protection. It also introduced a statutory duty to promote the well-being of carers and to consider them within the safeguarding context. It emphasises the need to consider well-being and independence alongside safety, to ensure that the person is fully included in any safeguarding process and to focus on individualised intended outcomes. The term 'vulnerable adult', which could be stigmatising and disempowering, has been replaced with the terms 'adult at risk' and 'adult with care and support needs' [9]. The act also updated the definitions of categories of abuse. The Care Act 2014 defines adult safeguarding duties as applying to a person aged over 18 who:

- has needs for care and support (whether or not the local authority is meeting any of those needs);
- is experiencing, or at risk of, abuse or neglect;
- as a result of those care and support needs is unable to protect themselves from either the risk or the experience of abuse or neglect.

Across the United Kingdom, devolved nations set out similar statutory principles and definitions of who is at risk or in need. The codes of practice set out the principles, definitions and formal arrangements for partnership collaboration between agencies including local authorities, police, health and social care agencies [8, 10–12]. These include local procedures for information-sharing, joint working, investigation, oversight and case review.

Many people served by mental health services may be at risk or in need, and mental health staff may be in a position of trust and confidence which leads to disclosure or help-seeking. Protection and safeguarding are therefore core organisational responsibilities, core clinical skills and core professional duties [13–15]. The Royal College of Psychiatrists (RCPsych) states [16]: 'Patients have a right to be free from all forms of abuse, neglect and exploitation by others, including from professionals. If any psychiatrist knows of any form of abuse being perpetrated on their patient, this should never be ignored and such concerns must be acted on' (p. 6). Mental health services must have appropriate governance arrangements, including accessible safeguarding leads responsible for advice and coordination, procedures for referral and multi-agency collaboration and appropriate training for all staff. Above all, this must be in an enabling culture underpinned by the principles of safeguarding and protection.

Preventive safeguarding can involve proactive community development – for example, provision of community facilities, resources and activities to minimise isolation and maximise participation, support networks and well-being. Preventive plans for a person at risk might include regular key working and monitoring, support for independent living, training and occupational support, review of treatment, involvement of advocacy services and, potentially, police and legal action to prevent criminal activity against a person [9]. Protective safeguarding interventions may include practical support, environmental modifications or legal and criminal justice interventions [17].

Categories of Violence and Abuse

Abuse and neglect may take many forms. Although this chapter focuses on violent abuse, readers should be aware of all categories of abuse that may constitute the need for safeguarding (Box 3.1). The list is not exhaustive. NHS England advises that 'Organisations and individuals should not be constrained in their view of what constitutes abuse or neglect, and should always consider the circumstances of the individual case' [18].

Institutional Abuse

Although people with mental disorders experience institutional violence and abuse at greater rates than others, the barriers to disclosure and corrective action mean that the actual prevalence of institutional abuse is unknown. Regular reports of sexual and physical violence perpetrated by mental health staff demonstrate that such abuse remains a persistent, contemporary and unacceptably widespread problem [19–26].

Box 3.1 Categories of violence and abuse

Listed in the Care Act

  Institutional (organisational) abuse
  Domestic violence and abuse
  Sexual violence and abuse
  Emotional or psychological abuse
  Physical violence and abuse, and use of force
  Modern slavery
  Neglects and acts of omission
  Self-neglect
  Financial or material abuse
  Discriminatory abuse

Not Listed in the Care Act

  Gangs and radicalisation
  Cyber bullying
  Disability hate crime
  Cuckooing
  Mate crime
  Forced marriage

Compared to people without disabilities, people with mental disorders are likely to have higher rates of institutional contact, including healthcare services, admission to locked wards, police social services and residential care. Care in locked and enclosed settings often means that people cannot escape or do not have the ability to complain or disclose abuse to outside bodies. When placed in distant placements, especially when combined with visiting restrictions and limited access to communications, help-seeking becomes even more difficult. Predatory abusers seek positions in institutions which give them respectable status and access to vulnerable victims, and the mental health system is no exception. [27–29]. People with a mental disorder are still viewed as less reliable or credible compared to staff, and so testimony and disclosures may either be disbelieved or not acted on [30, 31]. Patients who have a recorded history of childhood abuse are at particular risk of being targeted by predatory abusers who perceive that they are less likely to be seen as credible. This is compounded by previous negative experiences of seeking help for abuse, such that patients are less likely to disclose experiences of abuse or seek help [32]. Physical abuse which appears superficially similar to accepted restrictive interventions may not be addressed, and physical punishment may be justified under the guise of half-baked psychological theories, such as 'positive behavioural approaches' [33]. Staff may experience reprisal or intimidation for reporting concerns, so frequently regard raising concerns as pointless, or may have become so inured or depersonalised to what is being done that they no longer recognise it as abuse [34].

The term 'institutional abuse' does not mean that all staff in an institution are malicious or abusive. Gil describes a framework whereby institutional abuse can operate at different levels (Box 3.2) [35–37]. Some forms of institutional abuse do not involve violence perpetrated by staff but expose people to the risk of violence perpetrated by others. *Malignant alienation* is a progressive deterioration in the relationship between staff and a patient perceived as 'difficult', resulting in withdrawal of sympathy, support and treatment, and in some cases assumptions of deliberately assumed (factitious)

Box 3.2 Gil framework

Level 1: Direct acts of abuse carried out by one person against another, for example a healthcare professional who uses their role and status to gain access to and physically, sexually or emotionally abuse vulnerable patients, and to protect themselves from action when their conduct is challenged;

Level 2: 'Programme abuse', arising from an abusive regime or an indifferent culture within a team or institution – for example, when hospital staff repeatedly abuse inpatients or a mental health service vexatiously excludes a patient from treatment as a reprisal for having had complaints upheld;

Level 3: 'System abuse', where wider governance, safeguarding and protection systems fail to prevent and address abuse, thereby unknowingly enabling or enacting further abuse. This includes instances such as social services returning a child who has escaped from an abusive inpatient ward, or police fining or charging someone in response to repeated requests for protection.

disability. Such alienation is malignant because it can gain momentum and lead to a fatal outcome [38–40]. This can represent level 2 abuse, where individual staff may not intentionally be acting maliciously, but the overall impact is a deviation from professional standards, thereby causing significant harm. Patients who have had complaints about staff behaviour upheld may be deliberately or vexatiously excluded from mental health treatment by way of reprisal, potentially representing all three levels of institutional abuse. Both malignant alienation and vexatious exclusion can lead to a failure of safeguarding and protection from violence within and outside mental health services, and to self-injury or death by suicide [37, 41, 42].

Disability Hate Crime and Mate Crime

Assailants may target people with a mental disorder through fear or hostility, because they view them as a lesser person or simply because they think they can get away with violence towards them. Disability hate crimes are most commonly perpetrated by people who know their victims, such as neighbours or family members, and include physical and sexual violence, damage to property, theft and intimidation [43]. This type of violence can fracture social support, by causing people to avoid going outdoors and to fear making new friends [44].

Mate crime is an aspect of hate crime. Although there is no statutory definition of mate crime in UK law, the term is generally understood to refer to the befriending of vulnerable people for the purposes of taking advantage of, exploiting and/or abusing them. The perpetrator is likely to be perceived as a close friend, a carer or a family member and will use this relationship for exploitation [45]. Cuckooing is related to mate crime. It is a recently recognised type of crime where criminal gangs exploit vulnerable people by taking over their home, for example, to use it as a base for storing, selling or using drugs or weapons [46].

Domestic Violence and Abuse

The Domestic Abuse Act 2021 has created for the first time in England and Wales a statutory definition of domestic abuse and extended the forms of abuse recognised in law. The behaviour of person A towards person B is domestic abuse if:

a)   A and B are each aged 16 or over and are personally connected to each other, and
b)   the behaviour is abusive.

Abusive behaviours are recognised in the Act as 'physical, sexual, violent or threatening behaviour, controlling or coercive behaviour, economic abuse or psychological abuse, emotional or other abuse'. The term 'personally connected' encompasses a broader definition of the relationship between perpetrator and victim, including current and former partners, relatives and those with past or present shared parental responsibility, and applies regardless of gender or sexuality, encompassing the WHO definition of intimate partner violence and family violence. In addition, children up to age 18 who are related to the perpetrator or victim and 'see, hear, or experience the effects of domestic abuse' are now recognised in law as victims of domestic abuse.

Domestic violence and abuse affect people of any age, ethnicity, sexuality and socio-economic background. Compared to men, women experience domestic violence and abuse at higher rates, and this is further heightened when younger (16–24 years), during pregnancy or if they have certain characteristics, for example Black, Asian or minority ethnicity (BAME), socio-economic deprivation, and disabilities or long-term illness, including mental disorders and physical and drug-related conditions. Adults who were separated or divorced were more likely to have experienced domestic abuse compared with those who were married or civil partnered, cohabiting, single or widowed [47, 48]. Repeat victimisation occurs at higher rates in women than in men [49].

According to the Crime Survey for England and Wales for the year ending March 2020, an estimated 7.3% of women (1.6 million) and 3.6% of men (757,000) experienced domestic violence and abuse in the last year. Of crimes recorded by the police in the year ending March 2020, the victim was female in 74% of domestic-abuse-related crimes. Between March 2017 and March 2019, 77% of victims of domestic homicide were female, compared with 13% of victims of non-domestic homicide [47].

Worldwide, more than a quarter of women who have been in a relationship have suffered physical or sexual violence from an intimate partner at least once in their lifetime from age 15–49 [50]. These figures likely underestimate the extent of the problem given the context in which domestic violence and abuse occurs: behind closed doors, often not recognised or reported.

Lesbian, gay, bisexual, transgender, and queer or questioning (LGBTQ+) people experience domestic violence and abuse at higher rates than the general population, with transgender people estimated to suffer higher rates than any other section of the population [51, 52]. This highlights the importance of ensuring accessibility to services and support.

Forms of domestic violence and abuse may vary between ethnic groups: for example, forced marriage, abuse from extended family members, female genital mutilation and 'honour' based violence [53]. BAME victims report abuse later and at lower overall levels compared to victims who identify as white British or Irish [49, 54]. Difficulty accessing support and disclosing abuse may be related to poor knowledge of available services, fear of being shunned by their own communities, mistrust of the wider community and, for those seeking asylum, concern that reporting abuse will have a negative impact on their immigration status [55, 56]. There remains a need, as with other services for the BAME community, for community education, culturally specific services, suitably trained staff and specialist resources to support BAME women escaping violence [53].

There are complex associations between domestic abuse and mental disorders. Domestic violence is perpetrated against people with a mental disorder at higher rates [57, 58], and victims of violence are more likely to subsequently develop mental disorders [59, 60]. Domestic violence and abuse can lead to a number of adverse physical health outcomes including death [61]. People with mental disorders (men and women) are more likely to be victims than perpetrators [62]. Data on the prevalence of perpetration of violence by people with mental disorders are limited; however, there is some evidence that in men with mental disorders, comorbid diagnoses of substance use disorders or personality disorders are responsible for increased rates of domestic violence perpetration against women [63].

Domestic violence against women surged globally by 20% during the COVID-19 pandemic. In the United Kingdom, the charity Refuge reported a 61% increase in calls and contacts to the National Domestic Abuse Helpline, and a seven-fold increase in visits to their web-based helpline service following the first lockdown in March 2020 [64]. Restrictions on leaving the home, greater isolation of victims and reductions in support services all aggravated the potential for violence. In addition, on easing of lockdown a perceived loss of control could trigger a perpetrator to intensify abusive behaviour in an attempt to regain control. These factors have led to modified guidance on safeguarding and responses to domestic abuse [65, 66].

Stalking, Harassment and Sexual Violence

Sexual violence is perpetrated against people regardless of sexual orientation, gender identity and gender, though at higher rates against women than men [67]. Airway-related violence – strangulation, smothering or forced gagging through insertion of objects or body parts into the mouth – is a highly prevalent aspect of sexual violence [68]. As well as homicide, airway-related violence can cause hypoxic brain injury, sleep and breathing disorders, post-traumatic panic, dissociation and suicidality [69, 70]. The Domestic Abuse Act 2021 has created a new offence of non-fatal strangulation or suffocation of another person [71].

Perpetrators of stalking, harassment and repeated sexual assault may or may not have had an intimate relationship with their victim. After assaulting a stranger or acquaintance once, a perpetrator may repeatedly stalk or rape them because they realise that they can do so with impunity, either because the person is too unwell to report the abuse or because no action is taken when they do disclose it. Responses to being sexually assaulted include shame and humiliation, bewilderment at breach of trust, and fear about the impact on daily life, all of which may result in delays to disclosure [72]. There is often a two-way relationship between mental disorders and being victimised by stalking [73]. Perpetrators of institutional abuse may maintain contact with their victims to groom, further abuse, threaten or encourage them to kill themselves. Such harassment may intimidate a victim into maintaining silence and further harm their mental health, with the result that they are perceived as less credible [28].

Physical Violence and Use of Force

In addition to physical violence considered under other categories, people with mental disorders experience higher rates of community violence, including assault and robbery [4, 74].

Interventions for psychiatric emergencies in situations involving risk to life or injury commonly involve a degree of violence and the use of force. Hospital interventions may include physical restraint, confinement in seclusion rooms, non-consensual injection of medicines and forcible insertion of nasogastric tubes. Although the use of force by staff may be authorised by law, such force must be proportionate to the danger identified, and must go no further than what is immediately necessary to ensure safety. Consideration must be given to the psychological and emotional impact of being subject to such force, with respectful communication maintained and the opportunity for a patient who has been subjected to force to be debriefed and a post-incident review initiated [75, 76].

People are more likely to encounter violence in services when mental health assistance is diverted to the police and criminal justice system. Police officers are more likely than ambulance or mental health staff to use force: a police 'welfare check' may involve breaking down a person's door, distraction blows, use of tasers or firearms, physical restraint involving pain, mechanical restraint with handcuffs or leg restraints, and forcible confinement in a caged van or police cell [77–79]. Such displacement exposes people to the risk of further harm, such as prosecution for alleged offences related to suicidality, or victimisation by others [80, 81]. Visible police involvement, such as the sight of police vans outside one's house and being led out in handcuffs, may mark a person as a target for disability hate crime. Negative experiences of displacing mental health assistance to the police may make a person less likely to report crime or seek protection, and could lead to a greater risk of physical and sexual victimisation [77, 81].

Gangs and Radicalisation

There is a relationship between mental disorders and involvement in criminal gangs or terrorist groups. Gang members may be perpetrators, witnesses or victims of physical and sexual violence, as noted both in the United Kingdom and overseas [82]. Interventions such as the Navigator Programme and Project Future aim to support young people at risk of gang-related violence [83, 84].

The Prevent Strategy has been developed as a safeguarding framework to prevent people identified as vulnerable being drawn into terrorism, though its effectiveness and the role of psychiatrists has been controversial [85].

Child Abuse

Abuse of children is highly prevalent. The Crime Survey for England and Wales estimated that 20% of adults had experienced at least one form of child abuse, including physical or sexual violence and/or witnessing violence against parents or other household members, before the age of 16 years [86]. Most child abuse is perpetrated by adults in close relationships with the victim, and more than 90% of child sexual abuse is perpetrated by someone who knows the child [87]. Female genital mutilation is a specific type of sexual violence against girls which causes permanent physical damage and has profound psychological and sexual consequences, leading to increased rates of physical illnesses and mental disorders in later life [88]. Most children do try to disclose abuse or seek help at some stage, though a minority of victims may not disclose abuse until they reach adulthood; 15% of callers to a helpline for adult survivors said that they had not disclosed or sought help as a child. Although most parents with a mental disorder are able to care for their own children, either with or without additional support, living with a household member who has a long-term mental health condition or disability may be a risk factor for child abuse [86]. In 2019–20, there were 642,980 referrals to local authority children's services in the United Kingdom and 389,260 identified children in need, with the most common factor being domestic violence [89].

The impact depends on factors such as the severity and nature of violence, duration of exposure and the presence or absence of other supportive relationships. At least one child is violently killed every week in the United Kingdom [90]. Risk of physical injury may arise from neglect, through accidents or failure to protect from community violence or by being caught up in domestic violence. Witnessing the suffering of a victimised parent has considerable emotional impact. Exposure to parental conflict, regardless of violence, may arouse distressing feelings, such as anxiety, fear, sadness, loneliness, helplessness or despair, and may lead to deterioration in educational achievement, social withdrawal or aggression [91, 92]. Rates of substance abuse, depression, suicide, self-harm and physical health problems are higher in adults who were abused as children [93]. It is essential for health professionals to be alive to the inter-relationship between domestic abuse and harm to children [94].

Approaches to Preventing Violence

Societal measures to prevent violence form the first-line approach to protecting vulnerable adults and children. The WHO has published 'INSPIRE' and 'RESPECT': global strategies to address violence against children and violence against women. These emphasise the need for social change to recognise that violence is wrong, interventions to address poverty, and investment in services, education and safe environments [95, 96]. Effective early responses from social services and the criminal justice system are important for prevention, protection and justice [97–99]. Specific considerations for people with a mental disorder include access to treatment, preventing discrimination, addressing the use of force within services and measures to prevent institutional abuse.

Access to effective treatment, supporting community engagement and public campaigns to address discrimination may play a role in preventing disability hate crime and community violence. Measures to reduce the use of force in mental health services include access to early, preventive treatment, schemes such as 'First Response' to reduce displacement of mental healthcare to police, and inpatient schemes such as the RCPsych Reducing Restrictive Practices programme [100–102].

Within healthcare services, measures to prevent institutional abuse include [28, 33, 37, 38, 103–105]:

- Effective governance, including pre-employment checks, acting on concerns about staff and zero-tolerance policies for abusive and derogatory behaviour towards patients
- Interventions to facilitate respectful culture towards patients
- Education of staff about boundary violations: for example, awareness that derogatory and abusive language towards patients should always be addressed and reported
- Doors of consultation rooms should be unlockable from the outside, and should have windows or observation hatches
- The RCPsych Sexual Safety Collaborative, a programme designed to protect patients from rape and other forms of sexual violence within mental health services
- Action to reduce distant or out-of-area admissions many miles from friends and family, whereby visiting is limited and safeguards and scrutiny may be lessened.

With regards to out-of-area admissions, a whole-service perspective is essential to reducing the pressure on inpatient services. RCPsych believes 'a blended and complementary approach is required in the short, medium and long term', and is calling on the UK government to implement a package of measures [106]. The college calls for:

(a) priority areas with consistently high rates of inappropriate out-of-area placements and/or persistently high bed occupancy to immediately be given the resources to invest in additional local mental health beds that are properly staffed and resourced;

(b) mental health services, over the next two years, to maximise the therapeutic value of inpatient stays and undertake a local service capacity assessment. To reduce variation in inpatient care, the college suggests a national programme to support mental health providers to ensure time spent in hospital has clear clinical objectives and value. The college also believes local areas should undertake and publish a service capacity assessment and quality improvement programme;

(c) investment, over the next 2–5 years in high-quality community mental health services. The long-term focus should be to increase the capacity and capability of community mental health services in line with the NHS Long Term Plan, its mental health implementation plan and the new Community Mental Health Framework for Adults and Older Adults.

Although attention has been given to the use of video recording in clinical settings, this does not constitute a safeguard in itself [107]. There are several contemporary instances of abusive regimes in hospital, with acts of violence repeatedly captured on video but no action taken [23, 25].

For domestic violence, recognition of the need for collaborative working across health settings has led to joint campaign initiatives such as Whole Health London [108].

Local safeguarding children boards (LSCBs) consist of representatives from local partner agencies, such as housing, health, police and probation services. The LSCB operates at a strategic level, helping and protecting children in its area from abuse and neglect through coordinating and reviewing a multi-agency approach across all member organisations. The boards are charged with coordinating the functions of all partner agencies in relation to safeguarding children. Multi-agency safeguarding hubs (MASH) were developed by the police, local authorities and other agencies to co-locate safeguarding agencies and their data into secure research and decision-making units. This was in response to the inability of agencies, on occasions, to effectively share information which has been the comment of numerous serious case reviews and public enquiries [109].

Responding to Violence

Facilitating Disclosure

Victims of violence may face barriers to disclosure, including fears, past experiences and structural factors. They may feel shame or avoid contemplating what has been done to them. Healthcare services are often the first point of contact for people with experiences of domestic abuse, most commonly primary care, emergency departments, maternity, gynaecology, sexual health, addiction and mental health services. A survey found up to 1 in 4 women and 1 in 10 men attending community mental health services had experienced domestic abuse in the previous year [58].

Mental health staff may feel they lack the confidence or skills to respond effectively to a victim of violence and so avoid the topic or assume another agency will respond. People may fear, or have experience of, not being believed, seeing no effective action being taken, or suffering reprisal or worse violence for having disclosed or sought help [37, 99, 110]. Psychological theories, such as the wrong perception of the 'repetition compulsion', or incorrectly assuming that patients seek risky situations as an unconscious proxy for self-harm, may be used to blame victims rather than acknowledge that a person cannot escape from their situation [111]. Statutory services can respond to requests for help punitively, for example by fining or prosecuting a victim for wasting police time [112]. Even complaints that are upheld about abuse from staff may lead to vexatious exclusion from further mental health treatment by way of reprisal [31, 37]. Where the victim has also broken laws – for example, possession of drug or involvement in gangs – they may be at risk of prosecution and so avoid contact with the police. Refugees or people with insecure immigration status may be at risk of being detained or deported if they seek help. It is therefore essential to establish trustworthiness and consider how to address such barriers to disclosure [113–115].

Healthcare professionals are well placed to identify domestic abuse and other forms of violence, and to provide appropriate support. However, the opportunity is often missed: studies have found that domestic abuse may go undetected or unaddressed in primary and secondary care settings [114, 116, 117]. In the mental health setting, although service users find routine enquiry about domestic violence acceptable, only 10–30% of experience of recent violence is asked about and disclosed [115, 118]. People are more likely to disclose abuse when asked directly by someone whom they trust and who will understand them without judging. All mental health staff therefore need to understand the relationship between violence and mental health, and the procedures for protection and safeguarding, as a core element of professional training, and to incorporate routine inquiry into clinical assessment [119–122]. Healthcare services should consider displaying posters to raise awareness about protection from violence and ensure that private spaces are available to facilitate disclosure. Friends and family members may either support or inhibit disclosure, and so consideration should be given to enquiring in appropriate circumstances. All staff should have training in responding to intimations of violence, and should be aware of local procedures and support services [20, 121].

People with protected characteristics, including race, sexual orientation, gender identity, communication difficulties, mental disorders and physical disabilities, report specific additional barriers to access which result in needs being unmet by mainstream services. This has led to calls for more research and development of specialist services to reflect this – for example, the Galop National LGBT+ Domestic Abuse Helpline [123].

Where institutional abuse is disclosed or identified, professionals may identify organisational barriers to protecting victims and addressing harms. The Freedom to Speak Up Review made a range of recommendations to increase protections for whistle-blowers in 2015. Despite this, there are concerns that health and social care organisations are continuing to fail to listen to whistle-blowers and undermine them when concerns are raised [124, 125]. To facilitate disclosure, organisations should endeavour to create a culture that welcomes, supports and protects staff who raise concerns.

Characteristics and Warning Signs

Victims

While there is no 'typical' victim, there may be indicators that a person is being subjected to ongoing violence. The most prominent indicator is direct disclosure of having been a victim of violence. While outright false allegations are rare, inconsistencies in accounts may be expected and do not necessarily suggest that no incident occurred [126]. People who are perceived as less credible may be disbelieved or their testimony overlooked. These include people with mental disorders, women, children, transgender people and people at risk of racial discrimination. Clinicians should be aware of warning signs and risk factors for violent victimisation, which should prompt enquiry about physical and sexual violence (Box 3.3, Box 3.4) [4, 75, 121, 127–129]. A partial disclosure may be a means of testing the recipient's capacity for belief and whether he or she can be trusted. Details may be omitted for fear that a full disclosure may not be believed or may expose the person to greater danger.

Perpetrators

Healthcare staff may encounter perpetrators of violence against their patients where these are partners or family members, or other professionals. It is therefore necessary to be aware of the warning signs and characteristic behaviours of perpetrators as well as those of victims of

Box 3.3 Warning signs of possible abuse in victims

- Physical problems
  - Unexplained or recurrent injuries
  - Unexplained medical problems, such as gastrointestinal symptoms, headache, dizziness, persistent pain

- Mental health
  - Anxiety, panic or post-traumatic symptoms
  - Depressed or irritable mood
  - Self-harm or suicidality
  - Harmful use of alcohol or other drugs

- Sexual health
  - Genitourinary symptoms, including frequent bladder or kidney infections, vaginal bleeding, sexually transmitted infections, pelvic pain and sexual dysfunction
  - Consultations for emergency contraception, pregnancy, sexually transmitted diseases, miscarriage, anal fissures or tears, where the patient is a child, or is in a supervised environment such as an inpatient mental health ward or a care home
  - Adverse reproductive outcomes, including multiple unintended pregnancies or terminations, delayed pregnancy care, miscarriage, premature labour and stillbirth

- Behaviour
  - Repeatedly running away from a hospital or care setting
  - Reluctance to go home or reluctance to go to a placement
  - Reduced contact with friends or family
  - Missing appointments
  - Challenging or inappropriately sexualised behaviour
  - Partial or indirect disclosures, for example describing a care setting as 'harsh', a home environment as 'not safe' or a person known to them as 'rough'

Box 3.4 Risk factors for violent victimisation

Clinical Factors

Ongoing symptomatic mental illness

Harmful alcohol or drug use

Low self-esteem

Impaired decision-making capacity

Intellectual disability

Service-Related Factors

Recent psychiatric hospitalisation

Police involvement in mental health response

Box 3.4 (cont.)

Lack of access to health and social services

Dependent on others for support with physical, cognitive or mental-health-related disabilities

Negative experiences of disclosing abuse, such as failure to act or reprisal

Social Factors

Social isolation or exclusion

Unemployment

Homelessness and unstable housing

Household violence against others

Witnessing parental domestic violence

Association with gangs or extremist groups

Marginalised characteristics, including ethnicity, sexuality, gender identity

History of abuse or victimisation

violence. These include a history of previously perpetrating violence or abuse, harmful alcohol or drug use, expressed hostility, belittling, blame or negative attitudes towards a victim expressed in a consultation [27, 130, 131]. In institutional settings, additional characteristics and warning signs should be considered (Box 3.5) [27, 28, 33, 35, 99, 131–135].

Supporting and Responding to Disclosure

Response to a disclosure should follow local procedures and the principles of safe enquiry. A victim may be more at risk if a perpetrator is aware of disclosure. The WHO recommends the trauma-informed LIVES approach (Listen, Inquire, Validate, Enhance safety and Support) [136].

For domestic violence and abuse, UK intervention studies in primary and secondary care have found improvements in both identification and response to victims. The interventions include training healthcare staff, support of integrated specialist domestic violence advisors and a clear referral pathway to third-sector advocacy services. Training should cover safe enquiry, awareness of possible indicators of abuse, identification of domestic violence, response to disclosure and referral to appropriate specialist services for both victims and perpetrators [137, 138].

Linking Abuse and Recovery through Advocacy for Victims and Perpetrators (LARA-VP) is a highly commended online resource to support mental health professionals to identify and respond to domestic violence and abuse [139]. The National Institute for Health and Care Excellence (NICE) has published guidance to help identify, prevent and reduce domestic violence and abuse. Violence and abuse perpetrated against children by adults is not dealt with in the guidance, but it does include support for children who witness or are affected by domestic violence and abuse between adults [121]. The guidance should be read together with the quality standards, which cover services for adults and young people aged 16 and over [140].

Box 3.5 Warning signs for institutional abuse

Level One (Individual Staff) Signs

- Staff boundary violations aimed at grooming:
  - Disclosures about personal life and personal health problems.
  - Gifts or favours aimed at making patients feel special.

- Staff boundary violations aimed at objectifying or demeaning:
  - Sexualised comments about a patient's appearance, such as commenting on physical appearance, eye colour or attractiveness, particularly when made during physical examination or during physical restraint.
  - Derogatory or dismissive comments, particularly when made in front of patients, such as 'This one's a self-harmer'.
  - Verbal or emotional abuse towards patients.
  - Boasting about abusive and derogatory behaviour to colleagues.

- Physical or emotional separation of victim from carers, family or from oversight:
  - Undermining patients' credibility to other staff or to family and carers.
  - Informal 'fostering' arrangements whereby a staff member takes victims home at weekends or during holidays.
  - Locking consultation room doors during therapy sessions; no window or observation hatch in door.

- Directly witnessed physical or sexual violence towards patients.

Level Two (Team) Signs

- Persistent failure to follow good practice guidance. For example, consistently refusing to see a person after self-harm may indicate vexatious exclusion from treatment. High levels of physical force, such as prolonged prone restraint, may indicate a problematic or excessively violent ward culture.
- Incongruous stock orders of medicines or medical equipment. For example, orders for sedatives in excessive quantities, anaesthetic agents, contraceptives, hormone replacement therapy, mifepristone or vaginal speculums on a children's mental health ward.
- Separating patients physically and emotionally from their families: restricting visiting, removing phones, advising families that patients lie about physical or sexual assault just to get out of hospital.
- Inappropriate use of psychological formulations, particularly behavioural aversion approaches using 'reward' and 'attention-seeking', or punishment.
- Displacement of mental health assistance to police; encouragement of criminal sanctions for alleged offences related to suicidality.
- Use of derogatory language within the team: for example, 'She's just a PD', describing self-harm as 'attention-seeking' or 'manipulative'.

Level Three (Organisational and Governance) Signs

- Internal governance failings, such as repeated failure to follow complaints and incidents procedures within a reasonable timescale.

Box 3.5 (cont.)

- Repeated apologies in response to upheld complaints, in the absence of action plans to address the identified abuse or poor practice.
- Informally labelling complainants as 'vexatious' without informing them, and subsequently not responding to reports of abuse or misconduct.
- Use of unregistered providers for fostering or residential care.
- Operational policies which pre-emptively identify patients as malicious complainants.
- Failure to act on disclosures of abuse because of a lack of alternative hospital or residential placements.
- Prioritising loyalty to colleagues and reputational management over duty to patients.
- Delays or failure to co-operate with national inspectorates and professional regulators, such as responding to correspondence, providing requested information or carrying out required actions.
- Failure to act on independent reports identifying abuse or poor practice.
- Harassment of victims or people who provide evidence of concerns: for example, inappropriately contacting employers or professional bodies, silent phone calls, inappropriate deliveries and online threats of doxxing.
- Inconsistent disclosures to different regulators and inspectors: for example, failing to disclose to the Ombudsman that the organisation is also subject to regulatory action by a national inspectorate, or disclosing minimal information in response to requests.
- Prioritising surveillance of victims' social media and publications over actions required by inspectorate.

Staff should understand safeguarding and information-sharing responsibilities, including the role of multi-agency risk assessment conferences (MARAC) for people identified as at high risk, multi-agency safeguarding hubs (MASH) for children in need or at risk of harm, the Domestic Violence Disclosure Scheme (Clare's Law) and multi-agency public protection arrangements (MAPPA) for perpetrators [141–143]. MARACs are meetings where adults at high risk from domestic violence and abuse are discussed with representatives of social services, healthcare services, police, independent domestic violence advocates and other relevant agencies, such as housing key-workers and probation. The primary focus of a MARAC is the safety of the adult victim, though MARAC leads will liaise with other agencies to safeguard children and manage the behaviour of the perpetrator. MARAC referral criteria may include a high score on the Domestic Abuse, Stalking and Honour Based Violence (DASH) Checklist, increased frequency of domestic abuse or repeat domestic abuse within a year of last referral. Perception of high risk by a professional or the victim feeling unsafe is sufficient for referral. An analysis of a MARAC and independent domestic violence advocate intervention found that up to 60% of victims reported no further violence and it was cost effective [144].

The Survivors' Charter, developed to guide the criminal justice response to domestic and sexual violence, provides a useful framework for responding to disclosures of violence (Box 3.6) [99].

Respect

It should be explained in simple language that what was done was wrong, that it was not the victim's fault, that you will continue to believe and support them and that you are willing to

---

Box 3.6 The Survivors' Charter framework for response to disclosures of violence

Survivors of domestic violence should expect from the criminal justice system to be:
- respected
- believed
- protected
- supported
- updated
- heard
- safeguarded
- informed
- empowered

---

help ensure that they are safe from further violence. Explain the principles of clinical confidentiality and that you will respect these, within the bounds of any wider public protection duties. Explain that there may be a need to make referrals or share information with other agencies such as advocacy services or social services, with the person's consent.

Belief

A disclosure should be taken at face value and believed. Most disclosures of assault relate to real events, even if details are unclear or inconsistent, and most people with a mental disorder or a cognitive impairment are aware of, and able to give an account of, what was done to them. If an alleged perpetrator is a colleague or someone known to you, it is important to arrange for someone independent to respond to the disclosure. Care must be taken where a person is severely unwell or disabled and makes an allegation which appears implausible; they may be at risk of being targeted on the basis that they are unlikely to be believed or are unable to give a coherent account.

Protection

Following an initial disclosure, do not discharge a person back to an unsafe environment, whether this is the home environment, an inpatient unit or residential care. An inpatient may need to be kept in hospital until alternative accommodation or provision can be arranged. If you are concerned about immediate danger or you are not sure how to assess risk of further violence, ask for help urgently from a safeguarding advisor, social services or a specialist advocacy service. Consider whether there is a need to make a safety plan, and who can take the lead on this.

Support

In addition to mental health support, independent specialist advocacy or legal advice may be necessary [146]. People who do not have capacity to make decisions relating to safeguarding and protection procedures may have a statutory right to a specialist advocate. It may be necessary to review the care and support needs of a person with disabilities if they have changed following violence.

Updates

Follow through on actions, communicate regularly and stick to what you have agreed about confidentiality and information-sharing. Inform the person in advance if your position on this changes. If your action is to refer or hand over the concerns to another service or agency, ensure that they are acted on before ending your involvement.

Hearing the Person

Consider the impact of violence on a person, their concerns about the response and whether any further interventions are needed. For example, a person who has survived violence in healthcare settings may need support to access future health care and adjustments such as appointments in alternative venues, or remote video or phone appointments where possible.

Record what was disclosed. If your role involves physical examination, note any injuries. If a recent assault is disclosed, consider whether immediate medical attention is needed. This may include a specialist sexual assault referral centre. When making written notes, 'Disclosed' and 'disclosure' are more appropriate words than 'alleged' or 'allegations'. There is no need to use words such as 'alleged' in correspondence or clinical records, and doing so may imply that you do not believe their account, which is both invalidating to the individual and may jeopardise the credibility of a person who is already at risk of being disbelieved.

Safeguarding

Further actions in response to a disclosure may include support within services, referral to advocacy services, police reporting or referral to social services. Involvement of social services may be appropriate when the victim has care and support needs which mean that they are less able to protect themselves from violence or abuse.

Multi-agency working is consistently recognised as a vital element of protection and safeguarding, and this involves sharing information. Actions should be consistent with the principles of informed consent; decisions about disregarding or not seeking consent should be exceptional, made only in cases of danger or emergency, guided by professional codes of ethics and communicated to the person along with the reasoning for doing so. Where a person declines an offer of further action in response to a disclosure, decision-making capacity should not be used as an excuse not to engage with the person or with the issue of protection. Continued awareness, enquiry and discussion may help to establish a trusting relationship and explore and overcome barriers to further disclosure [14, 15, 146].

A victim must be able to disclose or ask for help at a pace that they feel is safe. While it may be tempting to encourage a victim to disclose the identity of a perpetrator or to make a report to the police, they may be making limited disclosures to evaluate whether you are trustworthy to receive further information. They may have reasons not to disclose, for example, protecting themselves from violent reprisal or from the re-traumatisation that may be associated with a police investigation. It is never appropriate to try to elicit disclosure by implying that a victim has a responsibility to protect others. Such pressure may reduce the likelihood of further disclosure. The responsibility for stopping further abuse lies primarily with the perpetrator and secondarily with regulators, inspectorates and protection services, not with the victim. Where a perpetrator of violence is a registered professional, colleagues may have a duty to report evidence of concerns to inspectorates or professional regulators [14, 147, 148].

Information

It is important to keep a victim informed of what actions are being taken, and to involve them in any ongoing processes [149]. Explain the meaning of confidentiality and information-sharing in detail. In response to a disclosure of violence, ensure a person has information about what can be done to protect them, what actions are being taken and the outcomes of any investigations. Victims should be provided with information about violence and abuse, support services and how to get help in an emergency.

Empowerment

Violence and consequent trauma involve abuse of power, lack of control, violation of consent and secrecy. Regaining control and power are vital elements of both the recovery from violence-related trauma and the prevention of institutional traumatisation caused by response to disclosures. A victim must feel that they have control over the process and their information, that consent is sought for any actions or sharing of information, and that they are consulted and informed throughout any protection or safeguarding process.

Conclusion

Violence is widespread. It is important to consider mental disorders as a risk factor for being a victim of violence, and to be aware of approaches to protection. Mental health staff have responsibilities for preventing violence and acting to protect victims of violence. This includes reducing the use of force within services, addressing institutional abuse and addressing the wider issue of community violence. There may be considerable barriers to disclosure or help-seeking, including a person with a mental disorder not being believed, shame and fear of reprisal. It is important to understand these barriers and to foster environments which facilitate disclosure; namely environments in which patients feel able to disclose concerns or abuse confident in the knowledge that they will not be judged and will be believed, treated with respect, and involved with, and in control of, any actions that may follow a disclosure. Multi-agency working with local authorities, non-statutory services and police is essential for effective safeguarding and protection, and clinical staff must be aware of local arrangements and professional duties regarding confidentiality and sharing of information.

References

1. TNS BMRB. Attitudes to mental illness 2014 research report [online]. London: Time to Change. Apr. 2015. www.bl.uk/collection-items/attitudes-to-mental-illness-2014-research-report#

2. Hughes, K., Bellis, M. A., Jones, L. et al. Prevalence and risk of violence against adults with disabilities: A systematic review and meta-analysis of observational studies. *The Lancet* 2012 Apr 28;379(9826):1621–9.

3. Khalifeh, H., Oram, S., Trevillion, K., Johnson, S., and Howard, L. M. Recent intimate partner violence among people with chronic mental illness: Findings from a national cross-sectional survey. *British Journal of Psychiatry* 2015 Sep;207(3):207–12.

4. Khalifeh, H., Johnson, S., Howard, L. M. et al. Violent and non-violent crime against adults with severe mental illness. *British Journal of Psychiatry* 2015 Apr;206(4):275–82.

5. World Health Organization. Global plan of action to strengthen the role of the health system within a national multisectoral response to address interpersonal violence, in particular against women and girls, and against children. Geneva: World Health Organization, 2016.

6. HM Government. Working together to safeguard children: A guide to inter-agency working to safeguard and promote the welfare of children [online]. London: HM Government, Jul. 2018. www.gov.uk/government/publications/working-together-to-safeguard-children–2.

7. Department of Health. No secrets: Guidance on developing and implementing multi-agency policies and procedures to

protect vulnerable adults from abuse. London: Department of Health, 2000.

8. HM Government. Care and support statutory guidance [online]. 28 May 2021. www.gov.uk/government/publications/car e-act-statutory-guidance/care-and-support -statutory-guidance.

9. Johnson, K. and Boland, B. Adult safeguarding under the Care Act 2014. *BJPsych Bulletin* 2019 Feb;43(1):38–42.

10. Department of Health, Social Services and Public Safety, Department of Justice. Adult safeguarding: Prevention and protection in partnership. Belfast: Northern Ireland Executive, 2015.

11. The Scottish Government. Adult Support and Protection (Scotland) Act 2007 Code of Practice. Edinburgh: The Scottish Government, 2014.

12. Welsh Government. Social Services and Well-being (Wales) Act 2014: Working together to safeguard people volume 1 – introduction and overview [online]. Cardiff: Welsh Government, 2018. https:// gov.wales/safeguarding-guidance.

13. General Medical Council. Protecting children and young people: The responsibilities of all doctors. London: General Medical Council, Jul. 2012.

14. Health and Care Professions Council. Standards of conduct, performance and ethics [online]. London: Health and Care Professions Council, 2016. www.hcpc- uk.org/standards/standards-of-conduct- performance-and-ethics/.

15. Nursing and Midwifery Council. The code: Professional standards of practice and behaviour for nurses, midwives and nursing associates [online]. London: Nursing and Midwifery Council, 2015. www.nmc.org.uk/standards/code/

16. Royal College of Psychiatrists. Good Psychiatric Practice Code of Ethics. London: The Royal College of Psychiatrists; 2014 Mar. Report No.: CR186.

17. British Medical Association. Adult safeguarding: A toolkit. London: British Medical Association, 2018.

18. NHS England North. Safeguarding adults: A guide for health care staff [online]. London: NHS England, 2017 [accessed 19 Sept. 2021]. www.england.nhs.uk/publica tion/safeguarding-adults-a-guide-for- health-care-staff/

19. Care Quality Commission. Sexual safety on mental health wards [online]. London: Care Quality Commission, 2018. www .cqc.org.uk/publications/major-report/sex ual-safety-mental-health-wards

20. Hughes, E., Lucock, M., and Brooker, C. Sexual violence and mental health services: A call to action. *Epidemiology and Psychiatric Sciences* 2019 Mar 11;28(6):594–7.

21. Kaplan, S., Busner, J., Chibnall, J., and Kang, G. Consumer satisfaction at a child and adolescent state psychiatric hospital. *Psychiatric Services* 2001 Feb 1;52(2):202–6.

22. Martin, H. Jailed nurse who raped patient with depression and PTSD is struck off [online]. *Mail Online.* 2019. www .dailymail.co.uk/news/article-7730999/Jail ed-mental-health-nurse-raped-patient- depression-PTSD-struck-off.html

23. BBC News. Muckamore Abbey Hospital: Timeline of hospital abuse allegations. [online]. 23 Jan 2020. www.bbc.com/news/ uk-northern-ireland-49498971

24. Murphy, G. CQC inspections and regulation of Whorlton Hall: Second independent report. London: Care Quality Commission, 2020.

25. Care Quality Commission. Cygnet Yew Trees Quality Report [online]. London: Care Quality Commission, Sept. 2020, p. 13. www.cqc.org.uk/location/1-5199037 51/reports

26. Thomas, R. Revealed: Hundreds of sexual assaults each year on mixed-gender wards. *Health Service Journal* [online]. 2020 Jan; www.hsj.co.uk/patient-safety/revealed- hundreds-of-sexual-assaults-each-year-on- mixed-gender-wards/7026629.article

27. Carter, P. Nurses as abusers: A career perspective. In F. Subotsky, S. Bewley and M. Crowe (eds.) *Abuse of the Doctor– Patient Relationship.* Cambridge: RCPsych Publications; 2010, pp. 127–37.

28. McKenna, A. and Hussain, T. An independent investigation into the conduct of David Britten at the Peter Dally clinic. London: Verita, 2008.

29. Zammit, J., Brown, S., Mooney, J. L., and King, S. Child sexual abuse in healthcare contexts [online]. London: Independent Inquiry into Child Sexual Abuse, Nov. 2020. Report No.: 978–1–5286–3088–7. www .iicsa.org.uk/reports-recommendations/pub lications/research/csa-healthcare-contexts

30. Crichton, P., Carel, H., and Kidd, I. J. Epistemic injustice in psychiatry. *BJPsych Bulletin* 2017 Apr;41(2):65–70.

31. Sullivan, P. Epistemic injustice and self-injury: A concept with clinical implications. *Philosophy, Psychiatry, & Psychology* 2019 Dec;26(4):349–62.

32. Wager, N. M. An experimental investigation of the perceived credibility of complainants of sexual revictimization: Disbelief and victim-blame. *Violence and Victims* 2019 Dec 1;34(6):992–1010.

33. Levy, A. and Kahan, B. J. *The Pindown Experience and the Protection of Children: The Report of the Staffordshire Child Care Inquiry 1990.* Stafford: Staffordshire County Council, 1991.

34. Strang, D. Trust and respect: Final report of the Independent Inquiry into Mental Health Services in Tayside. Dundee, 2020. https://independentinquiry.org/wp-content/uploads/2020/02/Final-Report-of-the-Independent-Inquiry-into-Mental-Health-Services-in-Tayside.pdf.

35. Gil, E. Institutional abuse of children in out-of-home care. *Child & Youth Services* 1982 Mar 10;4(1–2):7–13.

36. Penhale, B. Introduction. In J. Manthorpe, B. Penhale, and N. Stanley (eds.) Institutional Abuse: Perspectives Across the Life Course. London: Routledge; 1999, pp. 1–15.

37. Thomson, A. B. Testimonial and hermeneutical injustices in adult protection and patient safety: practical lessons for psychiatrists. In Philosophy Special Interest Group Biennial Conference. Online: Royal College of Psychiatrists; 2021. www .rcpsych.ac.uk/docs/default-source/events /faculties-and-sigs/philosophy-sig/2021/cal c--philsig-programme-final--sep-21.pdf? sfvrsn=fa0b2e56_6.

38. Gask, L. and Thomson, A.B. Suicide prevention in clinical practice. In Khan, M., Poole, R., and Robinson, C. (eds.) Preventing Suicide: An Evidence Based Approach. 1st ed. Cambridge: Cambridge University Press; in press.

39. Watts, D. and Morgan, G. Malignant alienation: Dangers for patients who are hard to like. *British Journal of Psychiatry* 1994 Jan;164(1):11–15.

40. Morgan, H. G. and Priest, P. Suicide and other unexpected deaths among psychiatric in-patients: The Bristol Confidential Inquiry. *British Journal of Psychiatry* 1991 Mar;158(3):368–74.

41. Palombini, E., Richardson, J., McAllister, E., Veale, D., and Thomson, A. B. When self-harm is about preventing harm: Emergency management of obsessive–compulsive disorder and associated self-harm. *BJPsych Bulletin* 2021 Apr;45(2):109–14.

42. Thomson, A. B., McAllister, E., and Veale, D. Frequent attendance with self-harm: What might you be missing? *Emergency Medicine Journal* 2020 Jun 1;37(6):331–44.

43. Clement, S., Brohan, E., Sayce, L., Pool, J., and Thornicroft, G. Disability hate crime and targeted violence and hostility: A mental health and discrimination perspective. *Journal of Mental Health* 2011 Jun 1;20(3):219–25.

44. Carr, S., Holley, J., Hafford-Letchfield, T. et al. Mental health service user experiences of targeted violence and hostility and help-seeking in the UK: A scoping review. *Global Mental Health* [online]. 11 Dec 2017;4. www .ncbi.nlm.nih.gov/pmc/articles/PM C5733370/ [Accessed 6.2.2021].

45. Association for Real Change. Mate crime: A challenge for the police, safeguarding and criminal justice agencies [online]. Chesterfield: Association for Real Change, 2013. (Real Change Challenges). https://ar cuk.org.uk/realchangechallenges/real-change-challenge-mate-crime/

46. The Centre for Social Justice, Justice & Care. Cuckooing: The case for strengthening the law against slavery in the home [online]. London: The Centre for Social Justice and Justice & Care, Nov. 2021. www.centreforsocialjustice.org.uk/library/cuckooing-the-case-for-strengthening-the-law-against-slavery-in-the-home. [Accessed 10.5.2022].

47. Office for National Statistics. Domestic abuse victim characteristics, England and Wales: Year ending March 2020 [online]. London: Office for National Statistics, Nov. 2020. www.ons.gov.uk/peoplepopulationandcommunity/crimeandjustice/articles/domesticabusevictimcharacteristicsenglandandwales/yearendingmarch2020. [Accessed 20.9.2022].

48. SafeLives. Getting it right first time [online]. Bristol: SafeLives, 2015. https://safelives.org.uk/policy-evidence/getting-it-right-first-time

49. Walby, S. and Allen, J. Domestic violence, sexual assault and stalking: Findings from the British Crime Survey. London: Home Office; 2004. Report No.: 276.

50. World Health Organization. Violence against women prevalence estimates, 2018: Global, regional and national prevalence estimates for intimate partner violence against women and global and regional prevalence estimates for non-partner sexual violence against women. Geneva: World Health Organization, 2021.

51. Magić, J. and Kelley, P. Recognise and respond: Strengthening advocacy for LGBT+ survivors of domestic abuse. London: Galop, the LGBT+ anti-violence charity, Oct.2019.

52. Scottish Transgender Alliance, LGBT Youth Scotland. Out of sight, out of mind? Transgender people's experiences of domestic abuse (report). LGBT Youth Scotland, 2010. www.scottishtrans.org/wp-content/uploads/2013/03/trans_domestic_abuse.pdf.

53. Thiara, R. K. and Roy, S. Vital statistics: The experiences of Black, Asian, Minority Ethnic & Refugee women and children facing violence and abuse [online].

London: Imkaan; 2010. www.imkaan.org.uk/resources

54. Penny, G. Supporting B&ME victims – what the data shows [online]. Safelives. 2015. https://safelives.org.uk/practice_blog/supporting-bme-victims-%E2%80%93-what-data-shows [Accessed 20.9.2021].

55. Baillot, H. and Connelly, E. Women seeking asylum: Safe from violence in the UK? [online]. London: Asylum Support Appeals Project, June 2018. www.asaproject.org/resources/reports [Accessed 20.9.2021].

56. Thiara, R. K. and Roy, S. Vital statistics 2: Key findings report on Black, minority ethnic and refugee women's and children's experiences of gender-based violence [online]. London: Imkaan, 2012. www.imkaan.org.uk/resources [Accessed 20.9.2021].

57. Trevillion, K., Oram, S., Feder, G., and Howard, L. M. Experiences of domestic violence and mental disorders: A systematic review and meta-analysis. *PLOS One.* 2012 Dec 26;7(12):e51740.

58. Khalifeh, H., Moran, P., Borschmann, R. et al. Domestic and sexual violence against patients with severe mental illness. *Psychological Medicine* 2015 Mar;45 (4):875–86.

59. Bacchus, L. J., Ranganathan, M., Watts, C. and Devries, K. Recent intimate partner violence against women and health: A systematic review and meta-analysis of cohort studies. *BMJ Open* 2018 Jul 1;8(7): e019995.

60. Chandan, J. S., Thomas, T., Bradbury-Jones, C. et al. Female survivors of intimate partner violence and risk of depression, anxiety and serious mental illness. *British Journal of Psychiatry* 2020 Oct;217 (4):562–7.

61. Stubbs, A. and Szoeke, C. The effect of intimate partner violence on the physical health and health-related behaviors of women: A systematic review of the literature. *Trauma Violence Abuse* 2021 Feb 5;1524838020985541.

62. Anderson, F., Howard, L., Dean, K., Moran, P., and Khalifeh, H. Childhood

maltreatment and adulthood domestic and sexual violence victimisation among people with severe mental illness. *Social Psychiatry and Psychiatric Epidemiology* 2016;51:961–70.

63. Yu, R., Nevado-Holgado, A. J., Molero, Y. et al. Mental disorders and intimate partner violence perpetrated by men towards women: A Swedish population-based longitudinal study. *PLOS Med.* 2019 Dec 17;16(12):e1002995.

64. Refuge. COVID: Refuge's National Domestic Abuse Helpline service review 2020/21 [online]. London: Refuge; 2021 Mar. www.refuge.org.uk/a-year-of-lockdown/ [Accessed 20.9.2021].

65. IRISi. Guidance for general practice teams – responding to domestic abuse during telephone and video consultations. [online]. Bristol: IRISi; 2020. https://irisi.org/wp-content/uploads/2020/06/IRISi-COVID-19-Doc-and-info-sheets-11.pdf [Accessed 4.8.2021].

66. Oxford Health Biomedical Research Centre. Domestic violence and abuse: How to prevent, assess and manage the risk of domestic violence and abuse in the context of the COVID-19 pandemic. Oxford: University of Oxford, 2020. https://oxfordhealthbrc.nihr.ac.uk/our-work/oxppl/domestic-violence-and-abuse/.

67. Office for National Statistics. Sexual offending: Victimisation and the path through the criminal justice system [online]. London: Office for National Statistics; 2018. www.ons.gov.uk/peoplepopulationandcommunity/crimeandjustice/articles/sexualoffendingvictimisationandthepaththroughthecriminaljusticesystem/2018-12-13

68. White, C., Martin, G., Schofield, A. M., and Majeed-Ariss, R. 'I thought he was going to kill me': Analysis of 204 case files of adults reporting non-fatal strangulation as part of a sexual assault over a 3 year period. *Journal of Forensic and Legal Medicine* 2021 Feb 16;79:102128.

69. Bichard, H., Byrne, C., Saville, C. W. N, and Coetzer, R. The neuropsychological outcomes of non-fatal strangulation in domestic and sexual violence: A systematic review. *Neuropsychological Rehabilitation* 2021 Jan 12;1–29.

70. Spencer, C. M. and Stith, S. M. Risk factors for male perpetration and female victimization of intimate partner homicide: A meta-analysis. *Trauma Violence Abuse.* 2020 Jul;21(3):527–40.

71. HM Government. Policy paper: Strangulation and suffocation [online]. www.gov.uk/government/publications/domestic-abuse-bill-2020-factsheets/strangulation-and-suffocation [Accessed 20.9.2021].

72. Melville-Wiseman, J. Professional sexual abuse in mental health services: Capturing practitioner views of a contemporary corruption of care. *Social Work and Social Sciences Review* 2011;15(3):26–43.

73. Dreßing, H., Gass, P., Schultz, K., and Kuehner, C. The prevalence and effects of stalking. *Deutsches Ärzteblatt International* 2020 May;117(20):347–53.

74. de Mooij, L. D., Kikkert, M., Lommerse, N. M. et al. Victimisation in adults with severe mental illness: Prevalence and risk factors. *British Journal of Psychiatry* 2015 Dec;207(6):515–22.

75. Care Quality Commission. Out of sight – who cares? A review of restraint, seclusion and segregation for autistic people, and people with a learning disability and/or mental health condition [online]. London: Care Quality Commission; 2020 Oct. www.cqc.org.uk/publications/themed-work/rssreview

76. Mental Welfare Commission for Scotland. Rights, risks and limits to freedom [online]. Edinburgh: Mental Welfare Commission for Scotland; 2021 Mar. www.mwcscot.org.uk/sites/default/files/2021-03/RightsRisksAndLimitsToFreedom_March2021.pdf.

77. DrEm_79. Commentary: 'I've lost count of the times my door has been broken by the police'. *BMJ* [online]. 2017 Mar 15;356. www.bmj.com/content/356/bmj.j1165 [Accessed 11.2.2020].

78. Hallett, N., Duxbury, J., McKee, T. et al. Taser use on individuals experiencing mental distress: An integrative literature

review. *Journal of Psychiatric and Mental Health Nursing*. 2021 Feb;28(1):56–71.

79. J O'Brien, A., Thom, K., Gordon, S. et al. The nature of police shootings in New Zealand: A comparison of mental health and non-mental health events. *International Journal of Law and Psychiatry* 2021 Feb;74:101648.

80. Thomson, A. B., Eales, S., McAllister, E., and Molodynski, A. Criminal sanctions for suicidality in the 21st Century UK. *British Journal of Psychiatry* 2022;221(5):653–654.

81. Eales, S., Molodynski, A., McAllister, E., and Thomson, A. B. Responsibility, judgement and ethics: Suicide and criminal justice [online]. *Royal College of Psychiatrists International Congress*; 2022 Jun; Edinburgh. www.rcpsych.ac.uk/events/congress

82. Public Health England. The mental health needs of gang-affiliated young people [online]. London: Public Health England; 2015. www.gov.uk/government/publications/mental-health-needs-of-gang-affiliated-young-people

83. Goodall, C., Jameson, J., and Lowe, D. J. Navigator: A tale of two cities [online]. Glasgow: SC Violence Reduction Unit; 2020. www.svru.co.uk/wp-content/uploads/2020/02/Navigator-12-month-report-2_0.pdf

84. Stubbs, J. and Durcottishan, G. Unlocking a different future: An independent evaluation of Project Future [online]. London: Centre for Mental Health; 2017. www.centreformentalhealth.org.uk/publications/unlocking-different-future

85. Royal College of Psychiatrists. Ethical considerations arising from the government's counterterrorism strategy [online]. London: Royal College of Psychiatrists; 2017. Report No.: PS04/16S. www.rcpsych.ac.uk/docs/default-source/improving-care/better-mh-policy/position-statements/ps04_16s.pdf?sfvrsn=f00cad70_4.

86. Office for National Statistics. Child abuse extent and nature, England and Wales [online]. London: Office for National Statistics; 2020 Jan. www.ons.gov.uk/peoplepopulationandcommunity/crimeandjustice/articles/childabuseextentandnatureenglandandwales/yearendingmarch2019.

87. Radford, L., Corral, S., Bradley, C. et al. Child abuse and neglect in the UK today [online]. London: National Society for the Prevention of Cruelty to Children; 2011. https://learning.nspcc.org.uk/research-resources/pre-2013/child-abuse-neglect-uk-today.

88. Klein, E., Helzner, E., Shayowitz, M., Kohlhoff, S., and Smith-Norowitz, T. A. Female genital mutilation: Health consequences and complications – A short literature review. *Obstet Gynecol Int* [online]. 10 Jul.; 2018. www.ncbi.nlm.nih.gov/pmc/articles/PMC6079349/.

89. Department for Education. Characteristics of children in need, reporting year 2020 [online]. https://explore-education-statistics.service.gov.uk/find-statistics/characteristics-of-children-in-need/2020.

90. National Society for the Prevention of Cruelty to Children. Statistics briefing: Child deaths due to abuse or neglect [online]. London: National Society for the Prevention of Cruelty to Children, Sep. 2020. https://learning.nspcc.org.uk/research-resources/statistics-briefings/child-deaths-abuse-neglect.

91. Cleaver, H., Unell, I. and Aldgate, J. *Children's Needs – Parenting Capacity. Child Abuse: Parental Mental Illness, Learning Disability, Substance Misuse, and Domestic Violence*. 2nd ed. London: The Stationery Office; 2011.

92. Onyskiw, J. E. Domestic violence and children's adjustment: A review of research. *Journal of Emotional Abuse* 2003;3(1–2):11–45.

93. Felitti, V. J., Anda, R. F., Nordenberg, D. et al. Relationship of childhood abuse and household dysfunction to many of the leading causes of death in adults: The adverse childhood experiences (ACE) study. *American Journal of Preventive Medicine* 1998 May 1;14(4):245–58.

94. Welsh Government. Social Services and Well-being (Wales) Act 2014: Working

together to safeguard people volume 5 – handling individual cases to protect children at risk [online]. Cardiff: Welsh Government; 2018. https://gov.wales/site s/default/files/publications/2019-05/work ing-together-to-safeguard-people-volume -5-handling-individual-cases-to-protect- children-at-risk.pdf.

95. World Health Organization. INSPIRE: Seven Strategies to End Violence Against Children. Geneva: World Health Organization, 2016.

96. World Health Organization. RESPECT Women: Preventing Violence Against Women. Geneva: World Health Organization, 2019. Report No.: WHO/ RHR/18.19.

97. Crown Prosecution Service. Key facts about how the CPS prosecutes allegations of rape [online]. 2020. www.cps.gov.uk/p ublication/key-facts-about-how-CPS- prosecutes-allegations-rape [Accessed 15.3.2021].

98. Faulkner, A. and Sweeney, A. Prevention in Adult Safeguarding: A Review of the Literature. London: Social Care Institute for Excellence, 2011.

99. Hawkins, S. and Laxton, C. Women's Access to Justice: From Reporting to Sentencing. London: All-Party Parliamentary Group on Domestic and Sexual Violence, 2015.

100. Molodynski, A., Puntis, S., Mcallister, E., Wheeler, H. and Cooper, K. Supporting people in mental health crisis in 21st-century Britain. *BJPsych Bulletin* 2020 Dec;44(6):231–2.

101. Shah, A., Ayers, T., Cannon, E. et al. The mental health safety improvement programme: a national quality improvement collaborative to reduce restrictive practice in England. *British Journal of Healthcare Management* 2022 May 2;28(5):128–37. https://doi.org/10 .12968/bjhc.2021.0159.

102. Trainer, M. Mental health joint response car pilot – evaluation report [online]. London: NHS England and NHS Improvement, Aug. 2020. https://aace .org.uk/initiatives/mental-health-joint- response-car/

103. National Collaborating Centre for Mental Health. Sexual Safety Collaborative: Standards and Guidance to Improve Sexual Safety on Mental Health and Learning Disabilities Inpatient Pathways. London: National Collaborating Centre for Mental Health, 2020.

104. Royal College of Psychiatrists. Exploring mental health inpatient capacity: response from the Royal College of Psychiatrists [online]. London: Royal College of Psychiatrists; 2019. www.rcpsych.ac.uk/d ocs/default-source/improving-care/bet ter-mh-policy/policy/exploring-mental- health-inpatient-capacity-report-- rcpsych-response-final-(002).pdf?sfvrs n=12df7d14_2 [Accessed 20.9.2021].

105. Stone, J. Regulation and its capacity to minimise abuse by professionals. In F. Subotsky, S. Bewley, and M. Crowe (eds.) Abuse of the Doctor-Patient Relationship. Cambridge: RCPsych Publications; 2010, pp. 177–89.

106. Wyatt, S., Aldridge, S., Callaghan, D., Dyke, A. and Moulin, L. Exploring mental health inpatient capacity across sustainability and transformation partnerships in England [online]. Birmingham: NHS Midlands and Lancashire Commissioning Support Unit; 2019. www.strategyunitwm.nhs.uk/publica tions/exploring-mental-health-inpatient- capacity [Accessed 25.9.2021].

107. Mental Welfare Commission for Scotland. Advice notes: Hidden surveillance. Edinburgh: Mental Welfare Commission for Scotland, Dec. 2015.

108. SafeLives. 'We only do bones here'. Why London needs a whole-health approach to domestic abuse. Bristol: SafeLives, Mar 2021.

109. Home Office. Multi-agency working and information sharing project: Final report [online]. London: Home Office, 2014. www.gov.uk/government/publica tions/multi-agency-working-and- information-sharing-project [Accessed 20.9.2021].

110. Carr, S., Hafford-Letchfield, T., Faulkner, A. et al. 'Keeping Control': A user-led exploratory study of mental health service

user experiences of targeted violence and abuse in the context of adult safeguarding in England. *Health and Social Care in the Community* 2019;27(5):e781–92.

111. Herman, J. L. *Trauma and Recovery.* New York: BasicBooks, 2015.

112. Independent Office for Police Conduct. Police contact with a man and a woman before he murdered her – Sussex Police, August 2016, Independent Office for Police Conduct [online]. Sale: Independent Office for Police Conduct; 2019 Aug. Report No.: 2016/071948. www .policeconduct.gov.uk/recommendations/ police-contact-man-and-woman-he-murdered-her-sussex-police-august-2016 [Accessed 9.2.2021].

113. Calcia, M. A., Bedi, S., Howard, L. M., Lempp, H. and Oram, S. Healthcare experiences of perpetrators of domestic violence and abuse: A systematic review and meta-synthesis. *BMJ Open.* 2021 May;11(5):e043183.

114. Rose, D., Trevillion, K., Woodall, A. et al. Barriers and facilitators of disclosures of domestic violence by mental health service users: Qualitative study. *British Journal of Psychiatry* 2011 Mar;198(3):189–94.

115. Trevillion, K., Howard, L. M., Morgan, C. et al. The response of mental health services to domestic violence: A qualitative study of service users' and professionals' experiences. *Journal of the American Psychiatric Nurses Association* 2012 Nov;18(6):326–36.

116. Richardson, J., Coid, J., Petruckevitch, A. et al. Identifying domestic violence: Cross sectional study in primary care. *BMJ* 2002 Feb 2;324(7332):274.

117. Howard, L. M., Trevillion, K., Khalifeh, H. et al. Domestic violence and severe psychiatric disorders: Prevalence and interventions. *Psychological Medicine* 2010 Jun;40(6):881–93.

118. Howard, L. M., Trevillion, K. and Agnew-Davies, R. Domestic violence and mental health. *International Review of Psychiatry* 2010;22(5):525–34.

119. Fiennes, S., Ingram, R., Quigley, L., Pell, J. and Robinson, J. *Safeguarding Adults: A National Framework of Standards for Good Practice and Outcomes in Adult Protection Work.* London: Association of Directors of Adult Social Services, 2005.

120. Howard, L. M. Routine enquiry about violence and abuse is needed for all mental health patients. *British Journal of Psychiatry* 2017 Apr;210(4):298.

121. National Institute for Health and Care Excellence. Domestic violence and abuse: Multi-agency working. London: National Institute for Health and Care Excellence; 2014 Feb. Report No.: PH50.

122. Equality and Human Rights Commission. Survival, recovery and justice: specialist services for survivors of domestic abuse. London: Equality and Human Rights Commission, Nov. 2020.

123. SafeLives. Free to be safe: LGBT+ people experiencing domestic abuse. Bristol: SafeLives, Sep. 2018.

124. Francis, R. Freedom to speak up: An independent review into creating an open and honest reporting culture in the NHS [online]. London, Feb. 2015. http://free domtospeakup.org.uk/the-report/

125. NHS England. Freedom to speak up: Raising concerns (whistleblowing) policy for the NHS [online]. London: NHS England; 2016. http://freedomtospeakup.org.uk/wp-content/uploads/2014/07/F2SU_web.pdf.

126. Saunders, C. L. The truth, the half-truth, and nothing like the truth: Reconceptualizing false allegations of rape. *British Journal of Criminology* 2012 Nov 1;52(6):1152–71.

127. Public Health Scotland. Gender-based violence and learning disability: guidance for practitioners. Edinburgh and Glasgow: Public Health Scotland, 2019.

128. Yakubovich, A. R., Stöckl, H., Murray, J. et al. Risk and protective factors for intimate partner violence against women: Systematic review and meta-analyses of prospective–longitudinal studies. *American Journal of Public Health* 2018 Jul;108(7):e1–11.

129. Boland, B., Burnage, J. and Chowhan, H. Safeguarding adults at risk of harm. *BMJ* 2013 May 14;346:f2716.

130. Henning, K., Jones, A. R. and Holdford, R. 'I didn't do it, but if I did I had a good reason': Minimization, denial, and attributions of blame among male and female domestic violence offenders. *Journal of Family Violence* 2005 Jun 1;20(3):131–9.

131. Kamavarapu, Y. S., Ferriter, M., Morton, S. and Völlm, B. Institutional abuse – Characteristics of victims, perpetrators and organsations: A systematic review. *European Psychiatry* 2017 Feb 1;40:45–54.

132. Anonymous. What it feels like to be compulsorily detained for treatment. *BMJ* 2017 Aug 16;358:j3546.

133. DrEm_79. Self harm and the emergency department. *BMJ* 2016 Apr 13;353:i1150.

134. Manthorpe, J., Penhale, B. and Stanley, N. (eds.) *Institutional Abuse: Perspectives Across the Life Course.* London: Routledge, 1999.

135. Mental Welfare Commission for Scotland. A recipe for abuse? Findings and recommendations from our investigation into the care and treatment of residents of a Supported Landlord Scheme. Edinburgh: Mental Welfare Commission for Scotland, Nov. 2009.

136. World Health Organization. *Caring for Women Subjected to Violence: A WHO Curriculum for Training Health-Care Providers.* Geneva: World Health Organization; 2019.

137. Feder, G., Davies, R. A., Baird, K. et al. Identification and referral to improve safety (IRIS) of women experiencing domestic violence with a primary care training and support programme: A cluster randomised controlled trial. *The Lancet.* 2011 Nov;378 (9805):1788–95.

138. Trevillion, K., Byford, S., Cary, M. et al. Linking abuse and recovery through advocacy: an observational study. *Epidemiology and Psychiatric Sciences* 2013 Apr 30;23(1):99–113.

139. Yapp, E. J., Oram, S., Lempp, H. K. et al. LARA-VP: A resource to help mental health professionals identify and respond to Domestic Violence and Abuse (DVA) [online]. London: King's College London; 2018. https://kclpure.kcl.ac.uk/portal/en/p ublications/laravp-a-resource-to-help-mental-health-professionals-identify-and-respond-to-domestic-violence-and-abuse-dva(f552c9e9-762e-4475-96b6-896632a4 d06a).html [Accessed 20.9.2021].

140. National Institute for Health and Care Excellence. Domestic violence and abuse [online]. London: National Institute for Health and Care Excellence; 2016. (Quality standards). Report No.: QS116. www.nice.org.uk/guidance/qs116 [Accessed 20.9.2021].

141. National MAPPA Team. Multi-agency public protection arrangements (MAPPA): Guidance [online]. London: HM Prison and Probation Service, 2021. www.gov.uk/government/publications/m ulti-agency-public-protection-arrangements-mappa-guidance [Accessed 20.9.2021].

142. Home Office. Domestic violence disclosure scheme: Guidance [online]. London: Home Office, 2016. www.gov.uk /government/publications/domestic-violence-disclosure-scheme-pilot-guidance [Accessed 20.9.2021].

143. Safelives. Resources for MARAC meetings [online]. https://safelives.org.uk /practice-support/resources-marac-meetings [Accessed 20.9.2021].

144. Howarth, E., Stimpson, L., Barran, D., and Robinson, A. *Safety in Numbers: A Multisite Evaluation of Independent Domestic Violence Advisor Services.* London: The Henry Smith Charity, 2009.

145. Pettitt, B., Greenhead, S., Khalifeh, H. et al. *At Risk, Yet Dismissed: The Criminal Victimisation of People with Mental Health Problems.* London: Mind, 2013.

146. General Medical Council. Confidentiality: Good practice in handling patient information [online]. London: General Medical Council. 2017. www.gmc-uk.org /ethical-guidance/ethical-guidance-for-doctors/confidentiality

147. General Medical Council. Raising and acting on concerns about patient safety [online]. London: General Medical Council, 2012. www.gmc-uk.org/ethical-guidance/ethical-guidance-for-doctors/raising-and-acting-on-concerns.

148. Nursing and Midwifery Council. Raising concerns: Guidance for nurses, midwives and nursing associates [online]. London: Nursing and Midwifery Council, 2019. www.nmc.org.uk/standards/guidance/raising-concerns-guidance-for-nurses-and-midwives/

149. Montgomery, L., Hanlon, D., and Armstrong, C. 10,000 Voices: Service users' experiences of adult safeguarding. *Journal of Adult Protection* 2017 Oct 9;19 (5):236–46.

Anticipation and Reduction of Violence: Implications of the NICE 2015 Guideline

Peter Tyrer and Tim Kendall

Introduction

In many chapters in this book, reference is made to the National Institute of Health and Clinical Excellence (NICE) updated guideline: 'Violence and aggression: short-term management in mental health, health and community settings' (NG10) published on 25 May 2015 [1]. The previous guideline [2] needed review, but we recognised right from the beginning that good studies of data, preferably in the form of randomised controlled trials, would be relatively limited in number. But the subject was important, and whereas the 2005 guideline confined itself to the management of violence in people over 16 and in only two settings (psychiatric settings and emergency departments), we needed to extend the enquiry to other settings, including the community.

So, our published guideline covered the short-term management of violence and aggression in adults (aged 18 and over), young people (aged 13 to 17) and children (aged 12 and under), and considered management in mental health, general hospital and other health and community settings. Violence in those with intellectual disability, discussed in Chapter 15, was felt to be sufficiently different to require a separate guideline [3]. We did not include older people, and have been taken to task for this by Jonathan Waite and Juliette Brown (Chapter 14); in retrospect, we should have done so.

A large section of the guideline was concerned with the prevention of violent situations and the safeguarding of both staff and people who use services (and the reader is reminded of this many times elsewhere in this book). The guidance also included the management of violence when it did occur. Although service users and carers were valuable members of the guideline group they were not authors of any part – that is corrected in the last section of this book.

This review was carried out in the period just before and just after the first edition of this book was published in 2013. We would like to think that we covered much of the subject matter described in this new edition but we clearly did not, and there have been several important developments since 2015 that will require updating of the guideline. For the first time we had a police officer on a NICE guideline committee and were surprised to be informed that there were no equivalent guidelines in the police force, but after reading Eric Baskind's chapter at the beginning of this book this becomes better understood. Perhaps unsurprisingly, the police are generally advised to use 'whatever means were necessary to prevent or manage the violent situation', without precise specification of what these means should be. We hope that this situation will change in the not too distant future.

In this chapter we update the principles behind the NICE guidance and, where necessary, expand on some of the recommendations we made in the guideline, but we try not to repeat advice from the guideline covered elsewhere in this book.

Principles of NICE Guidance

There are a few misconceptions about NICE that need to be cleared up. First, NICE guidelines are not legally enforceable and so are not mentioned in Chapter 2 of this book. They are only guidelines, not orders. Second, they concentrate on guidance from evidence, and this is always changing. Third, those who produce the guidelines are truly independent, as great care is taken in selecting only those who have no conflict of interest in the subject and in including all relevant groups (commonly called stakeholders) in developing the guidelines. One of the critics of NICE says they mean nothing as they just follow 'eminence-based guidelines' (Timimi, personal communication); this facile interplay of words is clever but nonsensical.

The 13 principles described in the latest NICE document are:

- Prepare guidance and standards on topics that reflect national priorities for health and care.
- Describe our approach in process and methods manuals and review them regularly.
- Use independent advisory committees to develop recommendations.
- Take into account the advice and experience of people using services and their carers or advocates, health and social care professionals, commissioners, providers and the public.
- Offer people interested in the topic the opportunity to comment on and influence our recommendations.
- Use evidence that is relevant, reliable and robust.
- Base our recommendations on an assessment of population benefits and value for money.
- Support innovation in the provision and organisation of health and social care services.
- Aim to reduce health inequalities.
- Consider whether it is appropriate to make different recommendations for different groups of people.
- Propose new research questions and data collection to resolve uncertainties in the evidence.
- Publish and disseminate our recommendations and provide support to encourage their adoption.
- Assess the need to update our recommendations in line with new evidence. [4]

The whole idea behind the guidelines is to help those who care for patients in any setting to reassure them that they are following best-known practice.

Reducing the Use of Restrictive Interventions

In the guideline, restrictive interventions were defined as those that 'may infringe a person's human rights and freedom of movement, including observation, seclusion, manual restraint, mechanical restraint and rapid tranquillisation' (p. 17).

One of the main requirements of the guideline was the need for each trust to have a 'restrictive intervention reduction training programme'. This is a complicated set of syllables and does not trip off the tongue, but the essential message we wanted to convey is to 'concentrate more of your efforts on preventing rather than managing violence'. During our review we became very aware of the large number of violence reduction programmes across the country, almost all of which are provided by private organisations. Some of these are very good, some mediocre, but far too many of them are preoccupied with restraint procedures once violence had been manifest. It is often difficult to determine which refer to restraint and which to prevention or defusion of violence, but it concerned us that

Trusts seemed more interested in commissioning these programmes rather than trying to change policies and training so that restrictive interventions could be avoided.

The programme for reducing restrictive practices is simple at one level but complicated at another. It should include seven elements, and these are worth dissecting in more detail so that they do not just come over as jargon.

Avoiding Restrictive Interventions

1. *Ensure effective service leadership.* A good therapeutic unit has a good leader who is reliable, consistent and respected by their colleagues. Conversely, a poor leader with a controlling mien and little empathy or interest will convey that same message to others in the team. So, choosing the right person to lead is a critical decision for those in authority, as the best policy will be undermined if the key decision maker does not have the right philosophy of care and readily jumps to meeting displayed aggression with an equally aggressive response.

2. *Address environmental factors likely to increase or decrease the need for restrictive interventions* (see recommendation 1.2.7)

   > This is a very important element of violence reduction. It is particularly important when patients are kept in restrictive environments for other reasons, such as psychiatric intensive care units (PICUs) (see also Chapter 8). In discussing environmental factors one needs to consider all aspects of the environment: its physical properties and its social and personal qualities, including interactions with staff.
   >
   > To illustrate the importance of the physical environment we describe the 'Sheffield experience'. The former PICU in the main psychiatric hospital was small and cramped. If a patient started lashing out or was otherwise extremely disruptive, it was impossible for others to escape the turmoil. If the behaviour was completely out of control the only place to house the patient was a small seclusion room. In other parts of this book it is noted that seclusion is not a desirable option (see Chapter 8); it is one of last resort.
   >
   > It was also difficult for patients to escape the confines of the main part of the PICU. The only way to get outside was to climb some stairs and travel along a walk-way within a cage to a small outdoor area. Change was needed.
   >
   > The importance of the environment was taken into account when planning the new PICU in the hospital. This was constructed to be considerably larger and so there was space for others to find a quiet place away from the disturbed person. There was also a 'green room' added – green has been found to be the most calming background colour, as anyone who has visited the old asylums will know. The outside area was safe and purpose built, having a leisurely appearance with secure seating and an abundance of plant life.
   >
   > The consequence of this planned environmental change was that physical restraint and rapid tranquillisation were halved when the new unit opened. Staff also prefer this new environment, and this improves therapeutic interaction. In a formal study of different PICUs, it was found that 'service users' satisfaction with forensic services was strongly associated with their experiences of the therapeutic relationship with their key-workers and the social climate of the ward. The findings emphasise the importance of forming and maintaining effective therapeutic relations and reinforce the need to maintain a therapeutic environment free of aggressive tension and threats of violence [5].

3. *Working with Service Users*

   The term 'service users' is not always appropriate for many individuals who are being detained against their will and have no special interest in being involved in the service. However, this is the language of the NICE guidelines so we are continuing the tradition.

One of the big plusses of these guidelines is that service users are important members of the guideline group, and two had important experiences to relate about their experiences.

The guideline asks Trusts to

(a) work in partnership with service users and their carers, (b) adopt approaches to care that respect service users' independence, choice and human rights, (c) increase social inclusion by decreasing exclusionary practices, such as the use of seclusion and the Mental Health Act 1983, (d) involve and empower service users and their carers, (e) include leisure activities that are personally meaningful and physical exercise for service users, (f) use clear and simple care pathways, (g) use de-escalation and (h) use crisis and risk-management plans and strategies to reduce the need for restrictive interventions.' [1, p. 21]

Violence is the offspring of coercion. Most people who are violent are subject to external control by others, most of which they can do nothing to reverse. Staff need to be aware of this difference in power when in coercion territory. Sadly, despite better understanding of mental illness at all levels of society, compulsory psychiatric admissions are increasing at the rate of 5% every year [6]. This is why the social climate in psychiatric settings is so important. It is always difficult to develop a collaborative relationship with someone who knows that 'the system' (as it is so frequently labelled) has the upper hand.

How is it possible to implement all eight of these NICE recommendations in ordinary NHS settings?

Work in Partnership with Service Users

There is not a particularly well-known form of management for much of mental illness called nidotherapy [7]. This was first piloted in a study of patients with multiple pathologies, mainly schizophrenia, substance misuse and severe personality disorder (more often in combination than separate), and was shown to reduce hospital bed use in a randomised trial [8]. Nidotherapy is a systematic and collaborative way of working in partnership with service users to change physical, social and personal environments. It has ten principles:

1. All people have the capacity to improve their lives when placed in the right environment.
2. Everyone should have the chance to test themselves in environments of their own choosing.
3. When people become distressed without apparent reason the cause can often be found in the immediate environment.
4. A person's environment includes not only place but also other people and self.
5. Seeing the world through another's eyes gives a better perspective than your eyes alone.
6. What someone else thinks is the best environment for a person is not necessarily so.
7. All people, no matter how handicapped, have strengths that can be fostered.
8. A person's environment should never be regarded as impossible to change.
9. Every environmental change involves some risk, but this is not a reason to avoid it.
10. Mutual collaboration is required to change environments for the better.

For those working in environments where violence is commonplace, this list of MAAP (Mom-And-Apple-Pie) recommendations may seem a long way from realisation. But this is not exactly true. Positive environmental change can be achieved in every setting. The contributors to an important book, *Transforming Environments and Rehabilitation* [9], illustrate this well. The changes are recent. O'Rourke et al. [10] point out that whilst there is growing acceptance in the National Health Service that involving service users in the delivery and planning of interventions is an effective model for change, Her Majesty's Prison Service is only recently beginning to recognise and value the importance for its population, with, for example, the setting up a prison councils and greater prisoner involvement in their environment and regime. (p. 275)

This complements the suggestions made in Chapter 12, and prisons are places where NICE guidelines apply.

Good research evidence is hard to come by, mainly because violent episodes are badly recorded, but the policy of enabling environments at the heart of these developments, headed at the Royal College by Rex Haigh, has now being widely used in prisons. This has extended further, to become psychologically informed environments (PIPEs) under the enthusiastic tutelage of Nick Benefield, former lead for personality disorders at the Department of Health. He summarises the essentials of PIPEs as:

1. Maintaining the intention to support personal and relational experience.
2. Staff to always make meaning from everyday interaction.
3. Supporting communication and exchange and dialogue.
4. The recognition and acknowledgement of the importance of relationships.
5. Supporting thoughtfulness and thinking.
6. Encouraging choice appropriate to the person's capacity.
7. Recognising the importance of interdependence. [11]

What relevance has this for psychiatrists treating people in NHS hospitals? One might conclude 'very little' for the average patient who spends only a short time in hospital, albeit much more for those in rehabilitation. Benefield et al. [11] end their title, 'a new optimism for criminal justice provision' with a question mark, and the continued increase in prisoner numbers may prevent many of these aims being realised. In all situations where there is an imbalance of control it is impossible to set up a genuine collaborative framework. In a recent qualitative study of prisoners' attitudes towards psychologists, a common view was that they (the psychologists) were 'the quiet ones with the power', so to get on well you had to agree with them. Being entirely honest was not necessarily a good policy [12].

Adopt Approaches to Care that Respect Service Users' Independence, Choice and Human Rights

There is a real danger that the words of this section title may be perceived as empty when dealing with people in potentially violent situations. But they are not. Holding on to a few trappings of independence is very important to those who have been stripped of everything else. Thus, it is necessary to point out what rights and options are available to people who are prone to violence, preferably at times apart from those when violence is presumed to be imminent (see also Chapter 3). 'Choice' is another 'politically correct' word that is used so frequently that it has become almost meaningless, and in the case of detained patients it seems to be in very short supply. But it is not absent, and emphasising to people that they do have choices in many areas is a good way of defusing violence.

Two examples of choice were given in the NICE guideline: advance decisions and advance statements. An advance decision is 'a written statement made by a person aged 18 or over that is legally binding and conveys a person's decision to refuse specific treatments and interventions in the future'; an advance statement is 'a written statement that conveys a person's preferences, wishes, beliefs and values about their future treatment and care. An advance statement is not legally binding' [1, p. 16]. These may be easily ignored, especially in acute episodes of violent confrontation when the person is seen for the first time, but for longer-term patients they should be considered, and organising them in advance may be a curious way of thwarting violence. One of the service users on our NICE guideline group did not actually write out an advance statement but let us know that he had made it clear, both in prison and in hospital, that if he was to be given any form of emergency medication it should not be in the form of haloperidol. He confirmed that this request was followed.

Increase Social Inclusion by Decreasing Exclusionary Practices and Involve and Empower Service Users and Their Carers

This again can often be ignored as a MAAP recommendation, but it is highly relevant. Our NICE guideline group was particularly critical of the ready use of seclusion in many psychiatric units. There is a place for seclusion, but it should be used late in the management of violence, not as a reflex reaction to any disturbed episode. If appropriate treatment is given early, the period in seclusion is greatly reduced [13], thereby emphasising that seclusion should not be an excuse for leaving the person concerned unattended. Locking a secure room should only be necessary for very short periods, and should never considered when secluding children (recommendation 8.7.2.23) [1].

Include Leisure Activities that are Personally Meaningful and Physical Exercise for Service Users

Leisure activities are an essential part of the social environment. If you are forced to spend all your time surrounded by people, often perceived to be enemies as they themselves are angry, in confined areas, there is great propensity to violence. Appropriate leisure activities are a way of escaping from potentially toxic environments.

The COVID-19 pandemic is going to have a big impact on prisoners because of the resultant changes in the environment. It is difficult to predict what might happen as a consequence of social/physical distancing and limitations on visiting. According to a recent report, during the fourteen-week lockdown at one prison episodes of violence were much lower than for the previous two quarters [14]. This trend is continuing. Perhaps with fewer people visiting, the environment has the potential to be more stable, leisure activities more actively sought, and with what could be described as less hassle. In Norway, where prisoners are given a great deal more respect than in most other countries, and where outdoor activities are manifold and attractive, episodes of violence are reported to be lower and, according to one key statistic, reoffending rates in the year after release are only 20% (compared with 45% in England) [15].

Actions to be Taken after Episodes of Violence

Violence in any setting is often the precursor for more violence, and so it is wise to evaluate each episode and determine policies for the future. For this reason, our NICE guideline recommended strongly a set of post-incident actions. In general enquiries we have found that post-incident reviews are commonplace in forensic settings, and less common in other settings, but they are important. Perhaps the ideal requirement of a 'service user experience monitoring unit' hosting such a review is the stumbling block. Service users are usually involved in such reviews but not in leading them, although this may change (see Chapter 21), and many units do not have such monitoring units. But the principle behind them is important because it makes the review an independent one, not a rubber-stamped exercise that is unlikely to identify systemic failings.

Our NICE guideline recommends that such reviews should take place within 72 hours of an incident. This is sometimes difficult to arrange and emphasises the need for a standard procedure to be put in place. If the review is delayed it is likely that important memories will be distorted, particularly if they reflect badly on those involved. It is also valuable to have detailed notes completed immediately after the incident, in which the time lines are a very important component. The review should always be conducted in a neutral format that helps staff to learn and improve rather than get tied up in the useless assignation of blame.

A good post-incident review will cover six areas:

1. the physical and emotional impact of the incident on everybody who was present,
2. clear identification of the precursors of the incident and what might have been done in terms of pharmacological (see Chapter 6) and psychological (see Chapter 7) intervention that could have defused the violence,
3. determine whether interventions were given at the right time and what warnings might have been detected earlier,
4. identify any existing barriers, protocols or constraints that might have contributed to the incident and whether these should be changed to reduce the likelihood of repeat episodes,
5. offer a wider look at the service's philosophy, education and training to see these if these were still appropriate,
6. make recommendations to avoid a similar incident happening in future, if possible.

To give an example of this, one of us (PT) was involved in investigating a unit where there had been an unacceptably high rate of violent episodes extending over more than a year. This enquiry showed that service users were not involved in any post-incident reviews, that the tolerance level of the staff was low, with a policy that involved calling a nearby unit whenever violence was expected, and that the staff who then descended on the unit (all men) had been specially trained in violence reduction. All six of the post-incident priorities needed to be changed and a completely new regime introduced.

Use Crisis and Risk-Management Plans and Strategies to Reduce the Need for Restrictive Interventions

The principles of risk assessment and management were described by Ruth McAllister and Sachin Patel in chapter 3 of the first edition of this book. In their chapter, they relied a great deal on the advice of the 2008 Royal College of Psychiatrists Report *Rethinking Risk to Others in Mental Health Services*. This emphasised that all risk assessment should be evidence based and also made the statement that 'accurate risk assessment is impossible at the individual level'.

Since this time, there has been a considerable number of research studies demonstrating that risk assessment instruments are very poor at identifying risk of violence. Put more bluntly, most of the measures that assess risk are no better than the single piece of knowledge 'this individual has been violent before'. Jeremy Coid and his colleagues compared people at greater risk of violence (all offenders) using three commonly used instruments (HCR-20, VRAG, OGRS-II) in individuals with different diagnoses

[16]. Moderate-to-good predictive accuracy for future violence was achieved for released prisoners with no mental disorder, and low-to-moderate accuracy for clinical syndromes and personality disorder, but accuracy was no better than chance for individuals with psychopathy.' They concluded that 'comprehensive diagnostic assessment should precede any assessment of risk and that risk assessment instruments cannot be relied upon when managing public risk from individuals with psychopathy'.

Manual Restraint

One of the most important components of guidance in the 2015 guideline was the recommendations on the use of manual restraint:

> 2.1 This guideline recommends that taking service users to the floor during manual restraint should be avoided, but that if it is necessary, the supine (face up) position should be used in preference to the prone (face down) position. The Winterbourne View Hospital Department of Health Review reported that restraint was being used to abuse service users. Mind's Mental health crisis care: physical restraint in crisis found that restrictive interventions were being used for too long, often not as a last resort, and sometimes purposely to inflict pain, humiliate or punish. MIND also reported that in 2011/12 the prone position was being used, in some trusts as many as 2 to 3 times a day. This position can, and has, caused death after as little as 10 minutes, by causing a cardiac event. Consistent implementation of these recommendations will save lives, improve safety and minimise distress for all involved. [1; internal references removed]

The major reason for avoiding manual restraint in the prone position is simple: there is real danger of death. This is because for the person who is held down and whose breathing cannot be seen, there is a real danger of asphyxiation. There are dozens of examples of patients in secure care and prisoners in correctional institutions dying under such circumstances. Although more staff may be necessary for the use of manual restraint in the supine position, only under exceptional circumstances and when no other staff are around should the prone position be used.

Norman Lamb, MP, was a health minister in the coalition government (2010–15) and argued a strong case for banning face-down restraint after it was found that this was being used hundreds of times a year in some mental health trusts. He raised the profile of this problem, and there was an immediate fall in the recorded incidents of this type of restraint, but they still accounted for nearly 70% of cases of restraint in 2015–16.

The NICE guideline has reinforced the importance of avoiding restrictive interventions wherever possible when dealing with imminent violence. It is asking all trusts to have in place programmes to reduce restricted interventions, and for these to be both implemented and regularly reported. One of the issues that concerned members of the NICE group was the large number of providers offering 'violence management' programmes to NHS trusts, most of them lacking any evidence base or peer review. Without a corresponding emphasis on violence reduction there was cause for concern, but we were unable to acquire hard evidence that physical restraint techniques were being used more often because staff had been trained in these to a greater extent than in psychological methods of defusing violence.

We are fully aware that with increased pressure on the NHS, and longer waiting times, there is potentially a greater risk of violence because of greater frustration with services. It is impossible to know whether the NICE guideline has had a positive impact but the trend is unfortunately in the wrong direction, at least in England, albeit less so in Scotland and Wales (The Guardian, 7 Oct 2017) [19]). The number of incidents of mental health staff being involved in attacks in England increased from 33,620 in 2013 to 42,692 in 2016–17. Data on deaths following manual restraint are more difficult to come by, but it is pleasing to know that there is no evidence of any marked increase and, if anything, the publicity created by previous concerns has had a positive effect.

Reciprocity of Reducing Violence for both Patients and Staff

National newspapers and other media outlets tend to highlight violent episodes in mental health settings in black-and-white terms. We read two types of accounts. One describes rampaging and bullying inmates, often described as psychopathic and out of control, dominating and intimidating staff. The converse account is of similarly aggressive and violent staff, who lose no opportunity to exercise physical restraint and who frighten the patients under their care.

But such accounts are slanted for the purposes of the journalists concerned. In practice, both staff and patients suffer if violence is endemic in a hospital setting. To take one example: in Muckamore Abbey Hospital in Northern Ireland, between 2014 and 2017, 53 incidents of assaults on patients by staff were reported; five of these incidents were investigated and substantiated and the news item was reported under the headline 'Five patients assaulted by staff'. [20] But hidden in the substance of the report were data showing that there were 4,546 incidents of physical abuse, assault or violence by patients on staff reported over the same time period and 193 instances of staff sickness relevant to these [19].

We think the important message here is that, in a single individual, the comprehensive diagnostic assessment is much more valuable than an on-paper risk assessment and other advice in the college guidance. To take one example, none of the many risk instruments predicting violence in people who qualify for the diagnosis of psychopathy provide data on prediction greater than chance [16]. If, however, more attention is paid to dynamic factors rather than static ones in individual cases, this can change. In a recent study the main recommendation was that causal factors were the most important in violence prevention programmes [21].

Dynamic Risk Assessment

The continuous assessment of risk in the rapidly changing circumstances of an operational incident, in order to implement the control measures necessary to ensure an acceptable level of safety' [22].

The third element of defusing aggression – the 'aim to build emotional bridges and maintain a therapeutic relationship' – can really only be achieved if a good (or at least a working) relationship has been established with the potential aggressor before the aggressive incident. Previous knowledge and understanding can achieve marvels when it precedes the episode.

We give one personal example. PT is a monozygotic twin, and his brother Stephen, also a psychiatrist, worked in New York for a short time. One afternoon he decided to visit a patient with bipolar disorder, whom he had met before and who had missed an appointment. When he called at the patient's apartment, the door was opened and he was quickly let in. The patient then picked up a samurai sword and grabbed Stephen, holding the sword at his neck. As Stephen knew the patient well he – almost automatically – said 'Don't be silly; put that sword down.' The man released him and they had, under the circumstances, a reasonably friendly conversation, from which my brother concluded that he was beginning to have elevated mood again. This particular outcome might have been very different had the patient been a complete stranger. Whatever bond had been established previously had been re-established by the response, essentially defusing the threat.

Conclusion

This chapter, and others in this book, show that we can never be complacent about the management of violence in mental health and hospital settings. What is clearly needed is an integrated set of guidelines to manage violence in all types of setting, ranging from hospitals, general practice surgeries, community settings of all types, and high-risk areas such as aeroplanes and moving vehicles. Even though the settings may differ, the principles for management of violence are essentially the same. What is needed is proper training to deal with risks effectively.

References

1. National Institute of Health and Clinical Excellence (2015). Violence and aggression: short-term management in mental health, health and community settings (NG10). London: Department of Health.

2. National Institute for Clinical Excellence (NICE) (2005). Violence: short-term management for over 16s in psychiatric and emergency departments. CG25. London: Department of Health.

3. National Institute of Health and Clinical Excellence (NICE) (2015). Challenging behaviour and learning disabilities: prevention and intervention is for people with learning disabilities whose behavior challenges. Nice Guideline [NG11]. London: Department of Health.

4. HM Stationery Office (2019). Surveillance of violence and aggression: short-term management in mental health, health and community settings (NICE guideline NG10).

5. Bressington, D., Stewart, B., Beer, D. and MacInnes, D. (2011). Levels of service user satisfaction in secure settings – A survey of the association between perceived social climate, perceived therapeutic relationship and satisfaction with forensic services. *International Journal of Nursing Studies* 48:1349–56.

6. Keown, P., Weich, S., Bhui, K. and Scott, J. (2011). Association between the provision of mental illness beds and rate of involuntary admissions in the NHS in England: Ecological study 1988–2008. *BMJ* 343:d3736.

7. Tyrer, P. and Tyrer, H. (2018). *Nidotherapy: Harmonising the Environment to the Patient*, 2nd ed. Cambridge: Cambridge University Press.

8. Ranger, M., Tyrer, P., Miloševska, K. et al. (2009). Cost-effectiveness of nidotherapy for comorbid personality disorder and severe mental illness: Randomized controlled trial. *Epidemiologia e Psichiatria Sociale* 18:128–36.

9. Akerman, G., Needs, A. and Bainbridge, C. (2018). *Transforming Environments and Rehabilitation: A Guide for Practitioners in Forensic Settings and Criminal Justice*. Abingdon: Routledge.

10. O'Rourke, R., Taylor, A. and Leggett, K. (2018). Establishing environment principals with young adult males in a custodial setting. In G. Akerman, A. Needs and C. Bainbridge (eds.), *Transforming Environments and Rehabilitation: A Guide for Practitioners in Forensic Settings and Criminal Justice*. Abingdon: Routledge, pp. 271–288.

11. Benefield, N., Turner, K., Bolger, L., and Bainbridge, C. (2018). Psychologically informed planned environments: a new optimism for criminal justice provision? In G. Akerman, A. Needs and C. Bainbridge (eds.), *Transforming Environments and Rehabilitation: A Guide for Practitioners in Forensic Settings and Criminal Justice*. Abingdon: Routledge, pp. 179–978.

12. Shingler, J., Sonnenberg, S. J., and Needs, A. (2020). Understanding indeterminate sentenced prisoners'

experiences of psychological risk assessment in the United Kingdom. *Psychology, Crime & Law* 6:571–92.

13. Tyrer, S., Beckley, J., Goel, D. et al. (2012). Factors affecting the practice of seclusion in an acute mental health service in Southland, New Zealand. *BJPsych Bulletin* 36:214–18.

14. Jenny, R. (2020). Coronavirus: Violence fears over longer lockdowns in prisons. British Broadcasting Corporation, 8 July. www.bbc.co.uk/news/uk-wales-53323771 [Accessed 8.9.2021].

15. Fazel, S. and Wolf, A. (2015). A systematic review of criminal recidivism rates worldwide: Current difficulties and recommendations for best practice. *Plos One* 10:e0130390.

16. Coid, J. W., Ullrich, S., and Kallis, C. (2013). Predicting future violence among individuals with psychopathy. *British Journal of Psychiatry* 203:387–8.

17. Department of Health (2012). Policy paper. Winterbourne View Hospital: DoH review and response. Published December 2012. Updated June 2013 [online]. www.gov.uk/government/publications/winterbourne-view-hospital-department-of-health-review-and-response [Accessed 8.9.2021].

18. MIND (2013). Mental health crisis care: Physical restraint in crisis [online]. www.mind.org.uk/media-a/4378/physical_restraint_final_web_version.pdf [Accessed 8.9.2021].

19. Campbell, D. (2017). Rise in violent attacks by patients on NHS mental health staff. *The Guardian* [online]. 7 October. www.theguardian.com/society/2017/oct/07/rise-in-violent-attacks-by-patients-on-nhs-mental-health-staff [Accessed 8.9.2021].

20. McCracken, N. (2018). Muckamore Hospital: Five patients assaulted by staff. *British Broadcasting Corporation* [online]. www.bbc.co.uk/news/uk-northern-ireland-45035899 [Accessed 8.9.2021]

21. Coid, J. W., Ullrich, S., Kallis, C. et al. (2016). Improving risk management for violence in mental health services: A multimethods approach. *Programme Grants for Applied Research* 4(16).

22. HM FIRE Service Inspectorate. (1998). *Dynamic Assessment of Risk at Operational Incidents*. London: HM FIRE Service Inspectorate.

Post-Incident Management

Ryan Kemp, Shaazneen Ali, Rachel O'Beney and Masum
Khwaja

Introduction

Violent incidents are part of working life in mental health services. How leaders respond to
them is critical in maintaining coherent and motivated teams. In this context, an incident is
defined as an event or near miss where significant harm or damage to persons or assets
either occurred or could have easily occurred. In this chapter, we will focus mostly on issues
of violence and aggression on inpatient units as it is here that the most common serious
incidents are found. At the time of writing, the world was in the grip of the COVID-19
pandemic, with staff facing unprecedented pressures and being at risk of trauma and moral
injury. While, not addressed directly, all the recommendations in this chapter are likely to
be useful for dealing with incidents related to COVID-19.

By initiating and coordinating post-incident review and support meetings, senior
members of staff are emphasising that violent incidents are taken seriously, and that
thinking and learning about their occurrence and impact is important. This can limit
further 'acting out' in both service users and staff [1]. Learning from 'facilitated debriefs'
[2] is now a mainstream concept in healthcare, and post-incident reviews are considered
helpful by staff and patients in minimising negative emotions [3].

Violence and aggression manifest in the form of anger, frustration and fear can be
enacted in many forms, ranging from a patient raising their voice during an argument to an
unprovoked attack involving a weapon. Evidence suggests that all types of aggressive
behaviour can pose a threat to the physical and psychological health of the individuals
involved [4]. Fear resulting from working in a climate of potential danger can also have
a damaging impact on patient care delivered by clinicians [5].

We argue that the immediate response to any incident takes place within a context that
will make that response more or less effective. We can broadly define that context as one
defined by a culture of psychological safety [6]. In addition, effective mental health teams
should be open to new learning and foster a culture of ongoing quality improvement. These
features of teams will be explored in some detail laster (see section 'Culture: Psychological
Safety, Learning and Team Cohesion'), but before that it is important to define terminology
and to situate post-incident management in relation to current clinical and legal guidance.

Definitions

The terms 'debrief', 'post-incident support' and 'post-incident review' are often used
interchangeably. But they are not the same, and this may lead to confusion. Debriefing
processes normally occur soon after the event, enable feedback and reflection and identify
areas for improvement. It is a mixture of support and teaching, aiming to understand

exactly what has happened and why. Sometimes this takes place several weeks after an incident, and is then referred to as a 'cold debrief' [7]. Clinical debriefing may be defined as a dialogue between two or more people that is focused on a discussion of the actions and thought processes involved in a particular patient care situation. The dialogue should encourage reflection on those actions and thought processes and incorporate improvement into future performance.

Psychological debriefing differs in that it is a formal version of providing emotional and psychological support immediately following a traumatic event. The goal of psychological debriefing is to prevent the development of post-traumatic stress disorder and other negative sequelae. It should be noted that the efficacy of this practice has been essentially disproved by evidence [8].

In the context of a seclusion and restraint reduction process, debriefing is considered a tertiary prevention strategy as it is designed to prevent further occurrences of coercion and is consistent with trauma-informed care and quality improvement principles [9]. Post-incident support is not the same as debriefing. It usually occurs immediately after an incident, is a way of 'checking in' with all those involved and taking stock of the situation, can often include dealing with practicalities, such as injuries, helps to identify necessary actions and basically consists of a genuine enquiry into all the key issues [7].

Post-incident review may be defined as a formal evaluation of the events that led to a serious incident: what happened and how it was managed. It tends to be reserved for major incidents. The aim is to understand whether (i) the incident could have been responded to differently and possibly avoided, and (ii) changes in practices need to be made to improve care and avoid a repetition [9]. Establishing all the facts in the context of an incident should be undertaken as part of a timely and factual debrief, reported according to local organisational guidelines. This part of the review needs to be less emotional and more factual.

The extent of the post-incident review will depend on the seriousness of the incident. Ideally, staff teams should have access to regular reflective practice meetings so there is an ongoing thinking space to digest the repercussions of incidents and a place to discuss changes to service delivery, enabling care to continue to be responsive to patient needs. Individual post-incident review sessions should also be made available if required, sometimes with individual staff members. The summary of learning should be escalated to the required care quality forum for noting and should ideally be shared with other teams as appropriate.

Guidance in Relation to Post-Incident Management

The importance of post-incident support is highlighted in the Department of Health's Positive and Proactive Care [10] guidance. The guidance states that 'service providers must ensure that appropriate lessons are learnt when incidents occur where restrictive interventions have had to be used' (p. 23). It also usefully describes the aims of post-incident reviews. The 'Safe Wards' model [11] proposed ten core interventions aimed at reducing conflict and restrictive practices ('containment') on the wards. Reflection on practice and review of interventions is integral to the model, which underpins post-incident debrief, support and review [12].

The National Institute for Health and Care Excellence (NICE) guidelines, *Violence and aggression: Short-term management in mental health, health and community settings, 2015* [13], outlines best practice in relation to managing aggression and violence. The guidance stipulates that health and social care provider organisations should ensure that wards have sufficient skilled staff to enable them to conduct an immediate post-incident debrief, respond to ongoing risks and contribute to formal external post-incident reviews.

In addition, NICE's *Violent and aggressive behaviours in people with mental health problems: Quality standard* [14] recommends an immediate post-incident debrief for people with a mental health problem who experience restraint, rapid tranquillisation or seclusion.

The Royal College of Psychiatrists' *Standards for Community-Based Mental Health Services* [15] stipulates that community mental health teams (CMHTs) should learn from incidents and share this learning with staff and service users alike. Employers are also mandated to ensure there are systems to support staff affected by an incident, under the Health and Safety at Work, Act 1974 [16] and the Management of Health and Safety at Work Regulations 1999 [17].

The post-incident review serves two broad purposes: to allow staff to process the emotions that the incident may have evoked, and to learn from the incident so that services can limit or prevent recurrence. The immediate post-incident debrief should involve both nursing and medical involvement, as well as any other involved parties. There should be a discussion with the service user involved in the incident, and with any other service users involved or resident on the ward concerned.

Culture: Psychological Safety, Learning and Team Cohesion

When an incident occurs, it is never in isolation. In mental health, incidents are almost always processed in relation to the overall effectiveness and cohesion of the team in which they occur. Incidents often evoke fear in clinicians, and in some dysfunctional cultures this leads to denial, downplaying or even cover-up. Such was the culture in the Mid-Staffordshire Hospitals, which experienced a scandal that led to many deaths and national outrage. In his review and recommendations, Don Berwick noted that 'fear is toxic to both safety and improvement' [18, p. 4]. Any team or organisational culture that exhibits fear as a prominent emotion is going to struggle to improve safety and will not learn from its mistakes.

There is growing evidence that psychological safety is critical to thriving teams, in both the commercial and the public sector [19]. Leadership incompetence and hierarchical structures in teams have been found to affect negatively the creation of psychological safety. Teams that create such safety exhibit the following qualities:

- Leaders are accessible and approachable
- Leaders acknowledge the limits of their knowledge
- Leaders are willing to display fallibility
- Leaders invite participation
- Failures are seen as learning opportunities
- Teams and leaders use direct language
- Leaders set and maintain boundaries
- Leaders hold people to account

The opposite of this are aloof, arrogant leaders who maintain their own safety at the expense of their teams, often finding ways to blame junior staff for errors or failures. If we are honest, we all know clinical and operational leaders who act in this manner. In teams such as these, wherein fear predominates, staff avoid reflecting on their mistakes as they fear being made the scapegoat for what are usually systemic failures. These sorts of teams, together with the structural problem of chronic underfunding, often lead to structures that are unable to perform adequately or that treat individual service users in a manner that accords with acceptable standards. This damages staff, and its continuation often leads to burnout. However, latterly this is being thought of as moral injury to the innocent people involved in a dysfunctional system.

Responding to Moral Injury

When clinicians find themselves in positions which mean that they are forced to make decisions and act in a manner which violates their moral or ethical code, they sustain a moral injury [20]. These injuries accumulate over time, although one-off events, if severe enough, can also injure. The effect is to create negative cognitions about self or the system; these cognitions particularly include guilt, shame and depression. These effects do not constitute a mental illness, but in vulnerable individuals they can contribute towards the onset of such illnesses. The best way to mitigate the effects of moral injury is a combination of (a) understanding the context of service delivery, (b) reflective practices (such as Schwarz rounds or Balint Groups), (c) new leadership that does not allow teams or members to avoid discussions of difficult circumstances, (d) routine peer support, and (e) compassionate supervision. In the context of post-incident management, the key dynamic is to ensure that teams are not overwhelmed by the consequences of moral injury, such as avoiding post-incident review meetings.

Emotional Processing

A crucial function of post-incident review, which is an element missing from the debriefing literature [20], is the importance of 'emotional processing'. This is where feelings such as shock, shame and anxiety can be voiced and processed, rather than defended against through further 'enactments' which fuel more anxiety or fear [1]. To defend against such overwhelming feelings of vulnerability after an incident, staff can, for example, implement extra rigid rules, 'stay away from' particular service users or subtly punish them, for example by forbidding requests for a 'second cup of tea'. Eventually they can become cynical about their work.

Purely focusing on 'facts' in a post-incident review, or keeping technical and emotional debriefing separate, may leave feelings and emotions unattended to and neglected. This can leave participants locked in a detached state of mind as a way of defending themselves against feeling overwhelmed, vulnerable and distressed [21]. Once feelings of shock, anxiety, vulnerability and anger have been acknowledged and discussed, the need to retreat into a detached and 'cut off state of mind' lifts and facilitates greater capacity, for more balanced and rational thought [21]. In this state of mind, it may then be much easier to effectively evaluate the incident, to determine exactly what happened and what could have been done differently, with this feeding into new learning and any changes that need to be made to service delivery.

In many instances it is important to give space to the feelings and reactions of everybody by discussing the problems in a group format, and to suggest, where appropriate, that strong feelings in one person might be shared with the team rather than being solely located in one person, who then remains alone in their distress [9]. Feelings of being isolated and alone after a traumatic event have been linked to the development of post-traumatic stress disorder (PTSD) [22]. Sharing in this way increases the care team's cohesiveness and can reduce discomfort and tension, providing immediate and continuing support. It can also serve as a basis for reconciliation and enable staff to resume their therapeutic relationship with a service user by whom they felt 'under attack' during the incident [9].

Poor evidence has been reported for people who are seen alone. This meant that participants failed to experience the therapeutic benefits of a group, including a sense of cohesion and the feeling their distress was shared [24]. The NICE guidelines for PTSD state that individual interventions are not indicated in the first instance and recommend watchful waiting [8], and that individual trauma-focused cognitive behavioural therapy should only be offered in the first month to those with severe post-traumatic symptoms. Systematic provision to individuals of brief, single-session interventions focusing on the traumatic incident should not be routine practice.

Another effect of not having the space to think and reflect about an incident is chronic detachment, manifest in staff sickness, avoidance of patients or leaving the post or profession entirely [1]. Bion [25] described the importance of 'emotional containment', pointing to the need to look after and contain staff, so they may have sufficient resources to care effectively for their service users. If staff distress is not attended to via post-incident reviews or debriefs, their undigested feelings may indirectly adversely affect patients. Feelings, if not properly expressed, can end up being unconsciously enacted against service users [1]. Individuals involved in incidents (patients, staff, carers) often report being grateful for the opportunity to express feelings and achieve some understanding of what happened [26, 27].

How to Conduct a Post-incident Review

A post-incident review should take place as soon as possible after the incident, and if possible before the end of a shift or working day. If this cannot be achieved, the review must be conducted within 72 hours. For learning purposes, it is important that events and facts are accurately recalled and recorded, and recollection degrades as time passes.

After an incident in which a restrictive intervention may have been used, and when the risks of harm have been contained, an immediate post-incident debrief should be conducted. The NICE quality standard [14] states that:

> The debrief should include a nurse and a doctor and identify and address physical harm to service users or staff, ongoing risks and the emotional impact on service users and staff, including witnesses. The incident should only be discussed with service users, witnesses and staff involved after they have recovered their composure. The debrief should use a framework for anticipating and reducing violence and aggression to determine the factors that contributed to an incident that led to a restrictive intervention, identify any factors that can be addressed quickly to reduce the likelihood of a further incident and amend risk and care plans accordingly. (p. 26)

It may be helpful for the team psychologist to facilitate the meeting, although any skilled person could lead the process. Attendance and support from the ward medical consultant and matron are also essential to reinforce the importance of the process. The meeting is not only to understand and address what happened to both service users and staff and consider ongoing risks, but also to gauge the emotional impact on service users, staff and witnesses. If anyone was physically hurt, this will have been dealt with immediately.

It is very important to consider the needs of other service users as it is often assumed that they 'did not notice' or 'are used to' incidents, when in fact they may be highly sensitive to their environment and may feel intensively vulnerable, thereby exacerbating their mental symptoms [28]. It is important to identify any factors that can be addressed quickly, to reduce the likelihood of a further incident and amend risk and care plans accordingly [13]. During incidents, service users often feel vulnerable, frightened, confused and exposed. These experiences can intensify 'defences' such as manic behaviour and delusional symptoms [29], and can generally unsettle service users. It is helpful if some staff involved in the incident can be present at the service users' review, to give some consistency and reassurance that they have 'weathered' the incident. However, it should not be assumed that involved staff would facilitate the meeting, especially if they are still working through their own feelings. It is important for service users (and carers who may join) to be offered their own contained space, enabling them to process anxieties and concerns, protected from staff expressing distress in an undigested way.

It is also important for the facilitator to ask for the 'story' of what happened from those involved. This narrative would hopefully include contributing factors, possible triggers and antecedents for the incident, how each person was involved and affected, how they felt during the incident and how they feel at the time of the review. Agreement over immediate actions that need to be taken to address continuing concerns that may emerge should be established.

When conducting a post-incident review, points to remember include:

- To ensure everyone involved is invited and everyone who wants to attend can, in their respective staff and service user groups.
- Allow adequate time for review (e.g. an hour).
- Participation is voluntary but may be actively encouraged.
- Remind participants that the meeting is strictly confidential.
- Everyone is equal in being invited to contribute.
- This is not a criticism or investigation.
- This is not counselling or therapy.
- Expect anger to be expressed, which may well be the result of participants feeling filled with stress and anxiety.
- The facilitator should offer a summary at the end of the review, including the next steps.

Immediate post-event review with staff facilitates safety on the unit and a return to pre-crisis functioning. Digestion of feelings of shock and trauma can enable resolution of upset feelings that generally should aid clear thinking and the consideration needed to work out the appropriate detail required for serious incident (SI) documentation [9].

Based on Mitchell and Everly [30], we outline several phases that a post-incident review should go through:

1. Introduction

   The review leader allows team members to introduce themselves and explains the purpose of the review. This helps create an environment conducive to participation, reduces resistance and gains the participants' cooperation. The team answers questions and this hopefully alleviates anxiety, which encourages mutual help and openness to learning. If the team feels 'psychologically safe' then this could be a short part of the process. If the team is fearful or undergoing other change processes, more time might be needed to prepare for the further stages of the review.

2. Factual Description of Incident

   Members of the team describe what they observed. This should be brief and factual. This allows participants to describe the event from their perspective, their role during the incident and what happened from their point of view. Those leading the review should try to prevent any blaming of individuals or conclusions being drawn prematurely.

3. Thoughtful Reactions Described

   The review leader asks participants to state what their first or most prominent thoughts were during the incident and then again during the review. This begins the transition from thoughts to emotional reactions (or from the external, factual level to a more internal, personal level).

4. Emotional Reactions Described

   Each member is invited to identify the most personally upsetting aspect of the incident and their emotional reactions. This should be done in a 'then and now' manner, as emotional reactions develop over time. For example, they may have initially felt fearful, but this could have altered into guilt and remorse. This phase tends to be the most emotionally powerful time of the meeting. It can be useful to encourage an emotionally articulate member of the team to speak early in the process; this illustrates that vulnerability is both acceptable and useful.

5. Stress-Related Reactions Described

   Ending the review at this point could possibly leave participants in a charged emotional state that could prove detrimental without appropriate support and closure. The review leader should ask the individuals to describe any affective, behavioural, cognitive or physical reactions they may have encountered during the incident or afterwards that continue to distress them. The review leader may need to give several examples of stress-related symptoms (such as angry feelings, trembling hands, difficulty making decisions, or severe fatigue) to get the group moving in this direction. Past problems might be raised, and discussion of how they were resolved can also help.

6. Coping Strategies Described

   The entire team is then involved in discussing the teaching of symptoms of stress usually encountered and providing a variety of stress management strategies. These do not have to involve formal technology-driven ideas (as these could be overly psychiatric), but could involve practical support, such as suggesting more time with family, increasing life's usual pleasures and team-building activities. This phase is cognitive in approach, designed to bring staff further away from the emotional content in the reaction phase. This phase continues until the topics that are most important for the particular group of individuals are exhausted.

7. Preparing for Returning to Work

   This allows the opportunity to clarify issues, answer questions and summarise the interventions just undertaken. This phase brings closure to the discussions that have transpired in the review and allows for the opportunity to end on a positive note. It may be necessary to outline what will happen next, for both staff and service users.

Formal External Post-Incident Review

A formal, external, post-incident review may also need to take place, depending on the seriousness of the incident. This, according to NICE guidelines (2015), should be done by the service-user experience-monitoring unit or its equivalent service user group, who should undertake a formal, external, post-incident review as soon as possible (and no later than 72 hours after the incident). The unit should ensure that the formal external post-incident review is led by a service user and includes staff from outside the ward where the incident took place, all of whom are trained to undertake investigations that aim to help staff learn and improve rather than assign blame.

Following the review, the physical and emotional impact on everyone involved should be evaluated to identify what led to the incident and what could have been done differently. This is to determine whether alternatives, including less restrictive interventions, were discussed, and whether service barriers or constraints make it difficult to avoid similar incidents occurring in the future. Changes to the service's policies, care environment, treatment approaches, staff education and training will be recommended where appropriate. The service-user experience-monitoring unit or equivalent service user group then give their report recommendations to the ward [13].

Perpetrator of Violent Behaviour

A medical review of the patient's mental and physical state should take place within two hours [31]. The review should include consideration of the Mental Health Act status of the patient, the observation level and the setting for further treatment. The risk assessment and care plan documentation should be updated.

Following each intervention for the short-term management of disturbed or violent behaviour, it should be established whether the service user understands why the intervention took place. They may be upset by the incident and how it was managed, or frightened about the consequences for them, and so should be given the opportunity to describe the incident from their perspective. Where possible, this interview should be carried out by a staff member who was not directly involved in the intervention. The discussion should be documented in the service user's notes.

The decision about whether or not to pursue criminal proceedings is discussed later in the chapter.

Victim of Violent Behaviour

Immediate first aid and medical treatment should be given to the injured person(s) where appropriate. A member of staff should be identified to stay with the injured person(s) until medical assistance is available.

It is important that victims know their rights – for example, the right to report a violent attack to the police. The individual's manager should discuss the issue of prosecution and offer to accompany the relevant service user(s) or staff member(s) to the police if necessary. A victim of violence may have the right to financial compensation from a government-funded scheme. A claim may be made to the Criminal Injuries Compensation Authority (CICA), a government organisation that may compensate people who have been physically or mentally injured because they were the blameless victim of a violent crime [31]. It offers a free service for processing applications and making financial awards.

Pursuing Criminal Proceedings

The Crown Prosecution Service (CPS), which is responsible for prosecuting criminal cases in England and Wales, provides guidance [32] in identifying the principles relevant to the decision to prosecute, and any prosecution which follows, of individuals who have:

- A mental disorder, as defined by the Mental Health Act 2007
- A learning disability
- A learning difficulty
- Autism spectrum disorder
- An acquired brain injury
- Dementia
- Other mental health, cognitive or neuro-diverse conditions.

Each case must be considered on its merits, taking into account all available information about any mental health problem and its relevance to the offence. There is a balance to be struck between the public interest in diverting a defendant with significant mental illness from the criminal justice system and other public interest factors, or the opposite option of prosecution, which may also address the need to safeguard the public. If there is significant evidence to establish that a defendant or suspect has a significant mental illness, a prosecution may not be appropriate unless the offence is serious or there is a real possibility that it may be repeated, although some commentators have advocated for the reporting of all acts of non-trivial violence to the police [33].

Conclusion

Violence may take many forms and impact on staff in a variety of ways. Clinical leaders need to instil a culture of care and learning to prevent trauma and moral injury. The effectiveness of a response to any incident takes place within a context of ongoing leadership. Environments which are psychologically safe have been found to facilitate team cohesion and a productive learning culture.

A post-incident management process is described where we argue that attending to and processing emotions is crucial to allow learning to take place. Careful and skilled facilitation is required, and we have described a process in detail. In some cases, an external review of incidents may be required, which again should be carefully implemented to avoid staff feeling they are under threat from the process. It should also be remembered that both victims and perpetrators of violence are likely to experience the incident as traumatising and need to be given opportunities to process events.

The CPS, which are responsible for prosecuting criminal cases in England and Wales, has published guidance on prosecution of individuals with a mental disorder, learning disability, dementia and other mental health, cognitive or neuro-diverse conditions.

References

1. Armstrong, D. R. *Social Defences Against Anxiety: Explorations in a Paradigm (The Tavistock Clinic Series)*. London: Karnac Books, 2014.

2. Dismukes, R. K. , Gaba, D. M. and Howard, S. K. So many roads: Facilitated debriefing in healthcare [online]. Vol. 1, *Simulation in Healthcare: Journal of the Society for Simulation in Healthcare*. 2006. https://journals.lww.com/simulationin healthcare/Fulltext/2006/00110/So_Many_ Roads__Facilitated_Debriefing_in.1.aspx.

3. Bonner, G., Lowe, T., Rawcliffe, D., and Wellman, N. Trauma for all: A pilot study of the subjective experience of physical restraint for mental health inpatients and staff in the UK. *Journal of Psychiatric and Mental Health Nursing* 2002 Aug;9(4):465–73. https://doi.org/10.1046/j.1365-2850.2002.00504.x. PMID: 12164909.

4. Mitchell, M. and Mitchell, G. Book reviews: *Violence and Mental Health Care Professionals.* Edited by Til Wykes. *International Journal of Social Psychiatry* 1997 Mar;43(1):76–7.

5. Foster, C. , Bowers, L. and Nijman, H. Aggressive behaviour on acute psychiatric wards: Prevalence, severity and management. *Journal of Advanced Nursing* 2007;58(2):140–9.

6. Edmondson, A. *Teaming: How Organizations Learn, Innovate, and Compete in the Knowledge Economy.* Hoboken: John Wiley & Sons, Incorporated, 2012

7. Burman, N. Debrief and post-incident support: Views of staff, patients and carers. *Nursing Times* 2018;114(9):63–6.

8. NICE Guidance. Post-traumatic stress disorder [online]. 2018. www.nice.org.uk/guidance/ng116 [Accessed 27.4.2022].

9. Te Pou Te Pou, the National Centre of Mental Health Research, Information and Workforce Development. Debriefing following seclusion and restraint: A summary of relevant literature [online]. 2014. https://openrepository.aut.ac.nz/bitstream/handle/10292/9084/debriefing-following-seclusion-and-restraint-281014.pdf [Accessed 27.4.2022].

10. Department of Health and Social Services. Positive and proactive care: Reducing the need for restrictive interventions. Social Care, Local Government and Care Partnership Directorate, 2014.

11. Safewards. Resources for Safewards implementation [online]. www.safewards.net/ [Accessed 27.4.2022].

12. Bowers, L. Safewards: A new model of conflict and containment on psychiatric wards [online]. *Journal of Psychiatric and*

Mental Health Nursing. 2014, 21 (6):499–508. https://doi.org/10.1111/jpm.

13. NICE Guidance. Violence and aggression: Short-term management in mental health, health and community settings [online]. NICE, 2015. www.nice.org.uk/guidance/ng10 [Accessed 27.4.2022].

14. NICE Guideline. Violent and aggressive behaviours in people with mental health problems: Quality standards [online]. NICE, 2017. www.nice.org.uk/guidance/qs154 [Accessed 27.4.2022].

15. Royal College of Psychiatrists, College Centre for Quality Improvement. Standards for Community-Based Mental Health Services. [online]. 3rd ed., 2019. www.rcpsych.ac.uk/docs/default-source/improving-care/ccqi/ccqi-resources/rcpsych_standards_com_2019_lr.pdf?sfvrsn=321ed2a3_2 [Accessed 27.4.2022].

16. Participation E. Health and Safety at Work etc. Act 1974 [online]. Statute Law Database; 1974. www.legislation.gov.uk/ukpga/1974/37/contents.

17. The Management of Health and Safety at Work Regulations 1999 [online]. Queen's Printer of Acts of Parliament; 1999. www.legislation.gov.uk/uksi/1999/3242/contents/made.

18. Berwick Review into Patient Safety. A promise to learn – a commitment to act. Improving the Safety of Patients in England. National Advisory Group on the Safety of Patients in England; 2013.

19. Edmondson, A., Higgins, M., Singer, S., and Weiner, J. Understanding psychological safety in health care and education organizations: A comparative perspective. *Research in Human Development* 2016 Jan 2;13:65–83.

20. Greenberg, N., Docherty, M., Gnanapragasam, S., and Wessely, S. Managing mental health challenges faced by healthcare workers during covid-19 pandemic. *BMJ* 2020 Mar 26;368: m1211.

21. Farrell, J., Reiss, N., and Shaw, I. *The Schema Therapy Clinician's Guide: A Complete Resource for Building and Delivering Individual, Group and Integrated*

Schema Mode Treatment Programs. London: Wiley-Blackwell, 2014.

22. Grey, N. A Casebook of Cognitive Therapy for Traumatic Stress Reactions. London: Routledge, 2009.

23. Rose, S., Bisson, J., Churchill, R., and Wessely, S. Psychological debriefing for preventing post-traumatic stress disorder (PTSD). Cochrane Database of Systematic Reviews. 2002;(2):CD000560. https://doi.org/10.1002/14651858.CD000560. PMID: 12076399.

24. Yalom, I. D. and Leszcz, M. The Theory and Practice of Group Psychotherapy, 6th ed. New York: Basic Books/Hachette Book Group, 2021.

25. Bion, W. R. Container and contained. In A. Colman and M. Geller (eds.), Group Relations Reader, Vol. 2. 1985. Saulsalito: AK Rice Institute, pp. 127–33.

26. McIvor, R. J., Canterbury, R., and Gunn, J. Psychological care of staff following traumatic incidents at work. Psychiatric Bulletin 1997;21(3):176–8.

27. Bonner, G. and Wellman, N. Post incident review of aggression and violence in mental health settings. Journal of Psychosocial Nursing and Mental Health Services. 2010 Jul 1;48(7):35–40.

28. Sherrer, M. V. The role of cognitive appraisal in adaptation to traumatic stress in adults with serious mental illness: A critical review. Trauma, Violence, & Abuse. 2011 Jul;12 (3):151–67.

29. Read, J., van Os, J., Morrison, A. P. and Ross, C. A. Childhood trauma, psychosis and schizophrenia: A literature review with theoretical and clinical implications. Acta Psychiatrica Scandinavica. 2005 Nov;112 (5):330–50.

30. Mitchell, J. T. and Everly, G. S. Critical Incident Stress Debriefing (CISD): An Operations Manual for the Prevention of Traumatic Stress Among Emergency Service and Disaster Workers. 2nd ed. Ellicott City: Chevron Publishing Corporation, 1997.

31. HM Government. Criminal Injuries Compensation Authority [online]. NICE; 2002. www.gov.uk/government/organisations/criminal-injuries-compensation-authority [Accessed 27.4.2022].

32. Crown Prosecution Service. Mental health: Suspects and defendants with mental health conditions or disorders. [online]. 2019. www.cps.gov.uk/legal-guidance/mental-health-suspects-and-defendants-mental-health-conditions-or-disorders [Accessed 27.4.2022].

33. Wilson, S., Murray, K., Harris, M. and Brown, M. Psychiatric in-patients, violence and the criminal justice system. The Psychiatrist 2012 Feb;36(2):41–4.

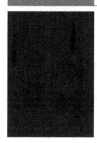

Introduction to Section 2

Section 2: The Treatment of Violence

Chapters 6, 7 and 8 cover the use of medication and psychological treatments in the management of violence; the section concludes with a pragmatic chapter on the prevention and management of violence in inpatient settings. When there is a degree of violence that represents a threat to others, medication of some nature is often necessary. The use of medication is fraught with risks, especially when high dosages are considered necessary in difficult cases. Rapid tranquillisation is sometimes necessary and, although there has to be some flexibility in the use of such drugs, it is very important for all practitioners to be aware of the protocols for such management in the settings where they work. Not all protocols are the same, but they are wisely chosen and illustrate the importance of pharmacists' advice, especially when many drugs have been or are currently being given simultaneously. Polypharmacy can be dangerous.

Psychological interventions are not usually emergency ones, but represent a background of a range of strategies that can prevent further episodes and provide an infrastructure for successful engagement. It is important to remember the single main piece of evidence coming from all reviews of antisocial behaviour: reward is more effective than punishment in responding to violence – a reminder that should be followed more assiduously in the criminal justice system.

This section ends with a discussion of management in the area where clinicians are most likely to experience violence: the inpatient ward. This is a microcosm of management described elsewhere in the book and one in which a good ward structure can be a major asset.

Use of Medication and Electroconvulsive Therapy in the Management of Violence

Peter Pratt, Caroline Parker, Masum Khwaja and Jonathan Waite

Our guidance will focus on the use of medication as an emergency response to the management of violence and disturbed behaviour. Where medication is used by the parenteral route for urgent sedation, we will use the term rapid tranquillisation (RT). We will also highlight the place of oral medication as part of de-escalation, pro re nata (PRN) (as required) or pre-RT, and briefly discuss the use of medication in the management of the risk of violence in the medium to longer term. Our guidance should be read in conjunction with the National Institute of Health and Care Excellence (NICE) 2015 guideline for the management of violence (NG10), and the 2018 British Association for Psychopharmacology (BAP) and National Association of Psychiatric Intensive Care and Low Secure Units (NAPICU) joint BAP NAPICU evidence-based consensus guidelines for the clinical management of acute disturbance: de-escalation and rapid tranquillisation [1, 2].

Clinical teams should adopt the national guidelines and key principles outlined in this chapter and use these to develop their local protocols for practice.

General Principles for Prescribing Medication to Prevent or Control Acute Violent Behaviour

The use of medication in the control of violence should be part of a comprehensive treatment plan to manage the risk of violence that includes an assessment of environmental factors and the use of other therapies. Medication should not be used to manage aggression caused by identifiable environmental factors (such as understaffing or lack of staff skills) that can be dealt with by other means.

The good practice principles in prescribing medication to prevent or control violence are:

- A multidisciplinary team should develop and document an individualised plan for the use of medication in patients who are at risk of violence. This should be reviewed at least every week. If PRN, pre-RT or RT medication has not been administered during the previous week, consideration should be given to stopping it.
- Medication should only be used when the risk of not using medication is judged to be greater than that arising from its use.
- The indication, dose, frequency and duration for which RT, pre-RT or PRN medication is to be used should be clearly stated as part of the prescription. In circumstances where

the outcome from RT is unknown, the initial dose should be prescribed as a single dose. The outcome from this initial dose will help prescribers individualise any subsequent prescribing of medication for RT that may be required.

- The lowest dose compatible with the desired outcome should be used.
- All doses should be individually tailored for each patient; for example, older patients generally require lower doses. Comorbid physical disorders and concomitant medication may influence the dose (and type) of medication prescribed. Pregnancy, the use of non-prescribed drugs and alcohol, medically frail or those whose physical health may be compromised (e.g. dehydrated), no previous exposure to psychotropic drugs, people already receiving regular psychotropic medication, people with a learning disability or autism and people at the extremes of age should all be taken into account when selecting dosage.
- The choice of medication used should be individualised and based on the patient's medical and treatment history, mental and physical state, any existing advanced directives and after an attempt has been made to establish a provisional diagnosis.
- The use of combined drugs from the same class of medicine is unnecessary and should normally be avoided.
- Following the use of RT, pre-RT or PRN medication, patients should be monitored in line with locally agreed protocols and the parameters of monitoring recorded in the clinical record.
- If RT medication is used, a senior doctor should review all medication at least daily.
- Side effects of all prescribed medication (including STAT doses, regular and pre-RT or PRN) should be reviewed regularly in line with locally agreed protocols.
- Following review, if prescribed medicines are unnecessary, ineffective or cause intolerable side effects, they should be reduced and/or discontinued.
- The use of medicines outside their licence, or above the maximum recommended dosage (either alone or in combination), is the responsibility of the individual practitioner, who should undertake the recommended safeguards in relation to documentation of indications and consent.

The 2018 BAP/NAPICU consensus guideline [2] also outlined a number of additional principles to guide best use of medicines in the management of behavioural disturbance. These provide a sound basis for individuals and their teams to build on the wider frameworks within NICE (2015) guidance in order to formulate their local plans and protocols for the management of disturbed behaviour.

- Effective interventions: Consider the strength of evidence which underpins the use of the intervention. Interventions should have an evidence base which confirms that they increase positive outcomes and/or reduce negative outcomes (harm) as a result of acute disturbance in the immediate to short term. The use of medication-related interventions should be individualised.
- Proportionality of intervention: The intervention for the management of behaviour should be proportionate to the acute severity of the risks associated with the disturbance. The least restrictive options available should always be considered in the first instance. RT should be used only when other pharmacological and non-pharmacological are not possible or have been exhausted.

- Treatment of any underlying disorders: Interventions should be considered within the context of achieving the longer-term desired outcomes for any underlying disorders.
- Continuous monitoring and review: the state of mental/physical health, risk to self/others, treatment effectiveness/harm and patient engagement level are all included here.

Review of the Management Plan

The last principle cited above highlights the need for continuous monitoring and regular review. During a period of disturbed behaviour, the clinical scenario and associated risks to self/others is likely to change with time. Therefore, interventions to reduce risk in the immediate or short term need to reflect this and not be maintained unnecessarily. Clinicians need to ensure that the right intervention is used for the right situation at the right time.

Consideration of a person's overall physical health is important when planning the management of an episode of behavioural disturbance. The acute disturbance and the interventions may both be associated with adverse physical health consequences. If combinations of medicines are administered, there may be additive or cumulative effects that lead to increased adverse outcomes.

It is possible that an intervention may lead to the recommended patient-centred approach to care being compromised. This can be offset by repeated assessment of the patient's level of engagement, enabling solutions to reduce harm and improve clinical outcomes.

The Use of Medicines Outside of Their Licence or Above Maximum Recommended Dosage (Either Alone or in Combination)

The 2006 Royal College of Psychiatrists consensus statement on the use of high-dose antipsychotics was updated in 2014 (CR190) [3]. This included a review of the use of high-dose antipsychotic medication in acute violence and emergency tranquillisation. Overall, this report concluded that there is a lack of evidence to support benefits of high-dose antipsychotic medication outweighing potential risks of harm.

The use of higher-than-licensed doses of antipsychotic medication is not generally supported by the 2015 NICE guideline for violence and aggression: short-term management in mental health, health and community settings [1] or the 2018 BAP/NAPICU consensus guideline [2] for the clinical management of acute disturbance.

However, NICE (2015) recognised that there may be exceptional circumstances where higher doses are sometimes prescribed. In situations where the doses of antipsychotic medicines prescribed exceed the licensed or BNF maximum daily dose (including PRN), then this should be considered as an individualised trial of medication and agreed wherever possible with the wider multidisciplinary team. High-dose antipsychotic prescribing should only occur if it is planned to achieve an agreed therapeutic goal that is well documented and carried out under the direction of a senior doctor. In 2014, the Medicines and Healthcare Products Regulatory Agency (MHRA) issued advice on the maximum dose of oral lorazepam (4mg per day). Although the guidance does not directly refer to the use of this drug in RT or pre-RT, prescribers should be aware of the increased risks of respiratory depression associated with high dosage of benzodiazepines. Where higher doses of benzodiazepine are used, clinical teams should be trained in the use of flumazenil to treat benzodiazepine-induced respiratory depression.

If a prescriber makes a judgement to knowingly exceed the licensed doses of medication, the decision should not be taken lightly or the risks underestimated. In such situations it is important to ensure that frequent and intensive monitoring of the patient takes place. Regular checks of airway, level of consciousness, pulse, blood pressure, respiratory effort, temperature and hydration should be undertaken, in line with local guidelines.

Use of Medication to Reduce the Medium- and Long-Term Risk of Violence

There are two major obstacles in using the evidence available to support the prescribing of medication to specifically control the medium- and longer-term risk of violence, as opposed to treating symptoms of the primary disorder that might be related to a risk of violence.

First, the aetiology of violence is complex, and a number of social and environmental factors might cause violence independently of the psychopathology of the patient [4]. For example, in individuals with psychotic disorders and symptoms, where the risk of violence is elevated, the risk may be unrelated to psychotic symptoms, such as delusions [5], and more likely linked to prospective predictors of violence, such as childhood conduct problems, victimisation history, economic deprivation, social living situation and substance misuse [4]. There is, nonetheless, some evidence to suggest increased risk of violence amongst patients experiencing delusions, especially if untreated [6]. A systematic review and meta-regression analysis of 110 studies found that dynamic (or modifiable) risk factors for violence included higher poor impulse control scores, hostile behaviour, non-adherence with psychological therapies, recent substance misuse, recent alcohol misuse and non-adherence with medication [7]. The strongest predictors of future violence were substance misuse and a history of assault and violence.

Second, the evidence base for prescribing medication specifically to reduce violence in the medium to longer-term is limited [8]. Fazel et al. (9) study of 82 627 patients prescribed antipsychotics and mood stabilisers over four years recorded an association between antipsychotic drugs and reductions in the rate of violent crime in the same people when they were on medication compared with when they were not. They also found a reduction in violent crime for mood stabilisers, especially in patients with bipolar disorder [9]. There is also evidence that clozapine reduces aggression in schizophrenia and schizoaffective disorder [10–14]. The reduction in hostility and anti-aggressive action of clozapine may be both independent and partly dependent on its antipsychotic and mood effects [13, 15, 16]. Clozapine has also been shown to markedly reduce aggressive behaviour in inpatients with schizophrenia over a twelve-week period [17]. A second twelve-week study indicated that clozapine was superior to olanzapine in reducing aggression, and olanzapine was superior to haloperidol [18]. Despite the overall limitations in the evidence base of pharmacological treatments, the review by Victoroff and colleagues [10] also found that clozapine may be more effective than olanzapine or haloperidol for reducing aggression amongst selected physically assaultive inpatients. They also suggest that propranolol, valproic acid and famotidine may be effective adjunctive therapy for reducing some aspects of hostility or aggression amongst inpatients with schizophrenia spectrum disorders

With regard to personality disorders, NICE guidelines for borderline personality disorder [19] recommend that 'drug treatment should not be used specifically for borderline personality disorder or for the individual symptoms or behaviours associated with the disorder' (p. 10). Similarly, NICE guidelines for the management of antisocial personality disorder [20] recommend that 'pharmacological interventions should not be routinely used for the treatment of antisocial personality disorder or associated behaviours of aggression, anger and impulsivity' (p. 28). NICE quality standard QS88 for borderline and antisocial personality disorder does allow prescribing for comorbid conditions and, for the cautious short-term (no longer than one week), use of antipsychotic or sedative treatment during a crisis and as 'part as part of the overall treatment plan' [21, p. 22]. If a drug is prescribed, then ideally it should be a drug (such as a sedative antihistamine) that has a low side-effect profile, low addictive properties, minimum potential for misuse and relative safety in overdose.

In practice, medication is often prescribed in the treatment of personality disorder to treat comorbid disorders or to target symptoms that may increase the risk of aggression, especially in those with high levels of arousal that cannot be reduced by environmental, behavioural or other therapeutic methods. If medication is to be prescribed, a sensible approach is to consider targeted symptom-specific prescribing and to weigh up the advantages versus disadvantages of prescribing [22, 23]. As with all prescribing, medication should be discontinued if it proves to be ineffective.

A recent analysis of systematic reviews of pharmacological and non-pharmacological behaviour-management interventions for adult patients in the acute hospital setting with traumatic brain injury or post-traumatic amnesia concluded that 'the current evidence for the management of challenging behaviours in patients with acute TBI/PTA is generally equivocal, potentially reflecting the heterogeneity of patients with TBI and their clinical behaviours' [24]. However, medication is widely used in the management of patients with aggression after a head injury, and the choice of medication to reduce aggression is often guided by the underlying hypothesised mechanism of action or by associated symptoms. The use of medicines should be considered in two categories: the treatment of the underlying disorder (e.g. depression), and the treatment of aggression. A partial response should lead to consideration of adjunctive treatment with a medicine that has a different mechanism of action [25].

Despite the lack of good evidence to support good outcomes, medication is used in the treatment of sexual deviancy disorders. The relationship of any coexisting mental disorder that may influence the risk of sexual offending is complex, but may establish a need for pharmacological treatment. The potential for violence is one of several factors taken into consideration when deciding whether to prescribe or not. Following their Cochrane review of pharmacological interventions for those who have sexually offended or are at risk of offending, Khan and colleagues [26] were unable to make any evidence-based treatment recommendations. They concluded that 'It is a concern that, despite treatment being mandated in many jurisdictions, evidence for the effectiveness of pharmacological interventions is so sparse and that no RCTs appear to have been published in two decades' (p. 2).

If medication is prescribed other than to treat a coexisting mental disorder that would normally require pharmacological treatment, it should be in addition to psychological treatment, and then in general only when other non-pharmacological treatments used alone have proved insufficient. If treatment involves hormonal implants, then it should be given in accordance with Section 57 of the Mental Health Act 1983.

Medication is used in the management of challenging behaviour in people with dementia. Of the different symptoms that constitute behavioural and psychological symptoms in dementia, only physical aggression has been shown to respond to medication [27]. The NICE guidelines for dementia state that antipsychotics should only be offered to people living with dementia when they are at risk of harming themselves or others and/or if they are experiencing agitation, hallucinations or delusions that are causing them severe distress [28]. Risperidone is the only antipsychotic licensed for the treatment of aggression in people with dementia.

Medication is also used in the management of challenging behaviour in people with intellectual disability. As mentioned in Chapter 15, angry and violent actions liable to harm self or others may require drug intervention, including RT in some cases, but most challenging behaviour is much milder in severity, and ways of managing it without recourse to drug therapy are now recognised to be more appropriate.

In summary, in prescribing medication to specifically target the medium- or long-term risk of violence, as opposed to symptoms of the patient's primary disorder that may be related to violence, the clinician should bear in mind the limited evidence base and the multifactorial aetiology of violent behaviour, and only prescribe medication following a careful multidisciplinary assessment and risk–benefit evaluation.

For interested readers, *Stahl's Illustrated Violence* [29] offers a simplified overview and highly illustrated guide to the underlying neurobiology, genetic predisposition and management of aggressive behaviours in patients with psychiatric disorders.

Use of Electroconvulsive Therapy to Control Violence

Electroconvulsive therapy (ECT) is not a practicable or a desirable measure to treat violence or the risk of violence in an emergency situation. The use of ECT in clinical practice is guided by the Royal College of Psychiatrists' *The ECT Handbook* [30] and NICE guidelines [31]. There is also a position statement on ECT (CERT01/17) [32].

Once an indication for ECT, in keeping with the above guidance, has been established, the potential for violence should be one of a range of factors to consider in terms of the risks versus benefits of giving ECT.

Although NICE does not recommend the use of ECT in the general management of schizophrenia, ECT remains an option rarely used for some patients with treatment-resistant schizophrenia when other treatments have failed or there is a known history of good response to ECT [33]. Furthermore, *The ECT Handbook* [30] recommends that ECT may be considered as a fourth-line option – that is, for patients with schizophrenia for whom clozapine has already proven ineffective or intolerable.

Valid consent for ECT must be obtained in all cases where the patient has capacity to do so. The decision to use ECT should be made jointly by the patient and the responsible clinician on the basis of an informed discussion. This discussion should be accompanied by the provision of full and appropriate information about the general risks associated with ECT and the potential benefits specific to that patient. Consent should be obtained without pressure or coercion, taking into account the circumstances and clinical setting, and the patient should be reminded of their right to withdraw consent at any point. There should be strict adherence to recognised guidelines about consent, and the involvement of patient advocates and/or carers to facilitate informed discussion is strongly encouraged. In all situations where informed discussion and consent is not possible, advance directives should be taken fully into account and the patient's advocate and/or carer consulted.

Section 58A of the Mental Health Act applies to ECT and to medication administered as part of ECT. It applies to detained patients and to all patients aged under 18 (whether or not detained). A patient who has capacity to consent may not be given ECT under Section 58A unless the approved clinician in charge, or a second opinion appointed doctor (SOAD) appointed by the Care Quality Commission, has certified that the patient has the capacity to consent and has done so. If the patient is under 18, only a SOAD may give the certificate, and the SOAD must certify that the treatment is appropriate.

A patient who lacks capacity to consent may not be given treatment under Section 58A unless a SOAD certifies that the patient lacks capacity to consent and that: treatment is appropriate; no valid and applicable advance decision has been made by the patient under the Mental Capacity Act 2005 refusing the treatment; no suitably authorised attorney or deputy objects to the treatment on the patient's behalf; and as long as the treatment would not conflict with a decision of the Court of Protection. The Care Quality Commission expects the clinical team making the referral to have checked that there is no conflict with a proxy decision maker or any advance decision to refuse treatment, as a condition of the SOAD visit [34].

In emergency situations, ECT may be given for two of the four situations mentioned in Section 62 of the Mental Health Act: treatment which (not being irreversible or hazardous) is immediately necessary to alleviate serious suffering by the patient; or which (not being irreversible or hazardous) is immediately necessary and represents the minimum interference necessary to prevent the patient from behaving violently or being a danger to themselves or to others.

Rapid Tranquillisation

The NICE 2015 guideline on violence [1] and aggression and the 2018 BAP/NAPICU consensus guideline [2] for the clinical management of acute disturbance use the term 'rapid tranquillisation' to describe the use of medication given by the parenteral route (usually intramuscular [IM] or, exceptionally, intravenous [IV]) if oral medication is not possible or appropriate and urgent sedation with medication is needed. Having such a clear-cut definition of what is meant by the term 'rapid tranquillisation' is helpful. In particular, this leaves no doubt or ambiguity about when the intervention has been used and what post-RT monitoring should be undertaken.

The prescribing and use of RT should be formulated in line with the principles outlined earlier and lead to an individualised plan of care. This should include details of how regular and PRN medication should be used, together with details of post-medication monitoring. The use of PRN medication as part of an individualised treatment plan may result in a reduction in the level of disturbed behaviour to the extent that RT is neither necessary nor indicated. In other situations, the use of PRN medication alongside other de-escalation interventions may not achieve the desired outcome and RT is required in order to prevent further harm.

The stages involved in RT and other drugs used in the course of RT (after NICE, 2015, and later evidence) are given in Table 6.1.

The 2015 NICE guidelines relied on the results of randomised controlled trials in recommending the drugs for RT. But here we were also aware of the difficulties of carrying out trials in this area (see Chapter 4) and were reminded frequently of the saying 'absence of evidence is not evidence of absence'. In other words, there were RT procedures based on less evidence but these were still of potential value as some enjoyed widespread use. BAP

Table 6.1 The stages involved in rapid tranquillisation

First phase: oral drugs to be given before RT (oral pre-RT) at time violence is suspected	Second phase where patient co-operates: (optional) for rapid oral action (buccal pre-RT)	Possible second phase where patient co-operates: (if drug) approved for oral administration
Lorazepam Promethazine Aripiprazole Olanzapine Haloperidol (baseline ECG advised) Quetiapine	Midazolam	Loxapine
Third phase: intramuscular monotherapy (RT)	**Fourth phase: intramuscular combined therapy (RT)**	**Fifth phase: intravenous monotherapy**
lorazepam promethazine olanzapine aripiprazole	promethazine + haloperidol	Injectable diazepam (Diazemuls)

recommends a range of drugs – promethazine, lorazepam, midazolam, clonazepam, diazepam, loxapine, aripiprazole, haloperidol, olanzapine, quetiapine, risperidone, droperidol and zuclopenthixol acetate – as potential sedative agents in RT [35] but not all of these are readily available. We advise great caution in the use of these drugs where evidence is limited but feel prescribers ought to be aware of them if first-line options are inappropriate/contraindicated or fail to achieve successful outcomes. Evidence of previous response to one or more of these drugs can be very valuable.

The use of RT should not be considered an inevitable consequence of managing an episode of disturbed behaviour. The BAP/NAPICU introduced the term 'pre-RT medication' as part of their consensus guideline for the clinical management of acute disturbance. Alongside the principle of using the least restrictive option, this highlights the importance of considering the use of oral PRN medication as part of a comprehensive plan of care, including de-escalation to manage an episode of disturbed behaviour before the use of RT becomes necessary.

Following the use of RT, the patient should be calm and still able to participate in further assessment and treatment. The aim of RT is not to induce sleep or unconsciousness, although there may be occasions when sedation is an appropriate goal. The patient should be able to respond to communication following the use of RT.

Environmental and situational factors can influence behaviour and should not be overlooked as part of an overall strategy or local protocol to manage behavioural disturbance. As highlighted earlier, consideration should also be given to any coexisting physical conditions, such as severe constipation, unmanaged pain, urinary tract infections and akathisia. Underlying and comorbid conditions should always be addressed as part of an individualised approach to the management of disturbed behaviour.

Prior to prescribing RT, account should be taken of any regularly prescribed medication (including depot formulations), and/or the recent use of any illicit substances or alcohol. Whilst it is not always possible to predict, prescribers should consider the possibility of pharmacokinetic or pharmacodynamic drug interactions which may lead to altered dose requirements and potential side effects.

If the patient's care plan includes their preference for the medication to be used in the event of an acute episode of illness (an advance directive), this should be followed if clinically appropriate. The Care Programme Approach co-ordinator should ensure that details of the patient's advance directive is available and notified to the prescribers during the acute phase of illness. In all cases, the patient must be informed that they are to be given RT prior to administration. If the level of disturbance subsides and no longer warrants the administration of RT, alternative interventions (including oral medication) should be considered as a more appropriate intervention.

Capacity and the Use of Medication and Rapid Tranquillisation

The capacity to give consent should also be assessed and documented clearly in the patient's clinical records. Wherever possible, patients should be given the opportunity to make an informed choice about medication, and consent to medical treatment should be sought (with consent or refusal recorded).

The Mental Capacity Act, the common law doctrine of necessity, the Mental Health Units (Use of Force) Act 2018 and an evaluation of 'best interests' are all relevant when considering the legality of administering RT to a patient who is refusing treatment or lacks capacity to consent to treatment. Subject to Mental Health Units (Use of Force) Act 2018, sections 5 and 6 of the Mental Capacity Act provide a defence against liability in relation to acts such as restraining mentally incapacitated adults using reasonable force or giving them medication without consent if considered to be necessary in their best interests. Where treatment or restraint is necessary not because it is in the patient's best interests but for the protection of others, defence would come from the common law doctrine of necessity.

Procedure for Determining the Best Interests of a Person With Impaired Capacity

This is laid down in section 4 of the Mental Capacity Act. It considers any valid advanced decisions and statements; the patient's past and present feelings, beliefs and values likely to influence their decision; and any other factors which they would be likely to consider if able to do so. If practicable and appropriate, the views of anyone named by the patient, such as a carer or person interested in their welfare, must also be consulted.

Detained Patients

For detained patients for whom Part IV of the Mental Health Act applies, Section 63 permits medication for mental disorder to be given to patients detained under certain sections of the Act (e.g. Sections 2, 3, 36, 37, 37/41, 38, 45A, 47 or 48), but only if the patient has given valid consent and has capacity to do so or, if the patient is incapable and/or refusing, medication is given by or under the direction of the approved clinician in charge of the treatment in question.

Medication can then be given for up to three months from the date it was first administered. Section 58 applies to the administration to a detained patient of medication for mental disorder once three months have passed from the date it was first administered: the so-called 'three-month rule'. This includes any time the patient has spent on a community treatment order (CTO). Medication can then only be given if the patient consents, treatment is approved by a SOAD or, in an emergency situation, under Section 62, and subject to one of the following conditions being met:

- treatment which is immediately necessary to save the patient's life
- treatment (not being irreversible or hazardous) which is immediately necessary to prevent a serious deterioration in their condition
- treatment (not being irreversible or hazardous) which is immediately necessary to alleviate serious suffering by the patient
- treatment (not being irreversible or hazardous) which is immediately necessary and represents the minimum interference necessary to prevent the patient from behaving violently or being a danger to himself or to others.

Detained persons not covered by Part IV of the Mental Health Act include:

- those detained on 'emergency' sections of the Act (e.g. Sections 4, 5, 135 and 136)
- those remanded to hospital for a report under Section 35, patients temporarily detained in hospital as a place of safety under Section 37 or 45A pending admission to the hospital named in their hospital order or hospital direction
- restricted patients who have been conditionally discharged (unless or until recalled).

These patients are in the same position as patients who are not subject to the Mental Health Act at all. They have the same rights in consenting to treatment as if they were not detained and therefore treatment can only be given, as described earlier, following an assessment of capacity, an evaluation of best interests, and the principles enshrined in the Mental Capacity Act and the common law doctrine of necessity.

Patients on Community Treatment Orders

If treatment is required as part of the management of violent behaviour, it is likely that the emergency provisions of the Mental Health Act (Sections 62A and 64G) will apply.

Patients With Capacity

For patients with capacity, the responsible clinician must complete Form CTO12 within one month of the CTO start date to certify that the patient both has capacity to consent to treatment and does consent to treatment (Mental Health Act Section 64C). There is no authority under the Act to give medication to a capacious patient on a CTO against their will in the community, even in an emergency. Treatment without their consent can only be given legally if they are recalled to hospital.

Patients Lacking Capacity

All treatment given in the community to a patient on a CTO lacking capacity (except in an emergency) after the first month must be certified by a SOAD and documented on Form CTO11.

Patients on a CTO who lack capacity to consent to treatment may be given medication without their consent in the community, provided they have not made an advance decision by which they refuse such treatment (Mental Capacity Act Section 24), and no proxy decision maker, such as a deputy appointed by the court (Mental Capacity Act Sections 16–20) or holder of a lasting power of attorney (Mental Capacity Act Sections 9–11), objects. Treatment may also be given in such circumstances if the patent does object, but force is not required in order to give the treatment (Mental Health Act Section 64D).

In an emergency, Section 64G of the Mental Health Act permits the administration of medicine which is immediately necessary to:

- save the patient's life
- prevent serious deterioration
- alleviate serious suffering by the patient
- prevent the patient behaving violently or being a danger to themselves or others, where the treatment represents the minimum interference necessary for that purpose, does not have unfavourable psychological consequences which cannot be reversed and does not entail significant physical hazard.

There is no requirement for the person giving treatment to be acting under the direction of an approved clinician. Force may be used provided that:

- the treatment is necessary to prevent harm to the patient
- the force used is proportionate to the likelihood of the patient suffering harm and to the seriousness of that harm.

Treatment under Section 64G might be considered where the possibility of recall to hospital before commencing treatment is not realistic or might exacerbate the patient's condition.

Treatment of Patients on a Community Treatment Order After Recall to Hospital

Such patients are 'detained patients' within the meaning of Part IV of the Mental Health Act. Their treatment is governed by Section 62A.

There are three circumstances in which medication may legally be given to recalled patients on CTO.

1   If the treatment has been specifically allowed on recall by the SOAD and documented on the Part IVA certificate (Section 62A(3)(a)).
2   If less than one month has elapsed since the CTO was made (Section 62A(3)(b)).
3   If the treatment was already being given on the authority of a Part IVA certificate and the person in charge of treatment believes that stopping the treatment would cause serious suffering (Section 62A(3)(b)).

Treatment may be continued in these circumstances while awaiting approval from a SOAD for a new treatment plan. In the absence of such circumstances, Part IV of the Mental Health Act resumes and Section 62 is applicable.

Route of Administration of Medicines Used As Part of the Management of an Episode of Severe Behavioural Disturbance

As outlined earlier, medication should be considered as part of a comprehensive and individualised plan which has been formulated by a multidisciplinary team. Consideration should be given to the role and place of all forms of pharmacological treatments, whether that be as regular or ongoing therapy, the place and role of PRN and pre-RT medication and whether RT is likely to be required.

The prescribing and use of medication to manage behavioural disturbance and violence should follow current guidance from NICE. Clinicians will also find the framework and guiding principles from BAP/NAPICU [2] helpful in formulating the medicines aspects of local protocols and individualised treatment plans.

In practice, the use of non-pharmacological interventions and/or oral PRN medication as part of de-escalation or pre-RT should reduce the need for RT. However, in some cases, the nature of disturbed behaviour may mean that it is not possible or appropriate to use oral medication. However, in all cases, the principle of ensuring the least restrictive option should be followed (i.e., consideration of oral medication as a first option).

During an episode of violent disturbed behaviour, the aim of RT is to rapidly calm or sedate the patient. Oral or inhaled medication is unlikely to be accepted. Forcible administration by these routes would be unacceptable and carry a high risk of injury or fatality. Medication administered via the oral route will generally take longer to achieve the desired effect. Novel routes of administration, such as inhalation, buccal or rectal routes, may offer the advantage of a more rapid absorption over the oral route, but as they all require a degree of cooperation by the patient to safely administer they would not normally be considered as alternatives for RT. This leaves the parenteral route as the only viable route for administration of medication for RT.

There are a number of antipsychotics that are available as soluble or disintegrating/dispersible tablets in the United Kingdom (aripiprazole, asenapine, risperidone and olanzapine) as well as liquid formulations (amisulpride, aripiprazole, clozapine, risperidone and haloperidol). Although absorption through the buccal mucosa is faster than the oral route and avoids problems associated with first-pass metabolism, it is important to note that the oro-dispersible formulations of aripiprazole, risperidone and olanzapine are not buccally absorbed. These tablets are designed to disperse in the saliva. It is only on swallowing that these formulations are absorbed via the gastrointestinal tract. In contrast, the buccal formulation of the antipsychotic drug asenapine is primarily absorbed from the buccal mucosa and largely inactivated if swallowed. Despite the limited evidence suggesting that asenapine may be associated with a reduction in hostility and agitation in patients with bipolar I disorder, it is unlikely to be a useful option as an alternative to RT because in these situations the collaboration of the patient is unlikely [36].

Confusion and 'wrong dose errors' can occur when prescriptions are handwritten using abbreviations such as 'p.o./i.m.' (oral/IM), as the dose associated with the particular route of administration may vary. Prescribing through a 'rule based' electronic system virtually eliminates the chances of ambiguous oral/IM prescriptions. Prescribers should ensure that there is absolute clarity about the intended dose/duration of treatment.

In all cases it is important that the prescriber specifies the intended dose, route, frequency and indication for all medicines as separate prescriptions. Where there is the opportunity to give multiple or additional doses, as is the case with PRN, pre-RT or RT, then the maximum total daily dose (including any regularly prescribed medication) must also be specified. Bioavailability and licensed indications for the same medication may vary according to the route of administration.

If medication is repeatedly refused, a multidisciplinary decision should be made about the need to administer medication by force. A decision to forcibly medicate should include consideration of the Use of Force Act 2018 and whether or not medication can be legally enforced under the Mental Health Act or other legislation.

If the decision has been made to forcibly medicate, the patient must be isolated from other patients on the ward. Nursing, medical and other staff involved in physically restraining the patient should be proficient in current 'control and restraint' techniques and have adequate immunisation against hepatitis B. Staff should ensure adequate physical restraint is in place so that parenteral administration of medication can be administered safely to a patient who is struggling to resist administration.

Following the administration of parenteral medication, further doses of medicines should be given orally in line with the clinical plan for care and to meet the desired outcomes from treatment.

The administration of RT through the intravenous (IV) route should only be considered in exceptional circumstances. There are considerable safety and practical issues associated with restraint and the administration of IV boluses. Administration by the IV route is not recommended in 'stand alone' or isolated psychiatric settings, especially when there is no provision to call an experienced medical resuscitation team. IV RT use is only suitable where there is a full crash team and medical support immediately available and on site (e.g. in an A&E setting in an acute hospital).

IV haloperidol may be associated with cardiac conduction abnormalities, such as Torsade de Pointes [37, 38]. In general, the use of intravenous IV RT and high doses of antipsychotics is of concern because of the potential to increase the QT interval and the associated risk of tachyarrhythmias. These are likely to be contributing factors in unexplained sudden deaths of acutely disturbed patients following the administration of antipsychotics.

The use of parenteral benzodiazepines may carry a risk of respiratory depression, and with IV diazepam there is a high risk of thrombophlebitis (reduced by using an emulsion formulation, Diazemuls). In routine practice, if parenteral administration is required there are few situations where IM injections would be inappropriate. It is also more difficult to forcibly administer an intravenous IV injection to a struggling and restrained patient as the injection site is specific and there is a risk of inadvertent intra-arterial administration. Administration by the IM injection does not require such a small injection site. The onset of action following an intramuscular IM injection is approximately 15 minutes, whereas onset of action following an intravenous IV injection is approximately 2–5 minutes. Administration of IV doses of diazepam or haloperidol as RT need to be given as slow boluses over at least 2–3 minutes.

Although the IV route may be appropriate to administer RT in exceptional circumstances, staff in many psychiatric units are unlikely to have the necessary training, skills or experience required to administer medicines safely by this route or manage the potentially serious side effects of IV RT should they arise. If IV benzodiazepines are administered as RT the risk of respiratory depression must not be underestimated. Although the benzodiazepine receptor antagonist flumazanil can reverse the respiratory depressants effects of benzodiazepine, it is important that staff are trained and competent to use this product.

Choice of Agent in Rapid Tranquillisation

As highlighted earlier (see 'General Principles for Prescribing Medication to Prevent or Control Acute Violent Behaviour'), the use of RT should be considered if oral medication is not possible or appropriate and urgent sedation with medication is needed. In such circumstances, PRN, pre-RT and other forms of de-escalation will either be inappropriate or will have failed to achieve the desired effect.

In 2015, NICE undertook a comprehensive review of the evidence for the use of medicines in the management of behavioural disturbance. Full details are available in appendix 15b of the NICE guideline NG10 [39].

Overall, the strength of evidence supporting the superiority of a particular medication over another is low. Given the potential for adverse effects from many of the medicines commonly used as RT, NICE 2015 advised lorazepam as a first option, in the absence of indications for an alternative. Despite the availability of a range of medicines that could be considered for use in RT (including a number of newer agents and formulations that were not included in the NICE review), there continues to be limited evidence to support a change from the 2015 NICE guidance.

NICE 2015 also advised consideration of the use of haloperidol in combination with promethazine as an alternative for RT. Concerns about the adverse experiences associated with the use of haloperidol, particularly the effect on cardiac conduction, may limit the place of this option, but for those without evidence of cardiac risk factors, when used in combination with promethazine there is a reasonable evidence base to support the combination as an effective intervention as RT [2, 40, 41].

Although the evidence supporting the use of IM olanzapine as RT was good, NICE 2015 was unable to recommend for it in the management of violence as the product was not marketed in the United Kingdom.

NICE make the following recommendations about the use of medication as RT in adults: When deciding which medication to use clinicians should consider:

- the service user's preferences or advance statements and decisions
- pre-existing physical health problems or pregnancy
- possible intoxication
- previous response to these medications, including adverse effects
- potential for interactions with other medications
- the total daily dose of medications prescribed and administered.

Lorazepam is advised as the first-choice option if:

- there is insufficient additional information to guide the first choice of medication for RT, or
- the service user has not taken antipsychotic medication before.

Haloperidol should be avoided if:

- there is evidence of cardiovascular disease, including a prolonged QT interval
- it has not been possible to confirm a satisfactory electrocardiogram

If there is a partial response to IM lorazepam, a further dose should be considered, but if there has been no response to lorazepam, clinicians should consider IM haloperidol combined with IM promethazine. If there is a partial response to this combination clinicians should consider a further dose.

In circumstances where there has been little or no response to IM haloperidol combined with IM promethazine, NICE 2015 advises that IM lorazepam should be considered if this has not been used already during the episode. However, if IM lorazepam has already been used, clinicians should arrange an urgent team meeting to carry out a review and seek a second opinion if needed.

When developing individualised care plans for patients, clinical teams should take account of the latest guidance from NICE. Findings from a large quality-improvement programme by the Prescribing Observatory for Mental Health POMH [42] found that the use of RT was not in line with the UK national guidance from NICE, with combinations of haloperidol and lorazepam commonly employed as RT despite evidence showing that this combination offers no offer additional benefits over the individual agents.

Clinical teams should also be mindful to consider strategies to manage episodes of violence that do not respond to their first- and second-line options. This should include the exclusion/treatment of any underlying physical/organic causes of ongoing violent behaviour. Clinical teams may also find the consensus guidelines from BAP/NAPICU [2] helpful when considering other options that fall outside of the scope of the guidance from NICE.

Pro Re Nata Medication

Commonly, inpatient prescription charts and electronic prescribing systems have the facility to prescribe medicines as PRN or 'as required'. This 'provision' enables prescribers to authorise the administration of certain medicines at the clinical discretion of the nursing staff. The prescriber should always specify the limits of discretion, such as the dose, route frequency, indication and maximum dose to be administered within a defined period. More details to help guide the safe use of medication as PRN should also be agreed and documented as part of the individual patient's clinical management plan.

Medicines commonly prescribed as PRN and used for the management or control of behaviour include lorazepam, haloperidol and promethazine. PRN may also be commonly used to prescribe analgesics, hypnotics and antimuscarinics.

Particular care is needed when prescribing any medication as PRN as this may lead to the inadvertent administration of greater than BNF maximum doses of medication [43]. The use of PRN may also lead to harmful use of combinations of drugs – or polypharmacy – if patients are already prescribed other regular psychotropics.

The prescribing and use of medication as PRN should be regularly reviewed (at least weekly) so that medication which is no longer required is discontinued.

Intramuscular Antipsychotics

Haloperidol

Haloperidol in combination with lorazepam was previously recommended as a preferred option by NICE in 2005 [44], particularly if violence was considered to be in the context of psychosis. This guidance has been updated and NICE no longer recommends this as a preferred option. Ostinelli [45] undertook a comprehensive review of the safety and efficacy of haloperidol for the management of psychosis-induced disturbed behaviour and concluded that where other options were available, the use of haloperidol alone could be considered unethical due to the high burden of side effects [46].

Despite these concerns, IM haloperidol (either alone or in combination with IM lorazepam) continues to be commonly used for RT within mental health settings in the United Kingdom [42] and is recommended in other national guidelines (BAP/NAPICU) [2].

Olanzapine

IM olanzapine has similar efficacy to IM haloperidol when used as a single agent for acute agitation [46, 47], but the incidence of extrapyramidal side effects (EPS) and QT prolongation was lower with olanzapine than haloperidol [48, 49], making it a preferable IM antipsychotic from a safety and tolerability perspective.

However, clinicians should be aware of the importance of using olanzapine as a monotherapy and that simultaneous administration with parenteral benzodiazepines should be avoided owing to concerns about safety [50]. The safety of this practice was not formally assessed prior to licensing [51], and a number of patient deaths occurred post-licensing, wherein IM olanzapine had been used in conjunction with several other agents, including benzodiazepines [52].

In trials, single doses of olanzapine commonly (1–10%) caused postural hypotension, bradycardia with or without hypotension or syncope, and tachycardia; and, more uncommonly (0.1–1%), sinus pause [47]. If a patient additionally requires a parenteral benzodiazepine, this should not be given until at least one hour after IM olanzapine [47] or vice versa.

The combination of olanzapine with promethazine has not been formally reported, and the use of IM olanzapine alone is not as effective as the combination of IM haloperidol and IM promethazine [41].

Aripiprazole

A recent Cochrane review compared the IM use of aripiprazole, placebo, haloperidol and olanzapine [53]. Although superior to placebo, aripiprazole was found to be less effective in controlling agitation than olanzapine after two hours and, when compared to haloperidol, patients required more doses of aripiprazole to produce the desired end point.

When comparing the IM use of lorazepam and aripiprazole for the management of acutely agitated patients, Zimbroff and colleagues found that lorazepam produced a greater improvement during the first two hours, although PANSS-EC scores (the positive and negative syndrome scale for recording outcome) were similar [54].

Loxapine

This antipsychotic is no longer marketed in the United Kingdom for oral and IM administration.

Other Licensed Intramuscular Agents in the United Kingdom

Lorazepam

This is the most widely used benzodiazepine for RT in the United Kingdom [42]. It is also available as a tablet that may be taken orally or sublingually as PRN or pre-RT, as well as being used for RT as IM administration.

It is readily and completely absorbed from the gastrointestinal tract after oral administration, reaches peak plasma levels at approximately two hours, and is quickly absorbed after IM injection. It is one of the shorter-acting benzodiazepines, it does not have any active metabolites and its hepatic metabolism is not significantly impaired by hepatic dysfunction. Like all benzodiazepines, lorazepam may cause respiratory depression [55].

In some countries, the practical requirement to store lorazepam injection in refrigerated conditions (2–8°C) to maintain stability of the product can prove to be inhibitory in medical settings.

Promethazine

Promethazine is a sedative antihistamine. It has been studied alongside IM haloperidol as an alternative agent to a parenteral benzodiazepine such as lorazepam [40]. A Cochrane review [56] concluded that the combination of promethazine and haloperidol was a safe and effective combination for use as RT. This confirmed the findings from the four large TREC trials [40, 41, 57, 58] which demonstrated the relative safety and efficacy of the promethazine–haloperidol combination versus IM midazolam, versus IM lorazepam, versus IM haloperidol alone and versus IM olanzapine, in a range of settings.

When used in combination with haloperidol, promethazine showed benefits as a sedative (the promethazine–haloperidol combination was more sedating than using haloperidol alone), with a relatively swift onset of action and potentially a protective effect against haloperidol-induced EPS [56]. As part of their comprehensive guidance for the management of behavioural disturbance, NICE advised consideration of a haloperidol/promethazine combination as a preferred option for RT in situations where there are no other factors that would indicate an alternative [1].

Other Licensed Products

Loxapine Adasuve (Breath-Actuated Inhalation)

This novel device is licensed in Europe as a product for inhalation from a breath-actuated device for use in the management of mild-to-moderate agitation in adult patients with schizophrenia or bipolar disorder. It has demonstrated superior efficacy to placebo with a quick onset of action [59, 60], but due to the need for cooperation by patients and the risks of bronchospasm (particularly in smokers), the use of this product is likely to have a limited place in the management of acute behavioural disturbance and should only be used in hospital settings.

Future Possible Developments

Intranasal Drug Delivery Systems

In a phase one study, a novel intranasal drug delivery system developed by Impel Pharmaceuticals has been reported to enable rapid delivery of olanzapine in healthy volunteers [61]. If further phase two and three studies confirm the safety and benefit of this type of drug delivery for the management of violent and disturbed behaviour, it could offer an alternative to the traditional way of administering medication for RT, pre-RT or PRN in future years.

Other Technologies

Other developments in technology may emerge in future years as alternatives to the traditional ways of administering medication to control violent or disturbed behaviours. This includes needle free injections [62].

Other Unlicensed Agents in the United Kingdom

If a prescriber decides to use a licensed treatment for an unlicensed indication, or a medication that is not licensed for use in the United Kingdom, the prescriber must be fully conversant with the risks and benefits of doing so. Prescribers should follow their relevant professional guidance – for example, guidance for doctors from the GMC [63]. The Royal College of Psychiatrists provides guidance on the use of licensed medicines for unlicensed use [64].

Further details of additional interventions can be found in the comprehensive consensus statement by BAP and NAPICU of their guidelines for the clinical management of acute disturbance: De-escalation and RT [2].

Midazolam: Intramuscular

The benzodiazepine midazolam is a schedule 3 controlled drug. It is licensed and commonly used in the United Kingdom as an IV sedative and induction anaesthetic. In the United Kingdom, midazolam injection is also licensed for use preoperatively as a premedication sedative.

IM use of midazolam has been investigated for RT. This is widely used in some countries where the requirement to store lorazepam injection in refrigerated conditions inhibits the use of IM lorazepam.

In some studies, midazolam has shown to have a faster onset of action than lorazepam [40, 65] and some antipsychotics [65, 66], and it has a shorter duration of action [65]. However, it can unpredictably lead to respiratory depression more frequently than other agents [57, 66, 67] and therefore it should only be used in scenarios where services are fully confident in observing for and managing the consequences of respiratory depression [56].

Midazolam: Buccal and Sublingual

Buccal and sublingual midazolam have been studied in a number of populations and scenarios, notably as an emergency anti-epileptic in paediatrics and intellectual disabilities as an alternative to rectal diazepam, where the route of administration is a key feature [68]. It has also been used for RT in adult psychiatric patients [69, 70].

Sublingual midazolam is quickly absorbed, including via the buccal mucosa, and gives high bioavailability (about 75%) and reliable plasma concentrations [71]. However, there is a minimal role for the use of buccal or sublingual midazolam in RT, as it requires the patient's cooperation with this oral formulation [69].

Droperidol

This butyrophenone antipsychotic drug was commonly prescribed for the management of acute behavioural disturbances in the 1990s, but following concerns about cardiac related fatalities, the oral formulation was withdrawn. The parenteral formulation was subsequently withdrawn by the manufacturer as they considered the drug to be uneconomic due to falling sales.

More recently, Panpharma has made the injectable formulation of droperidol available in the United Kingdom as a licensed treatment for IV use for the prevention and treatment of post-operative nausea and vomiting in adults and, as second line, in children and adolescents. The reintroduction of the IV formulation of droperidol has also led to calls for its use to be considered as an option in the management of behavioural disturbance in emergency departments and other areas [2, 72].

Other Agents Available Outside of the United Kingdom

Several other parenteral agents are licensed for RT and available outside of the United Kingdom.

Clonazepam

This drug is only licensed in the United Kingdom for IV administration in status epilepticus. It is a long-acting benzodiazepine and, like diazepam, has active metabolites with long half-lives. There is therefore a risk of accumulation. It has a higher risk of profound hypotension than lorazepam, and may be used in countries where IM lorazepam is not available.

Perphenazine

Perphenazine is a phenothiazine antipsychotic, similar to chlorpromazine. Its IM use is limited by its propensity to cause hypotension, sedation and EPS.

Ziprasidone

Both the oral and IM injection formulations of this second-generation antipsychotic are unlikely to be licensed in the United Kingdom, although it has been available in the USA since 2001 [47, 73], including in children and adolescents [74, 75], older adults [76, 77] and the medically unwell [66].

Unrecommended Agents in the United Kingdom

In addition to those already mentioned, the following agents are available in the United Kingdom but are not recommended for RT: zuclopenthixol acetate, IM diazepam, parental chlorpromazine, amylobarbitone (or 'amobarbital'), paraldehyde and IM depot antipsychotics [1, 78].

Familiarity With Responsibilities and Processes in Rapid Tranquillisation

All staff involved in the prescribing and administration of medicines for RT should be familiar with the practical arrangements and responsibilities in this regard.

Prescribers who prescribe RT should [44, 79]:

- Be familiar with the properties of benzodiazepines and their antagonists, antipsychotics, antimuscarinics and antihistamines
- Be able to assess the risks associated with RT, particularly when the patient is highly aroused and may have been misusing substances, may be dehydrated or may be physically ill
- Understand the cardiovascular effects of the acute administration of the tranquillising medications and the need to titrate the dose
- Recognise the importance of nursing in the recovery position

- Recognise the importance of monitoring pulse, blood pressure and respiration
- Be familiar with and trained in the use of resuscitation equipment
- Undertake regular resuscitation training
- Understand the importance of maintaining an unobstructed airway.

Seeking Advice in Rapid Tranquillisation

Any member of the professional team caring for a patient who requires RT should seek the advice of a senior colleague or a member of another profession (e.g. pharmacist, senior nurse or matron) at any stage in the RT process if they are at all unsure about the intended treatment plan. This may include situations when a patient does not respond as expected to the prescribed doses, if the maximum BNF dose has been given yet there is a clinical need for further pharmacological management, if the prescription is unclear/illegible or if the clinician is unfamiliar with the use of the prescribed medication (either formulation or dose).

Monitoring Post-Rapid Tranquillisation

After RT has been administered, it is essential to check the patient's physical well-being. If the patient has been given IM injections, this may have involved physical restraint. The injection of one or more medicines into a person who is physically stressed by the restraint process can lead to adverse physical sequelae.

Following the administration of RT, NICE [1] recommends that the patient is monitored for the emergence of side effects and that pulse, blood pressure, respiratory rate, temperature, level of hydration and level of consciousness is monitored at least every hour until there are no further concerns about the patient's physical health status.

In circumstances where the patient is considered to be at a higher risk, more frequent and intensive monitoring by appropriately trained staff is required. Particular attention should be paid to the patient's respiratory effort, airway and level of consciousness. NICE (2015) [1] recommends that monitoring of the aforementioned parameters should take place every 15 minutes until there are no further concerns if:

- the BNF maximum dose has been exceeded, or
- the service user/patient appears to be asleep or sedated, or
- has recently taken illicit substances or alcohol, or
- has any relevant significant pre-existing physical health problem, or
- experienced any harm as a result of any restrictive intervention.

Other circumstances that may warrant more intensive monitoring include:

- If an older adult's mobility is affected, or they are at high risk of falls, or
- Where the patient has a relevant medical disorder, or
- Concurrently prescribed additional medication that may exacerbate risk.

Monitoring following the use of RT should be documented in line with national guidance and the local organisation policies. In circumstances where staff are unable to carry out the monitoring of any of the parameters outline by NICE [1], the reasons for such omissions must also be documented and further attempts to monitor should be made, until there are no concerns about the patient's physical health status. Note that it is always possible to observe breathing and pallor, even if the patient is in seclusion.

In view of the higher risk of cardiac arrhythmias associated with the use of haloperidol in particular, some organisations also monitor with the electrocardiogram (ECG) and find this measure more practicable than trying to measure blood pressure in a resistive patient.

Pulse oximeters should be available and staff should be familiar with their use. Additionally, ECG machines should be available at all sites where RT is likely to be used. NICE guidance for the management of Psychosis and Schizophrenia in Adults: Prevention and Management [80] recommends that an ECG is obtained if the patient is being admitted as an inpatient, or if:

- Specified in the summary of product characteristics of the proposed treatment
- A physical examination has identified specific cardiovascular risk (such as diagnosis of high blood pressure)
- There is a personal history of cardiovascular disease

Risks and Complications Associated With Rapid Tranquillisation

There are specific risks associated with the different classes of medications that are used in RT. Staff using these medicines should be aware of these risks and competent in their use. Table 6.2 lists some common and some serious adverse effects following the administration of RT, and the recommended management.

When prescribing medication for RT, the specific properties of the individual medications should be taken into consideration; when combinations are used, risks may be compounded. The use of IV and high doses of antipsychotics is rarely justifiable. Their use may increase the possibilities of cardiac QT abnormalities and the associated risk of tachyarrhythmias. Other life-threatening reactions may include an acute laryngeal stridor. Respiratory depression (by accumulated doses of benzodiazepines or hypoxia) may also be implicated in fatal outcomes of acutely disturbed patients who have been prescribed medication to control behaviour.

The use of RT sedation may be a risk factor for venous thromboembolic disease [81], particularly in patients who are obese, dehydrated, have comorbid cardiac disease or diabetes or are taking oestrogen-containing contraceptives or hormone replacement therapy.

Circumstances for Special Care

Extra care should be taken when implementing RT in the following circumstances:

- The presence of congenital prolonged QTc syndromes;
- The concurrent prescription or use of other medication that lengthens QTc intervals both directly and indirectly;
- Prolonged QTc interval is a marker for cardiac arrhythmia: potential cardiorespiratory collapse and physical exertion, stress, illicit drug use (ecstasy and cannabis, and possibly other illicit substances) and metabolic factors are risk factors;
- The presence of certain disorders affecting metabolism, such as hypo-/ hyperthermia, stress and extreme emotions, and extreme physical exertion.

Older Adults and Rapid Tranquillisation

Although patients aged 65 years and older are generally cared for in separate services from working-age adults, it is generally accepted that frailty rather than age per se should be the distinguishing factor when considering the most appropriate service for a person. As with

Table 6.2 Common or serious adverse effects following rapid tranquillisation and recommended management

Complication	Symptoms/signs	Management
Acute dystonia	Severe painful muscular stiffness	Procyclidine 5–10 mg intramuscularly
Hypotension	Fall in blood pressure (orthostatic or <50 mmHg diastolic)	Lie patient flat and raise legs – tilt bed head down Monitor closely Seek medical advice
Neuroleptic malignant syndrome	Increasing temperature, fluctuating blood pressure, muscular rigidity, confusion/ fluctuating or altered consciousness	Neuroleptic malignant syndrome is a potentially serious, even fatal, side effect Medical advice should be sought immediately Withhold antipsychotics Monitor closely (temperature, blood pressure, pulse) Liaise with general medical team
Arrhythmias	Slow (<50/min), irregular or impalpable pulse	Monitor vital observations and electrocardiogram and liaise with general medical team immediately May require immediate defibrillation
Respiratory depression	Reducing respiratory rate, reducing consciousness	Give oxygen, and place the patient in the recovery position, instigating measures for basic life support If indicated, an oropharyngeal/nasopharyngeal airway should be inserted and the patient mechanically ventilated. This should only be undertaken when appropriately qualified and skilled staff are available If respiratory rate drops below 10 breaths/min, seek medical advice. If the patient has received benzodiazepines, if suitably trained give flumazenil: - 200 mcg intravenously over 15 s - if consciousness not resumed within 60s, give 100 mcg over 10 s. - repeat at 60 s intervals; maximum dose 1 mg/24 h. Continue to monitor after respiratory rate returns to normal. Flumazenil has a shorter duration of action than many benzodiazepines so repeated doses may be required. Patients may become agitated or anxious on waking. Flumazenil is best avoided in patients with epilepsy – start mechanical ventilation instead

all other medication, when prescribing RT medication for patients in this population, their age should not be the only deciding factor when determining a regimen.

The physical fitness of the individual must be considered. Particular care should be given to coexisting medical states and prescribed medication, the risk of accumulation of sedatives and the possibility of delirium. Both antipsychotics and benzodiazepines may affect mobility and increase the risk of falls. Patients should be monitored for signs of impaired mobility and unsteadiness. Older people are at increased risk of venous thromboembolic disease [81].

Lorazepam remains the first medicine of choice as RT in this population, but if two or more parenteral doses of ≥2 mg lorazepam during one episode are required, junior staff should seek advice from senior colleagues. Older adults may have poorer muscle perfusion than younger patients, which may produce erratic absorption of intramuscularly administered medicines into the blood stream. Therefore, a longer interval should be allowed between IM doses (at least one hour).

In 2004, the MHRA recommended that olanzapine and risperidone are not to be used in the treatment of behavioural symptoms of dementia due to the increased risk of stroke. However, from observational data, the European Pharmacovigilance Working Party [82] concluded that the likelihood of cerebrovascular adverse events associated with the use of first-generation antipsychotics in patients with dementia was not significantly different from that of olanzapine and risperidone. Therefore, it is recommended that antipsychotics for RT are only prescribed to patients with dementia or a history of cerebrovascular events after careful consideration and where lorazepam alone is insufficient or inappropriate. This decision to prescribe antipsychotics for RT should be documented in the notes, with the rationale clearly recorded.

Patients Under 18 Years of Age and Rapid Tranquillisation

Although the evidence base for the use of specific pharmacological therapies in the general psychiatric population is not very rigorous and is based on relatively small numbers, data in children and young people (CYP) are even more so and are predominantly collected from settings outside the United Kingdom [83]. When using medicines for RT in CYP and young people aged under 18 years, the same principles of good practice as outlined for adults should be followed [1]. When considering medication choice for RT in CYP, prescribers should take account of the following: lorazepam IM is the only pharmacological option that is listed by NICE 2015; young people's brains continue to develop beyond adolescence until around 25 years of age; and the physical size/BMI of the young person.

As with all patients receiving RT medication, a CYP must be informed that medication is going to be given, and they must be granted the opportunity at any stage to accept oral medication voluntarily. In CYP who are not Gillick competent, parents/carers should be informed of the situation and their consent sought for such treatment. It is good practice to inform both the CYP and their parents/carers.

When treating CYP, antipsychotics with a high potential for inducing EPS extrapyramidal side effects or reactions (EPSs) should be avoided. Younger people are more likely to be antipsychotic-naïve and sensitive to EPS. If the level of disturbance does not warrant the use of RT and oral medication is indicated as part of a de-escalation strategy or pre-RT/PRN, then risperidone (tablets or liquid or dispersible tablet) may be a more reasonable consideration for use. Other medicine options through the oral route for this population include the sedating antihistamine alimemazine.

If non-pharmacological interventions are ineffective and pre-RT or PRN medication is considered to be necessary for CYP with moderate, severe or profound intellectual disability and/or epilepsy, then even smaller doses of risperidone should be used [84, 85]. For some CYP or young people there may be a higher incidence of disinhibition or paradoxical reactions to benzodiazepines, which should be borne in mind if lorazepam is used.

In exceptional circumstances, if haloperidol IM is administered as RT then prophylactic procyclidine should also be given (oral or IM) because of the higher incidence of EPS.

In younger children, the formulation of the medicines may become even more pertinent and guide the choice of agent (Paediatric Formulary Committee, 2011: https://bnfc .nice.org.uk/). Several of the aforementioned medicines are available in liquid formulations or as dispersible tablets. It should also be noted that many of these medications are unlicensed in this age group for this indication.

Pregnancy and Rapid Tranquillisation

According to the latest NICE CG192 guidelines on antenatal and postnatal mental health [86], a pregnant woman requiring RT should be treated in accordance with the relevant NICE guidelines on the short-term management of disturbed behaviour, with the following provisos:

- She should not be secluded after RT.
- Restraint procedures should be adapted to avoid possible harm to the foetus.
- When choosing an agent for RT in a pregnant woman, an antipsychotic or a benzodiazepine with a short half-life should be considered; if an antipsychotic is used, it should be at the minimum effective dose because of neonatal extrapyramidal symptoms; if a benzodiazepine is used, the risks of floppy baby syndrome should be taken into account.
- During the perinatal period, the woman's care should be managed in close collaboration with a paediatrician and an anaesthetist.

Further information on the use of psychotropic medication preconception, in pregnancy and postpartum drug treatment has been published by the BAP [87] and the NAPICU/BAP [2].

Starting Regular Antipsychotic Treatment After Rapid Tranquillisation

After RT has been given, the continuation of medication in the medium to longer term is likely to be indicated in patients with an established psychiatric illness that would usually be treated by medication (e.g. a patient with a diagnosis of schizophrenia who has relapsed following cessation of antipsychotic treatment in the community). A similar scenario in a patient with bipolar affective disorder might indicate the need for the longer-term use of mood-stabilising medication (antipsychotic and/or mood stabiliser[s]).

In patients who do not have a mental illness that would usually require medium- to long-term prescribing, the prescribing of a short-term course of regular psychotropic medication after RT may still be indicated. For example, a highly aroused patient may require the use of regular anxiolytic medication for a few days or weeks following RT until their condition has stabilised and the risk of further violence significantly reduced. In such circumstances it is important to ensure than systems are in place to prevent the inadvertent long-term continuation of medication, beyond the initial post-RT period.

The final choice of agent and the formulation and route of administration should be guided by factors such as the patient's medication history and current medication regime, the patient's preference (including advanced directive if made), their response and their tolerance to treatment to date.

Monitoring and Audit of Medication Used in the Management of Behavioural Control

All psychiatric units should have policies and procedures to govern the use of medication for behaviour control, and the practice with regard to the use of medication for this purpose must be recorded and regularly audited in line with the requirements set out in the Mental Health Units (Use of Force) Act 2018. The term 'chemical restraint' is used within the act to describe the use of medication which is intended to 'prevent, restrict or subdue movement of any part of the patient's body'. The systems and processes to record the details of medication used as 'chemical restraint' should highlight the extent to which RT and other medication-related behavioural control interventions are used. This will enable regular and close monitoring of the use of medication for behavioural control at both the organisational and the national level.

Conclusion

The term 'rapid tranquillisation' refers to the use of parenteral medication, given by the IM (or, rarely, the IV) for urgent sedation to control violent behaviour. The use of RT should always be a considered, appropriate and proportionate response to a violent situation. Before using RT, alternative and less restrictive interventions should be considered and implemented where appropriate.

All organisations where RT may be used should develop and implement a policy for the use of RT. In England and Wales, this policy should be based on the latest guidance from NICE. Additional guidance from recognised professional bodies, such as BAP and NAPICU, may be useful to include as part of an organisation's RT policy development.

A multidisciplinary team should be responsible for overseeing the development of local guidance for the use of RT and this should be kept under regular review.

The evidence base for first-line medication choice as RT is limited. Previous response, patient/service user preference and medical comorbidities/contraindications should be taken into account when considering the choice of medication for an individual patient.

The advice from a specialist mental health pharmacist (where available) as part of a multidisciplinary team may be particularly helpful in optimising the use of medicines for RT.

References

1. National Institute for Health and Care Excellence. Violence and aggression: Short-term Management in Mental Health, Health and Community Settings. NICE Guideline NG10 [online]. 2015. www.nice.org.uk/guidance/ng10 [Accessed 25.9.2021].

2. Patel, M. X., Sethi, F. N., Barnes, T. R. et al. Joint BAP NAPICU evidence-based consensus guidelines for the clinical management of acute disturbance: De-escalation and rapid tranquillisation. *Journal of Psychopharmacology* 2018;32 (6):601–40.

3. Royal College of Psychiatrists. Consensus statement on high-dose antipsychotic medication. College Report CR190 [online]. 2014. www.rcpsych.ac.uk/docs/default-source/members/faculties/rehabilitation-and-social-psychiatry/rehab-cr190.pdf?sfvrsn=d8397218_4 [Accessed 29.4.2022].

4. Swanson, J. W., Swartz, M. S., Van Dorn, R. A. et al. Comparison of antipsychotic medication effects on reducing violence in people with schizophrenia. *British Journal of Psychiatry.* 2008;193(1):37–43.

5. Appelbaum, P. S., Robbins, P. C., and Monahan, J. Violence and delusions: Data from the MacArthur Violence Risk Assessment Study. *The American Journal of Psychiatry.* 2000;157(4):566–72.

6. Látalová, K. Violence and duration of untreated psychosis in first-episode patients. *International Journal of Clinical Practice* 2014 Mar;68(3):330–5. https://doi.org/10.1111/ijcp.12327. Epub 2014 Jan 28. PMID: 24471741.

7. Witt, K., van Dorn, R., and Fazel, S. Risk factors for violence in psychosis: Systematic review and meta-regression analysis of 110 studies. *PLOS One.* 2013;8(2):e55942. https://doi.org/10.1371/journal.pone.0055942. Epub 2013 Feb 13. Erratum in: *PLOS One.* 2013;8(9). https://doi.org/10.1371/annotation/f4abfc20-5a38-4dec-aa46-7d28018bbe38. PMID: 23418482; PMCID: PMC3572179.

8. Goedhard, L. E., Stolker, J. J., Heerdink, E. R. et al. Pharmacotherapy for the treatment of aggressive behavior in general adult psychiatry: A systematic review. *Journal of Clinical Psychiatry* 2006;67(7):1013–24.

9. Fazel, S., Zetterqvist, J., Larsson, H., Långström, N., and Lichtenstein, P. Antipsychotics, mood stabilisers, and risk of violent crime. *The Lancet* 2014 Sep 27;384(9949):1206–14. https://doi.org/10.1016/S0140-6736(14)60379-2. Epub 2014 May 8. PMID: 24816046; PMCID: PMC4165625.

10. Victoroff, J., Coburn, K., Reeve, A., Sampson, S., and Shillcutt, S. Pharmacological management of persistent hostility and aggression in persons with schizophrenia spectrum disorders: a systematic review. *Journal of Neuropsychiatry and Clinical Neurosciences* 2014;26(4):283–312.

11. Chengappa, K. N. R., Vasile, J., Levine, J. et al. Clozapine: Its impact on aggressive behavior among patients in a state psychiatric hospital. *Schizophrenia Research* 2002; 53(1–2):1–6.

12. Volavka, J., Czobor, P., Nolan, K. et al. Overt aggression and psychotic symptoms in patients with schizophrenia treated with clozapine, olanzapine, risperidone, or haloperidol. *Journal of Clinical Psychopharmacology.* 2004;24(2):225–8.

13. Krakowski, M. I., Czobor, P., Citrome, L., Bark, N., and Cooper, T. B. Atypical antipsychotic agents in the treatment of violent patients with schizophrenia and schizoaffective disorder. *Archives of General Psychiatry* 2006;63(6):622–9.

14. Frogley, C., Taylor, D., Dickens, G., and Picchioni, M. A systematic review of the evidence of clozapine's anti-aggressive effects. *International Journal of Neuropsychopharmacology* 2012;15(9):1351–71.

15. Kraus, J. E., and Sheitman, B. B. Clozapine reduces violent behavior in heterogeneous diagnostic groups. *Journal of Neuropsychiatry and Clinical Neurosciences* 2005;17(1):36–44.

16. Strassnig, M. T., Nascimento, V., Deckler, E. and Harvey, P. D. Pharmacological treatment of violence in schizophrenia. *CNS Spectrums* 2020;25(2):207–15.

17. Krakowski, M. I., Czobor, P. and Nolan, K. A. Atypical antipsychotics, neurocognitive deficits, and aggression in schizophrenic patients. *Journal of Clinical Psychopharmacology* 2008;28(5):485–93.

18. Krakowski, M. I. and Czobor, P. Neurocognitive impairment limits the response to treatment of aggression with antipsychotic agents. *Schizophrenia Bulletin* 2011;37 311–2.

19. National Institute for Health and Clinical Excellence. *Borderline Personality Disorder: The NICE Guideline on Treatment and Management (Clinical Guideline CG78).* London: The British Psychological Society & The Royal College of Psychiatrists, 2009.

20. National Institute for Health and Clinical Excellence. Antisocial Personality Disorder: Treatment, Management and Prevention Clinical Guideline CG77 [online]. 2009. www.nice.org.uk/guidance/ cg77/resources/antisocial-personality- disorder-prevention-and-management- pdf-975633461701 [Accessed 29.4.2022].

21. National Institute of Clinical Excellence (NICE). Quality standard [QS88]. Personality disorders: borderline and antisocial. www.nice.org.uk/guidance/q s88/chapter/Quality-statement-4-Pharmac ological-interventions [Accessed 24.9.2021].

22. Soloff, P. H. Algorithms for pharmacological treatment of personality dimensions: symptom-specific treatments for cognitive-perceptual, affective, and impulsive-behavioral dysregulation. *Bulletin of the Menninger Clinic* 1998;62 (2):195–214.

23. Tyrer, P. and Bateman, A. W. Drug treatment for personality disorders. *Advances in Psychiatric Treatment* 2018;10 (5):389–98.

24. Block, H., George, S., Milanese, S. et al. Evidence for the management of challenging behaviours in patients with acute traumatic brain injury or post-traumatic amnesia: An umbrella review. *Brain Impairment,* 2021;22 (1):1–19. https://doi.org/10.1017/BrImp .2020.5

25. Jacobson, R. R. Commentary: Aggression and impulsivity after head injury. *Advances in Psychiatric Treatment* 2018;3(3):160–3.

26. Khan, O., Ferriter, M., Huband, N., at al. Pharmacological interventions for those who have sexually offended or are at risk of offending. *Cochrane Database of Systematic Reviews* 2015;2015(2):Cd007989.

27. Ballard, C. and Waite, J. The effectiveness of atypical antipsychotics for the treatment of aggression and psychosis in Alzheimer's disease. *Cochrane Database of Systematic Reviews* 2006(1):CD003476.

28. National Institute for Health and Care Excellence. Dementia: Assessment, management and support for people living with dementia and their carers. Guideline NG97 [online]. 2018. www.nice.org.uk/gui dance/ng97/resources/dementia- assessment-management-and-support-for -people-living-with-dementia-and-their- carers-pdf-1837760199109 [Accessed 29.4.2022].

29. Stahl, S. M. and Morrissette, D. A. *Stahl's Illustrated: Violence: Neural Circuits, Genetics and Treatment.* Cambridge: Cambridge University Press, 2014.

30. Ferrier, I. and Waite, J. *The ECT Handbook,* 4th ed. Cambridge: Cambridge University Press, 2019.

31. National Institute for Health and Care Excellence. Guidance on the Use of Electroconvulsive Therapy. Technology Appraisal Guidance TA59 [online]. 2009. www.nice.org.uk/guidance/ta59 [Accessed 29.4.2022].

32. Royal College of Psychiatrists. Statement on Electroconvulsive Therapy (ECT), CERT01/17 London: R; 2017 www .rcpsych.ac.uk/docs/default-source/about- us/who-we-are/electroconvulsive-therapy– -ect-ctee-statement-feb17.pdf?sfvrsn=2f4 a94f9_2 [Accessed 29.4.2022].

33. Tharyan, P. and Adams, C. E. Electroconvulsive therapy for schizophrenia. *Cochrane Database of Systematic Reviews* 2005(2):Cd000076.

34. Commission CQ. Guidance for SOADS: Consent for Treatment and the SOAD Role under the Revised Mental Health Act. CQC, 2008.

35. Rogers, P., Leung, C. and Nicholson, T. R. J. *Pocket Prescriber Psychiatry.* Florida: CRC Press.

36. Citrome, L., Landbloom, R., Chang, C. T., and Earley, W. Effects of asenapine on agitation and hostility in adults with acute manic or mixed episodes associated with bipolar I disorder. *Neuropsychiatric Disease and Treatment* 2017;13:2955–63.

37. Hassaballa, H. A. and Balk, R. A. Torsade de pointes associated with the administration of intravenous haloperidol. *American Journal of Therapeutics* 2003;10 (1):58–60.

38. Hassaballa, H. A. and Balk, R. A. Torsade de pointes associated with the administration of intravenous haloperidol: a review of the literature and practical guidelines for use. *Expert Opinion on Drug Safety* 2003;2(6):543–7.

39. National Institute of Clinical Excellence. NICE guideline NG10 Appendix 15B: Clinical evidence – forest plots for review of rapid tranquillisation. [online] 2015. www.nice.org.uk/guidance/ng10/evidence/appendix-15b-pdf-2549889109 [Accessed 29.4.2022].

40. Huf, G., Coutinho, E. S., Adams, C. E. and TREC Collaborative Group. Rapid tranquillisation in psychiatric emergency settings in Brazil: Pragmatic randomised controlled trial of intramuscular haloperidol versus intramuscular haloperidol plus promethazine. *BMJ* 2007;335(7625):869.

41. Raveendran, N. S., Tharyan, P., Alexander, J., Adams, C. E. and TREC Collaborative Group. Rapid tranquillisation in psychiatric emergency settings in India: Pragmatic randomised controlled trial of intramuscular olanzapine versus intramuscular haloperidol plus promethazine. *BMJ* 2007;335(7625):865.

42. Paton, C., Adams, C. E., Dye, S. et al. The pharmacological management of acute behavioural disturbance: Data from a clinical audit conducted in UK mental health services. *Journal of Psychopharmacology* 2019;33(4):472–81.

43. Baker, J. A., Lovell, K. and Harris, N. A best-evidence synthesis review of the administration of psychotropic pro re nata (PRN) medication in in-patient mental health settings. *Journal of Clinical Nursing* 2008;17(9):1122–31.

44. National Institute for Health and Care Excellence. Violence: The Short-Term Management of Disturbed and Violent Behaviour in Inpatient Psychiatric Settings and Emergency Departments. NICE Clinical Guideline CG 25 [online]. 2005. www.ncbi.nlm.nih.gov/books/NBK305020/ [Accessed 29.4.2022]

45. Ostinelli, E. G., Brooke-Powney, M. J., Li, X. and Adams, C. E. Haloperidol for psychosis-induced aggression or agitation (rapid tranquillisation). *Cochrane Database of Systematic Reviews.* 2017;7:CD009377.

46. Hsu, W. Y., Huang, S. S., Lee, B. S. and Chiu, N. Y. Comparison of intramuscular olanzapine, orally disintegrating olanzapine tablets, oral risperidone solution, and intramuscular haloperidol in the management of acute agitation in an acute care psychiatric ward in Taiwan. *Journal of Clinical Psychopharmacology* 2010;30(3):230–4.

47. Baldaçara, L., Sanches, M., Cordeiro, D. C. and Jackoswski, A. P. Rapid tranquilization for agitated patients in emergency psychiatric rooms: A randomized trial of olanzapine, ziprasidone, haloperidol plus promethazine, haloperidol plus midazolam and haloperidol alone. *Revista brasileira de psiquiatria (Sao Paulo, Brazil: 1999)* 2011;33(1):30–9.

48. Belgamwar, R. B. and Fenton, M. Olanzapine IM or velotab for acutely disturbed/agitated people with suspected serious mental illnesses. *Cochrane Database of Systematic Reviews* 2005;2: CD003729.

49. Kishi, T., Matsunaga, S. and Iwata, N. Intramuscular olanzapine for agitated patients: A systematic review and meta-analysis of randomized controlled trials. *Journal of Psychiatric Research* 2015;68:198–209.

50. Eli Lilly. Zyprexa powder for solution for injection 2009. www.ema.europa.eu/en/documents/product-information/zyprexa-epar-product-information_en.pdf [Accessed 29.4.2022]

51. Wright, P., Birkett, M., David, S. R. et al. Double-blind, placebo-controlled comparison of intramuscular olanzapine and intramuscular haloperidol in the treatment of acute agitation in schizophrenia. *The American Journal of Psychiatry.* 2001;158(7):1149–51.

52. Eli Lilly. Important safety information: Reported serious adverse events following use of Zyprexa Intramuscular (28 September) 2004. www .palliativedrugs.com/download/SafetyLette rzyprexa.pdf [Accessed 29.4.2022].

53. Ostinelli, E. G., Jajawi, S., Spyridi, S., Sayal, K., and Jayaram, M. B. Aripiprazole (intramuscular) for psychosis-induced aggression or agitation (rapid tranquillisation). *Cochrane Database of Systematic Reviews* 2018;1:CD008074.

54. Zimbroff, D. L., Marcus, R. N., Manos, G. et al. Management of acute agitation in patients with bipolar disorder: Efficacy and safety of intramuscular aripiprazole. *Journal of Clinical Psychopharmacology* 2007;27(2):171–6.

55. Broadstock, M. The effectiveness and safety of drug treatment for urgent sedation in psychiatric emergencies. A critical appraisal of the literature. *NZHTA Report* 2001; 4(1):2001.

56. Huf, G., Alexander, J., Gandhi, P. and Allen, M. H. Haloperidol plus promethazine for psychosis-induced aggression. *Cochrane Database of Systematic Reviews* 2016;11:CD005146.

57. Trec Collaborative Group. Rapid tranquillisation for agitated patients in emergency psychiatric rooms: A randomised trial of midazolam versus haloperidol plus promethazine. *BMJ* 2003;327(7417):708–13.

58. Alexander, J., Tharyan, P., Adams, C. et al. Rapid tranquillisation of violent or agitated patients in a psychiatric emergency setting: Pragmatic randomised trial of intramuscular lorazepam v. haloperidol plus promethazine. *British Journal of Psychiatry* 2004;185:63–9.

59. Allen, M. H., Feifel, D., Lesem, M. D. et al. Efficacy and safety of loxapine for inhalation in the treatment of agitation in patients with schizophrenia: A randomized, double-blind, placebo-controlled trial. *Journal of Clinical Psychiatry* 2011;72(10):1313–21.

60. Lesem, M. D., Tran-Johnson, T. K., Riesenberg, R. A. et al. Rapid acute treatment of agitation in individuals with schizophrenia: Multicentre, randomised, placebo-controlled study of inhaled loxapine. *British Journal of Psychiatry* 2011;198(1):51–8.

61. Shrewsbury, S. B., Hocevar-Trnka, J., Satterly, K. H. et al. The SNAP 101 double-blind, placebo/active-controlled, safety, pharmacokinetic, and pharmacodynamic study of INP105 (nasal olanzapine) in healthy adults. *Journal of Clinical Psychiatry* 2020;81(4):19m13086.

62. Ravi, A. D., Sadhna, D., Nagpaal, D. and Chawla, L. Needle free injection technology: A complete insight. *International Journal of Pharmaceutical Investigation* 2015;5(4):192–9.

63. GMC. Prescribing unlicensed medicines. [online] 2021. www.gmc-uk.org/ethical-guidance/ethical-guidance-for-doctors/go od-practice-in-prescribing-and-managing-medicines-and-devices/prescribing-unlicensed-medicines [Accessed 29.4.2022].

64. Royal College of Psychiatrists. Use of licensed medicines for unlicensed applications in psychiatric practice. College report CR210. [online]. 2010. www .rcpsych.ac.uk/docs/default-source/improv ing-care/better-mh-policy/college-reports/ college-report-cr210.pdf?sfvrsn=60c7f2 d_2 [Accessed 29.4.2022].

65. Nobay, F., Simon, B. C., Levitt, M. A. and Dresden, G. M. A prospective, double-blind, randomized trial of midazolam versus haloperidol versus lorazepam in the chemical restraint of violent and severely agitated patients. *Academic Emergency Medicine: Official Journal of the Society for Academic Emergency Medicine.* 2004;11 (7):744–9.

66. Martel, M., Sterzinger, A., Miner, J., Clinton, J. and Biros, M. Management of acute undifferentiated agitation in the emergency department: A randomized double-blind trial of droperidol, ziprasidone, and midazolam. *Academic Emergency Medicine: Official Journal of the Society for Academic Emergency Medicine.* 2005;12(12):1167–72.

67. Isbister, G. K., Calver, L. A., Page, C. B. et al. Randomized controlled trial of intramuscular droperidol versus midazolam for violence and acute behavioral disturbance: The DORM study. *Annals of Emergency Medicine* 2010;56 (4):392–401 e1.

68. Sweetman, S. *Martindale: The Complete Drug Reference*. Medicines Complete Royal Pharmaceutical Society; 2009. www .medicinescomplete.com/mc/martindale/c urrent/ [Accessed 29.4.2022].

69. Taylor, D., Okocha, C., Paton, C., Smith, S. and Connolly, A. Buccal midazolam for agitation on psychiatric intensive care wards. *International Journal of Psychiatry in Clinical Practice* 2008;12:309–11.

70. Parker, C. Midazolam for rapid tranquillisation: Its place in practice. *Journal of Psychiatric Intensive Care* 2014;11(01):66–72.

71. Schwagmeier, R., Alincic, S. and Striebel, H. W. Midazolam pharmacokinetics following intravenous and buccal administration. *British Journal of Clinical Pharmacology* 1998;46(3):203–6.

72. Perkins, J., Ho, J. D., Vilke, G. M., and DeMers, G. American Academy of Emergency Medicine position statement: Safety of droperidol use in the emergency department. *Journal of Emergency Medicine* 2015;49(1):91–7.

73. Brook, S., Lucey, J. V., and Gunn, K. P. Intramuscular ziprasidone compared with intramuscular haloperidol in the treatment of acute psychosis. *Journal of Clinical Psychiatry* 2000;61(12):933–41.

74. Khan, S. S. and Mican, L. M. A naturalistic evaluation of intramuscular ziprasidone versus intramuscular olanzapine for the management of acute agitation and aggression in children and adolescents. *Journal of Child and Adolescent Psychopharmacology* 2006;16(6):671–7.

75. Barzman, D. H., DelBello, M. P., Forrester, J. J., Keck, P. E. and Jr., Strakowski, S. M. A retrospective chart review of intramuscular ziprasidone for agitation in children and adolescents on psychiatric units: prospective studies are needed. *Journal of Child and Adolescent Psychopharmacology* 2007;17(4):503–9.

76. Kohen, I., Preval, H., Southard, R. and Francis, A. Naturalistic study of intramuscular ziprasidone versus conventional agents in agitated elderly patients: retrospective findings from a psychiatric emergency service. *American Journal of Geriatric Pharmacotherapy* 2005 3(4):240–5.

77. Barak, Y., Mazeh, D., Plopski, I. and Baruch, Y. Intramuscular ziprasidone treatment of acute psychotic agitation in elderly patients with schizophrenia. *American Journal of Geriatric Psychiatry* 2006 14(7):629–33.

78. Ahmed, U., Jones, H. and Adams, C. E. Chlorpromazine for psychosis induced aggression or agitation. *Cochrane Database of Systematic Reviews* 2010 (4): Cd007445.

79. Royal College of Psychiatrists. Management of Imminent Violence: Clinical Practice Guidelines to Support Mental Health Services (Occasional Paper OP41). Royal College of Psychiatrists, 1998.

80. National Institute for Health and Care Excellence. Psychosis and Schizophrenia in Adults: Prevention and Management. Clinical Guideline CG178 [online]. 2014. www.nice.org.uk/guidance/cg178 [Accessed 29.4.2022].

81. National Institute for Health and Clinical Excellence. Venous Thromboembolism: Reducing the Risk Clinical Guideline CG 92 [online]. 2010. www.nice.org.uk/guidance/cg92 [Accessed 29.4.2022].

82. European Pharmacovigilance Working Party. Antipsychotics and Cerebrovascular Accident. 2005. https://assets .publishing.service.gov.uk/government/uplo ads/system/uploads/attachment_data/file/36 8871/Pharmacovigilance_Working_Party_P ublic_Assessment_Report_on_antipsychotic s_and_cerebrovascular_accident.pdf [Accessed 29.4.2022].

83. Sorrentino, A. Chemical restraints for the agitated, violent, or psychotic pediatric

patient in the emergency department: Controversies and recommendations. *Current Opinion in Pediatrics* 2004;16 (2):201–5.

84. Einfeld, S. L. Systematic management approach to pharmacotherapy for people with learning disabilities. *Advances in Psychiatric Treatment* 2018;7 (1):43–9.

85. Allington-Smith, P. Mental health of children with learning disabilities. *Advances in Psychiatric Treatment* 2018;12 (2):130–8.

86. National Institute for Health and Care Excellence. Antenatal and postnatal mental health: Clinical management and service guidance Clinical guideline CG192 [online]. 2020. www.nice.org.uk/guidance/cg192 [Accessed 29.4.2022].

87. McAllister-Williams, R. H., Baldwin, D. S., Cantwell, R. et al. British Association for Psychopharmacology consensus guidance on the use of psychotropic medication preconception, in pregnancy and postpartum 2017. *Journal of Psychopharmacology* 2017;31(5):519–52.

Psychological, Psychosocial and Psychotherapeutic Interventions for the Prevention and Management of Violence

Miriam Barrett, Joanna Dow, Sarah Devereux, Gabriel Kirtchuk and Hannah Crisford

Introduction

The reasons why a patient with mental disorder may present with violence are complex, reflecting biological, psychodynamic and social factors, and often a combination of these. This chapter will begin with an outline of psychological mechanisms that can underlie or give rise to violence, followed by a range of psychological, psychosocial and psychotherapeutic interventions for its prevention and management. This will complement reference to psychological interventions.

Psychological Mechanisms Which Can Give Rise to Violence

Walker [1] defines violence as 'the intended infliction of bodily harm on another person'. This definition confines violence to conscious acts on the body of one person by another, ignoring unconscious motivation. In a collection of papers, Cordess and Cox [2] stress the role of the psychodynamic psychotherapeutic process, with its emphasis on transference and countertransference, in the understanding of criminal acts.

It is important to distinguish between aggression in the broader sense, as an essential component of human behaviour necessary for self-preservation and the consequent achievement of goals, and violence itself as a destructive act. Psychoanalytic literature has debated whether aggression constitutes a drive or is a reaction to a failure in the environment, in particular deprivation and aggression.

Trauma is a useful concept in understanding the psychopathology of patients who are violent, as many of them have experienced significant trauma themselves. Violence may be an unconscious re-enactment of the person's own trauma in an effort to avoid or conquer unbearable feelings of powerlessness [3], gain mastery or communicate in a primitive way what has happened. In forensic populations perpetrators may be traumatised by their own violent offences [4] which, if the trauma is not addressed, could be a maintaining factor for other conditions such as psychosis, which together could increase the risk of aggression.

More recently, psychoanalysts have begun to consider violence from the perspective of mental representation, thereby placing a focus on internal processes which result in violent

---

We would like to dedicate this chapter to the late Prof. Gabriel Kirtchuk, Consultant Psychiatrist in Psychotherapy (Forensic) and a Fellow of the British Psychoanalytical Society, who was generous with his contributions to the last and inspired our thinking.

acts. Glasser [5, 6] distinguishes between aggression and sadism to describe two different types of violence: in aggression the aim is to negate a danger or destroy an object which is perceived as a threat, whereas in sadism the aim is to inflict pain and emotional suffering on the object. Research has looked to separate individuals using 'reactive' violence from those using 'instrumental' or goal-focused violence and to consider different interventions in those offending in mainly one domain. As a consequence, emotional dysregulation and problem-solving skills are addressed in the first of these, and the second examines the negative effects of the violence for the perpetrator. This is followed by examining the progress of their lives so that meaningful goals can be met without instrumental violence.

Furthermore, violence can be conceptualised in the context of insecure attachments and a failure to develop the capacity to mentalise. Mentalisation is the ability to understand the mental state of oneself and others, which underlies overt behaviour. Both insecure attachment and lack of mentalisation can be risk factors for increased interpersonal aggression and violence [7, 8, 9, 10].

There appears to be a close relationship between violence and suicide. When considering violence, it is important to define whether the object of instinctual satisfaction is external or internal. Thus, someone may be attacked because they have become identified with an internal fantasy object and the attack may be driven by an impulse to destroy this object within oneself. Conversely, a suicide attempt or act of self-mutilation may occur if the self or body becomes identified with the hated other.

There are suggestions that the motivation for, and manifestations of, violence may differ between the female and male gender. Males express instrumental attitudes for violence, such as the need to take control or as a means to an end, whereas females tend to view aggression as emerging from a loss of control [11]. Assaults by women appear to have a more unexpected or hidden quality, whereas men seem to show more of an intimidating posture as a display of power, followed by assault [12]. Copping [13] has written an interesting and useful chapter on gender differences between in violence and aggression.

It is beyond the remit of this chapter to give more than an initial outline of the complex psychological mechanisms which can give rise to violence. Please see the references for a fuller review of the literature: [3], [14], [15].

Psychological Interventions for the Prevention and Management of Violence

Psychological interventions and therapies make use of the therapeutic relationship as an agent for change. They can focus on the management of violence or its prevention. These points are important: a good knowledge of the patient and formulation of their violent behaviour, understanding the patient's background and predisposing factors, the history of aggression and the triggers, as well as any perpetuating factors, and a focus on understanding the relationships between mental health and risk of violence together with skills to assess when and why behaviour is likely to turn violent.

As regards staff training, the training manual 'Positive & Safe: Violence Reduction and Management Programme', endorsed by the National Institute for Health and Care Excellence (NICE) in their guidelines on violence and aggression [16], is intended for instructors to ensure that a standard programme of skills training is being delivered, with a view to sharing best practice and providing a coordinated approach to the prevention and management of conflict, including incidents of violence. It focuses on prediction, prevention and management of aggression and violence, before going on to discuss primary, secondary and tertiary interventions. Although written for use in high secure settings, much of the material is equally applicable to other settings within the NHS and elsewhere.

Work can either be with the patient (e.g. in order to develop greater self-control and techniques for self-soothing), the staff group (e.g. challenging behaviour awareness training) or on the interaction between staff and patient (e.g. in the form of reflective practice). The Department of Health and Social Care [17] has developed a model called Relational Security for use in secure mental health services to keep everyone safe. This uses a format whereby the multidisciplinary team considers the patient within the following four key areas: the role of 'the care team' (therapy, boundaries), 'other patients' (the mix, the dynamics,), 'personal world' (personal environment, physical environment) and the outside word (outside connections, visitor). These areas (and this format) could be relevant and used in a wider range of settings.

Relational security is based on having safe and effective relationships between staff and patients, which can lead to a reduction in procedural and physical security, and risk-averse practice. There are suggestions that increased collaboration between staff and patients, a shift towards greater patient agency and so-called 'red-teaming' can improve risk assessment and mobilise adaptive change in secure and forensic settings [18]. Doctor [19] investigates some of the inherent difficulties in risk assessment and provides an overview of current psychodynamic approaches to risk assessment and management.

In order to help reduce violence, a number of interventions may need to be used, together with a strategy that will be applicable in different settings. What follows are some of the different psychological models used most frequently for the prevention and management of violence.

Anger Management

O'Connor and Crisford [12] highlight meta-analyses [20, 21] that have found that cognitive behavioural therapy (CBT) was effective at reducing anger and violence recidivism. Anger is the most common precipitator to violence, and interventions have focused on working with this emotion. Novaco has written widely about anger and suggested a basic framework [22] highlighting the interaction between the environment, cognitions, physiological arousal and behavioural reactions. As with any intervention, engagement is core and motivational interviewing [23] can be a vital adjunct in the first stages of therapy to support someone who wants to change their behaviour. Davies [24] suggests a CBT model for anger and irritability, supporting a formulation that looks at triggers, appraisals/judgements, inhibitions and response in the context of pre-existing beliefs and current mood.

A closely related intervention widely used for anger management is stress inoculation [25, 26]. This has three main components: cognitive preparation, skills acquisition and rehearsal, and the practice of skills during role-played exposure to a hierarchy of personally relevant triggers. Whilst a useful model to use with aggressive patients, the model can also be used to support staff (Novaco has used this with the police force) to know and manage their own triggers to support effective de-escalation of situations involving abusive individuals in provocative situations.

Positive Behavioural Support

Positive behavioural support [27, 28, 29] is a multi-component framework for developing an understanding of challenging behaviour. It is based on the assessment of the broad social and physical context in which the behaviour occurs and is used to construct socially valid interventions with the aim of improving quality of life for the person and their carer. It involves a functional assessment, the idea that the behaviour that challenges has meaning, as well as development of appropriate proactive and reactive interventions to decrease problem behaviours, such as teaching new skills and making changes to the environment. Given that deficits in adaptive skills are often key contributing factors in behavioural challenges, teaching the patient new skills (e.g. communication, social, self-management and self-help skills) is a central intervention. The improvement of quality of life is seen as both an intervention and an outcome. There is a growing academic evidence base and body of research that supports the use of positive behavioural support, in particular in the reduction of restrictive practices.

This is in line with similar initiatives, such as the launch by NHS Protect of 'Meeting needs and reducing distress: Guidance for the prevention and management of clinically related challenging behaviour in NHS settings' [30]. This document outlines practical approaches for staff with a view to delivering high-quality, personalised care that meets the needs of patients and reduces their distress, including conflict resolution and challenging behaviour awareness training.

Mentalisation-Based Therapeutic Techniques

Poor mentalising function has been identified as a risk factor for violence. Reducing impulsivity by increasing a person's capacity to think before they act on a feeling is fundamental to therapeutic techniques such as dialectical behaviour therapy (DBT) and mentalisation-based treatment (MBT).

To 'mentalise' [31] is to consider simultaneously our own states of mind – motives, wishes, intentions, fears, perceptions, initiatives and responses – and those of others with whom we are interacting. This contributes to tolerance, an awareness of uncertainty and complexity, and an appreciation of nuance and surprise in human relationships.

The therapist's stance is one of 'not knowing', of trying to get alongside the patient in order to formulate in words what the patient is experiencing. The therapist does not give interpretations; rather, they ask questions, wonder how the patient felt about a particular event, especially an interaction, urging them to expand on the perceptions, thoughts and emotions involved: the focus becomes the patient's interpretations, not the therapists. When considering the perceived motives and behaviour of others, patients are encouraged to reflect and to try to understand the possible meanings of the interaction. They are supported to consider such perceptions and interpretations as products of their own minds, which may or may not accurately take account of the reality of others' intentions and behaviour.

Mentalisation-based therapeutic techniques have been shown to reduce affect storms, improve abilities to self-reflect and reduce self-harming behaviour in patients with borderline personality disorder [32].

In MBT, patients focus on what is going on in their mind and think about what may be going on in other people's minds, particularly in situations which may cause a strong emotional reaction or problematic behaviours. When patients focus on understanding their own and other people's thoughts and feelings, this can help them better understand and control their impulses, emotions and behaviours, and can improve their relationship with other people.

Bateman et al. [33] carried out a randomised controlled trial with patients who had comorbid borderline personality disorder and antisocial personality disorder. MBT was compared with structured clinical management (SCM). Patients treated with MBT showed a significantly greater reduction in the target symptoms of anger, hostility and paranoia than those in the other group.

DBT skills training [34] is now being increasingly used with angry and violent client groups. The skills taught are highly relevant to violence, encompassing modules on mindfulness, distress tolerance, emotional regulation and interpersonal effectiveness. These skills are often directly relevant to patients who have traumatic, neglected and angry backgrounds. The skills training component of this model helps clients to recognise emotions such as sadness or shame and, instead of short circuiting to anger and violence, supports them to manage stress pro-socially using skills such as self-soothing and effective problem solving. Myths about emotions (e.g. 'letting others know you are upset is showing a weakness') are explored, and angry responses are validated and worked through to meet objectives that are more useful to the patient than violent resolutions. These allow for relationships and other objectives to be maintained or achieved.

Application of a Psychoanalytic Perspective

Work with patients with a history of violence presents staff and organisations with particular challenges. Unable to put their pain or distress into words, these patients frequently communicate their feelings via violent acts. The extent of violence and human suffering of the 'index offence' can be such that it acts as a psychic assault, filling staff with terror and evoking a strong emotional response. Bion refers to this as 'nameless dread' [35, p. 116]. The violent situation may at times be too disturbing and frightening, thereby leaving clinicians with 'blind spots' for a patient's violent history, unable to remember or see this for what it is, or with a wish to react punitively.

Gordon and Kirtchuk write:

> To experience strong emotional responses to patients, let alone to do so regularly or to discuss them in staff meetings, is equivalent to professional suicide … Yet, to remain unaware, to render oneself oblivious, or to hide one's reactions from others, however understandable, deprives the worker of valuable information – not only about oneself but about the patient. [36, pp. 1, 3]

Listening to and exploring the worker's personal responses, feelings and sensibilities to the patient – so-called countertransference – can give significant clues to emotional meaning and the patient's internal world and provide understanding and containment for the staff. Importantly, risk assessment and management in forensic settings can be vitally informed by such countertransference-based understandings. This is the basis for psychoanalytically informed supervision, reflective practice and interpersonal dynamics consultations [37].

Psychoanalytic understanding and the practice of reflective practice can also provide vital support for staff working with patients with complex mental disorders. As Cooper and Lousada [38] remind us, '[f]or mental health clinicians the work, if done well, disturbs the practitioner'. The Five Year Forward View for Mental Health, from the Independent Mental Health Taskforce, highlights the high rate of sickness absence and levels of stress amongst mental health staff, whilst noting that 'the care they receive impacts on the care they are able to deliver' [39, p. 45]. It makes a case for every trust to become an 'enabling' environment where staff want to work, to monitor staff's well-being and to provide effective occupational health services.

Alison Vaspe, in her book *Psychoanalysis, The NHS, and Mental Health Work Today* [40, p.235], concludes that

> The relationship between staff, between patients, between staff and patients, staff and those who manage them, workforces and the various bodies and organisations that monitor and govern them – these are shown to be the key to the capacity of mental health staff to hold the

psychologically vulnerable patient in mind. This includes the capacity to experience disturbance, in order to offer a form of containment that allows the disturbed patient to feel understood, on a deep level. With this level of thoughtfulness built into the system within which they work, those staff who are sensitive and interested in the minds of their patients, and have not developed – or do not want to develop – thick skins and a rigid, task-based mentality, are less likely to leave full-time employment in mental health services, or to need time off for sickness because they are demoralised or burnt-out. This is good for the workforce as a whole, economically, also because it reduces disruption to teams, and, hence, interruptions to the continuity of patient care.

Individual or group psychoanalytic psychotherapy, if successful, may allow a person to gain a better understanding of and to take greater responsibility for their actions in the past, to develop more coherent narratives of their offending experience which will impact on their ability to plan a safer future [41].

In addition, the therapeutic community model [42, 43, 44, 45, 46] can be of benefit for this patient group, who frequently have fragmented states of mind and have experienced a breakdown in communication between carers. The central philosophy of therapeutic communities is that patients are active participants in their own and each other's treatment and share responsibility for the daily running of the community with staff, with the aim of producing durable, personal change. The communal setting, reflective space and culture of enquiry in a therapeutic community, including time for staff to meet on a regular basis to discuss and think about their patients, provides an opportunity for a therapeutic couple and a reflective mind to bring different aspects of the patient together, thereby allowing a more congruent picture to emerge and providing containment for patient and staff (if the split off aspects of the patient can be brought together and integrated in the staff's mind, this can help towards an understanding of the patient and their difficulty and ultimately contribute to the patient feeling more integrated). It also provides a social reality in which to address patients' problems in interpersonal relating.

The Millfield Unit, an NHS forensic therapeutic community based at the John Howard Centre in East London, is an example of a modified therapeutic community, providing intensive psychotherapy for personality disordered offenders and patients with a history of violence.

Having evolved from therapeutic community principles, The Royal College of Psychiatrists' Enabling Environments quality and accreditation scheme [47] is based on the idea that positive and enabling relationships promote the well-being of all participants. Its award is a quality mark given to a wide range of organisations (e.g. in health, education, the criminal justice system) who can prove that they are achieving excellence in providing a healthy relational environment for all their participants.

Psychosocial Interventions

Social isolation, the lack of a social network, as well as a number of factors such as low income, unemployment, economic stress, depression and emotional insecurity, are known to be risks factors for violence, including violence against partners [48, 49].

Work experience or placements, as a pro-social activity, are therefore important interventions, as is education. Of all the self-help programmes available to prisoners in Massachusetts, USA, the one most successful in preventing recidivism or reoffending after they were released from prison was gaining a college degree while in prison. National surveys in the USA have confirmed education, especially higher education, as the single most effective means of preventing violence and crime [50].

Studies point to the significance of **strategies to address substance misuse, given that it greatly increases the risk of a violent incident (with or without a comorbid mental illness).** Whiting et al. [51] reviewed evidence from a range of studies and found that 'past criminality and substance misuse are strongly predictive of future violence in many individual disorders' (p. 150). The NICE guidelines [52, 53] for substance misuse recommend person-centred interventions that provide options for abstinence-oriented, maintenance-oriented and harm-reduction support plans. Interventions should focus on the readiness for change of the patient and often start with motivational interviewing before moving on to develop coping strategies, consider cue exposure and then onto relapse prevention.

A great deal of research has focused on the environment as a risk factor for mental illness. The opposite approach, examining the environment as a therapeutic factor in mental illness, has received less attention and underlies the concept of nidotherapy. Nidotherapy [54, 55] is 'the collaborative systematic assessment and modification of the environment to minimise the impact of any form of mental disorder on the individual or the society' [56]. It consists of four phases: personal understanding (an in-depth understanding of the patient's reasoning and functioning), environmental analysis, development of a timetable of environmental change (the nidopathway), and monitoring and adjustment of the nidopathway. Importantly, nidotherapy needs to be patient-centred and genuinely collaborative (also see Chapter 4).

Family Therapy

Family and couples therapy can also be of benefit in the prevention and management of violence. Research shows that both men and women can perpetrate relationship violence, and both sexes can be victims. Systematic approaches, such as behavioural couples treatment or domestic-violence-focused couples treatment, show promise in couples who have chosen to stay together after violent incidents and have underlying issues such as substance misuse. The Ministry of Health, New Zealand provides useful information regarding Family Violence Assessment and Intervention Guidelines [57].

Family therapy in secure units is often carried out with the parents of the offender, their children, siblings, partner, etc., even if the violence was against someone they did not know at all as opposed to violence occurring within a relationship. Its benefits include supporting and maintaining community connections and links, gathering useful information about the patient for both therapeutic and risk assessment purposes and supporting healing or transitions within the family after the disruption of often lengthy admissions. The creation of a working collaboration or therapeutic alliance between patient, professional and carer – the 'triangle of care' [58] – also promotes safety, supports recovery and sustains well-being.

Conclusion

For all of the aforementioned psychosocial interventions, the relationship with the patient is key to preventing and managing the risk of violence and aggression. This is underpinned by the NICE guidance on violence and aggression (NG10) which recommends staff training in psychosocial methods to:

- enable staff to develop a person-centred, values-based approach to care in which the personal relationship, continuity of care and a positive approach to promoting health underpin the therapeutic relationship

- ensure that staff work as a therapeutic team by using a positive and encouraging approach, maintaining staff emotional regulation and self-management and encouraging good leadership
- ensure patients are offered appropriate psychological therapies and help.

References

1. Walker, N. *Crime and Punishment in Britain*. 2nd ed. Edinburgh: Edinburgh University Press, 1968.

2. Cordess, C. and Cox, M. *Forensic Psychotherapy: Crime, Psychodynamics and the Offender Patient, Vol. 1 Mainly Theory, and Vol. 2 Mainly Practice*. London/Bristol, PA: Jessica Kingsley, 1996.

3. Garland, C. *Understanding Trauma: A Psychoanalytical Approach*. Tavistock Clinic Series. London: Taylor and Francis, 1998.

4. Crisford, H., Dare, H. and Evangeli, M. Offence-related posttraumatic stress disorder (PTSD) symptomatology and guilt in mentally disordered violent and sexual offenders. *Journal of Forensic Psychiatry & Psychology* 2008; 19 (1):86–107.

5. Glasser, M. Aspects of violence. Paper given to the Applied Section of the British Psychoanalytical Society, 1985. See Perelberg, R. J. (ed.) 1999, *Psychoanalytic Understanding of Violence and Suicide*. The New Library of Psychoanalysis. Abingdon: Routledge.

6. Glasser, M. On violence: A preliminary communication. *The International Journal of Psycho-analysis* Oct 1998; 79 (Pt 5):887–902 PMID: 9871829

7. Allen, J. G. and Fonagy, P. *Mentalizing in Practice. The Handbook of Mentalization Based Treatment*. Chichester: Wiley & Sons, 2006.

8. Taubner, S., White, L. O., Zimmermann, J., Fonagy, F. and Nolte, T. Attachment-related mentalization moderates the relationship between psychopathic traits and proactive aggression in adolescence. *Journal of Abnormal Child Psychology*, 2013;41:929–938.

9. Ogilvie, C. A., Newman, E., Todd, L. and Peck, D. The relationship between attachment & psychopathy: A meta-analysis. *Aggression and Violent Behaviour.* 2014; 19(4):322–339.

10. Cassidy, J. and Shaver, P. *Handbook of Attachment: Theory, Research & Clinical applications*. New York: Guildford Press, 2016

11. Driscoll, H., Zinkivskay, A., Evans, K. and Campbell, A. Gender differences in social representations of aggression: The phenomenological experience of differences in inhibitory control? *Br J Psychol.* 2006 May;97(Pt 2):139–53. https://doi.org/10.1348/000712605X63073. PMID: 16613646.

12. O'Connor, J. and Crisford, H. *Assessment and Interventions for Anger*. Presentation at Royal Holloway, University of London, for the Doctorate in Clinic Psychology Training,England, 2017.

13. Copping, L. (2017). Gender differences in violence and aggression. In Sturmey, P. (ed.), *The Wiley Handbook of Violence and Aggression*. Chichester: John Wiley & Sons. https://doi.org/10.1002/9781119057574.whbva005.

14. Perelberg, R. *Psychoanalytic Understanding of Violence and Suicide*. The New Library of Psychoanalysis. London: Routledge, 1998.

15. Yakeley, J. Psychodynamic approaches to violence. *British Journal of Psychiatric Advances*, 2018; 24(2):83–92.

16. National Institute for Health and Care Excellence. Violence and aggression. Short-term management in mental health, health and community settings. Updated edition. Nice Guideline NG10. 2015.

17. Royal College of Psychiatrists. See Think Act. 2nd ed. 2015. https://assets.publishing.service.gov.uk/government/uploads/system/uploads/attachment_data/file/320249/See_Think_Act_2010.pdf [Accessed 24 April 2022].

18. Markham, S. Red-teaming the Panopticon (mobilising adaptive change in secure and forensic settings). *Journal of Forensic Psychiatry and Psychology*, 2017; 29 (1):16–36.

19. Doctor, R. *Dangerous Patients: A Psychodynamic Approach to Risk Assessment and Management*. Forensic Psychotherapy Monograph Series, London: Routledge, 2003.

20. Beck, R. and Fernandez, E. Cognitive-behavioral therapy in the treatment of anger: A meta-analysis. *Cognitive Therapy and Research*, 1988; 22(1):63–74.

21. Henwood, K. S., Chou, S. and Browne, K. D. A systematic review and meta-analysis on the effectiveness of CBT informed anger management. *Aggression and Violent Behaviour* 2015; 25B:280–92.

22. Novaco, R. W. Anger and coping with stress: Cognitive behavioural interventions. In Forest, J. A. P. A. N. and Rathjen, D. P. (eds.), *Cognitive Behaviour Therapy: Research and Application*. New York: Plenum Press, 1978, pp. 135–73.

23. Miller, W. R. and Rollnick, S., *Motivational interviewing: Helping people change*. New York: Guilford Press, 2013

24. Davies, W. *Overcoming Anger and Irritability: A Self-Help Guide Using Cognitive Behavioural Techniques*. 2nd ed. London: Robinson, 2009

25. Meichenbaum, D. Stress inoculation training: A preventative and treatment approach. In Lehrer, P. M., Woolfolk, R. L. and Sime, W.E. (eds.), *Principles and Practice of Stress Management*, 3rd ed. New York: Guilford Press, 2007, pp. 497–516.

26. Novaco, R. W., Stress inoculation: A cognitive therapy for anger and its application to a case of depression. *Journal of Consulting and Clinical Psychology*, 1977;45(4):600–8.

27. Horner, R. H., Dunlap, G., Koegel, R. L. et al. Toward a technology of 'non-aversive' behavioural support. *Journal of the Association for Persons with Severe Handicaps* 1990; 15(3):125–32.

28. Allen, D., James, W., Evans, J., Hawkins, S., and Jenkins, R. Positive behavioural support: Definition, current status and future directions. *Learning Disability Review*, 2005; 10(2):4–11.

29. Gore, N. J. , McGill, P. , Toogood, S. et al. Definition and scope for positive behaviour support. *International Journal of Positive Behaviour Support* 2013;3(2):14–23.

30. NHS Protect. Meeting needs and reducing distress: Guidance for the prevention and management of clinically related challenging behaviour in NHS settings. 2013. Available at www.crisisprevention.com/CPI/media/Media/Blogs/Meeting-needs-and-reducing-distress-NHS-Protect-CB.pdf [Accessed 24 April 2022].

31. Bateman, A. W. and Fonagy, P. Mentalization-based treatment of BPD. *J Pers Disord*. 2004 Feb;18(1):36–51. https://doi.org/10.1521/pedi.18.1.36.32772. PMID: 15061343.

32. Bateman, A. and Fonagy, P. *Psychotherapy for Borderline Personality Disorder. Mentalization Based Treatment*. USA. Oxford University Press. 2004.

33. Bateman, A., O'Connell, J., Lorenzini, N., Gardner, T. and Fonagy, P. A randomised controlled trial of mentalization-based treatment versus structured clinical management for patients with comorbid borderline personality disorder and antisocial personality disorder. *BMC Psychiatry*. 2016 Aug 30;16(1):304. https://doi.org/10.1186/s12888-016-1000-9. PMID: 27577562; PMCID: PMC5006360.

34. Linehan, M. *DBT Skills Training Manual*. New York: Guilford Press, 2015

35. Bion, W.R. *Learning from Experience*. London: Tavistock, 1962

36. Gordon, J. and Kirtchuk, G. (eds.) *Psychic Assaults and Frightened Clinicians: Countertransference in Forensic Settings*, London: Karnac Books, 2008.

37. Ching, L., Hillen, T., Reiss, D., Kirtchuk, G., Scott, S. and Maier, M. The interpersonal dynamics consultation in physical health settings: A model for reflective practice. *BJPsych Advances* 2013; 25(2):122–30.

38. Cooper, A. and Lousada, J., *Borderline Welfare: Feeling and Fear of Feeling in Modern Welfare.* London: Karnac, 2005

39. NHS England. The Five Year Forward View for Mental Health. 2016. www.england.nhs.uk/publication/the-five-year-forward-view-for-mental-health/ [Accessed 25 April 2022].

40. Vaspe, A. *Psychoanalysis, The NHS, and Mental Health Work Today: Psychoanalytic Ideas.* London: Karnac, 2017.

41. Adshead, G., Ferrito, M., and Bose, S. Recovery after homicide narrative shifts in therapy with homicide perpetrators. *Criminal Justice and Behaviour*, 2015; 42 (1):70–81.

42. Main, T. The hospital as a therapeutic institution. *Bulletin of the Menninger Clinic* 1946; 10:66–70.

43. Rapoport, R. N. *Community as Doctor.* London: Tavistock Publications, 1960.

44. Rutter, D. and Tyrer, P. The value of therapeutic communities in the treatment of personality disorder: A suitable place for treatment? *Journal of Psychiatric Practice* 2003 Jul;9(4):291–302. https://doi.org/10.1097/00131746-200307000-00004. PMID: 15985944.

45. Lees, J., Manning, N. and Rawlings, B. A culture of enquiry: Research evidence and the therapeutic community. *Psychiatric Quarterly* 2004 Fall;75(3):279–94. https://doi.org/10.1023/b:psaq.0000031797.74295.f8. PMID: 15335230.

46. Pearce, S., Scott, L., Attwood, G. et al. Democratic therapeutic community treatment for personality disorder: randomised controlled trial. *British Journal of Psychiatry* 2017 Feb;210(2):149–56. https://doi.org/10.1192/bjp.bp.116.184366. Epub 2016 Dec 1. PMID: 27908900.

47. Royal College of Psychiatrists. Enabling Environment Awards. www.rcpsych.ac.uk/quality/qualityandaccreditation/enabling environments.aspx [Accessed 25 April 2022].

48. Kalvin, C. B. and Bierman, K. L. Child and adolescent risk factors that differentially predict violent versus nonviolent crime. *Aggressive Behavior* 2017 Nov;43(6):568–77. https://doi.org/10.1002/ab.21715. Epub 2017 Jun 8. PMID: 28597509; PMCID: PMC5640463.

49. Evans, D. P. COVID-19 and violence: A research call to action. *BMC Women's Health* 2020 Nov 10;20(1):249. https://doi.org/10.1186/s12905-020-01115-1. PMID: 33172466; PMCID: PMC7653443.

50. Gilligan, J. Can psychoanalysis help us to understand the causes and prevention of violence? *Psychoanalytic Psychotherapy* 2016;30(2):125–37.

51. Whiting, D., Lichtenstein, P. and Fazel, S. Violence and mental disorders: A structured review of associations by individual diagnoses, risk factors, and risk assessment. *Lancet Psychiatry* 2021 Feb;8 (2):150–61. https://doi.org/10.1016/S2215-0366(20)30262-5. Epub 2020 Oct 20. PMID: 33096045.

52. National Institute for Health & Clinical Excellence. Drug misuse – Psychosocial Interventions. NICE CG 51. Issued July 2007. www.nice.org.uk/guidance/cg51/evidence/drug-misuse-psychosocial-interventions-full-guideline-195261805 [Accessed 25 April 2022].

53. National Institute for Health & Clinical Excellence. Coexisting severe mental illness and substance misuse: Community health and social care services. NICE Guideline NG58. Issued 2016. www.nice.org.uk/guidance/NG58 [Accessed 25 April 2022].

54. Tyrer, P. Nidotherapy: A new approach to the treatment of personality disorder. *Acta Psychiatrica Scandinavica* 2002 Jun;105 (6):469–71; discussion:471–2. https://doi.org/10.1034/j.1600-0447.2002.01362.x. PMID: 12059852.

55. Tyrer, P. The importance of nidotherapy and environmental change in the management of people with complex mental disorders. *International Journal of Environmental Research and Public Health* 2018;15(5):972.

56. Tyrer, P., Sensky, T. and Mitchard, S. Principles of nidotherapy in the treatment of persistent mental and personality

disorders. Psychother Psychosom 2003, Nov–Dec, 72(6):350–6.

57. Ministry of Health New Zealand. Family Violence Assessment and Intervention Guideline. Child abuse and intimate partner violence. 2016 www.health.govt.nz/publication/family-violence-assessment-and-intervention-guideline-child-abuse-and-intimate-partner-violence [Accessed 25 April 2022].

58. Carerstrust. The Triangle of Care. Carers Included: A Guide to Best Practice in Mental Health Care. 2013. https://carers.org/downloads/resources-pdfs/triangle-of-care-england/the-triangle-of-care-carers-included-second-edition.pdf [Accessed 24 April 2022].

Chapter

8

Prevention and Management of Violence in Inpatient Psychiatric Settings

Mehtab Ghazi Rahman, Masum Khwaja and Shanika Balachandra

Introduction

Ensuring wards are safe for patients, staff and visitors is a basic requirement for any inpatient unit. Exposure to violence and aggression has a deleterious impact on patient and staff safety, treatment outcomes, staff morale and performance, and the therapeutic environment.

Violence and aggression remain common reasons for admission to psychiatric wards, and violence and aggression commonly occur in inpatient psychiatric units. In the United Kingdom, the National Audit of Violence for working age adults 2006–7 found that 46% of nursing staff working in an inpatient mental health setting said that they had been physically assaulted, 72% that they had been threatened or made to feel unsafe and 58% that they had experienced violence that had upset or distressed them. In the case of patients, 45% had experienced violence that had upset or distressed them, 34% had felt threatened or unsafe and 18% had been physically assaulted. The likelihood of visitors being exposed to violence of any type was understandably lower than for the other groups, but there was a consistent pattern that the 'threat of violence' was more common than 'actual assault' and 'evident across all respondent groups' [1].

The audit identified areas where improvement is required:

- Life on the ward: administration of medication; involving patients in decisions; activities and therapies; provision of information;
- Ward staffing: staff ratio and skill mix; flexible staffing in relation to resident population;
- Training and support for staff: undertaking searches; recording incidents; observation and rapid tranquillisation;
- Environmental safety: basic safety features (i.e. de-escalation area and an effective alarm system); ensuring privacy and dignity; lack of space and overcrowding;
- Being supported in relation to actual incidents: proactive measures; post-incident support; reporting of less severe incidents.

The Royal College of Psychiatrists (RCPsych) College Centre for Quality Improvement (CCQI) has developed comprehensive standards for inpatient mental health services [2]. Each area of practice (see Table 8.3) for which a standard has been set is subdivided into standards, classed as either:

a. essential standards: Failure to meet these would result in a significant threat to patient safety, rights or dignity and/or would breach the law. These standards also include the fundamentals of care, including the provision of evidence-based care and treatment;

b. expected standard that most services should meet; and

c. desirable standards that high performing services should meet.

In this chapter we will discuss the clinical management of acutely disturbed behaviour in inpatient units and touch on clinical governance, the RCPsych Standards and the areas of concern identified by the National Audit of Violence 2006–2007.

Clinical Governance

Inpatient wards should refer to the seven pillars of clinical governance to monitor their clinical performance: clinical effectiveness, risk management, patient experience and involvement, communication, resource effectiveness, strategic effectiveness and learning effectiveness.

Policies and Guidance

Organisations must ensure that effective and monitored policies and practices are in place to manage and reduce the likelihood of violence.

Providers should be mindful of the Care Quality Commission (CQC) Key Lines of Enquiry and follow guidance from bodies such as the National Institute for Health and Care Excellence (NICE), RCPsych (see standards mentioned earlier), and the National Association of Psychiatric Intensive Care and Low Secure Units (NAPICU) in order to ensure they are delivering high-quality, evidence-based care to their patients [3, 4, 5].

Providers should also be aware of models of inpatient care aimed at reducing incidents of violence on inpatient wards (e.g. Safewards [6] and Star Wards [7]). Safewards was developed following research that showed an up to ten-fold variation in incidents of violence, restraint and seclusion between different acute mental health wards with similar patient populations. An impact review of Star Wards in 2013 found that 60% of participating wards reported a decrease in aggression following implementation of their activity and well-being-based programme [7].

Quality Assurance

The reduction in bed capacity over the last decade with an associated increase in the threshold for admission, has added to the pressure inpatient units face. Unless there is careful monitoring quality of care may slip and the principle of person-centred care replaced by the need to find a bed [8].

Robust local quality-assurance mechanisms and active participation in accredited quality initiatives, such as those run by the RCPsych Quality Network, are important to ensure the consistent delivery of high-quality clinical care [9]. The quality of clinical care delivered by inpatient units can be assessed using specific key performance indicators (KPIs). KPIs include patient-related outcome measures (PROMs) (e.g. patient satisfaction surveys), clinician rated outcome measures (CROMs), Health of the Nation Outcome Scales (HoNOS), patient safety measures (e.g. adverse events), audit of restrictive interventions (audit of rapid tranquillisation [RT] administration, seclusion occupancy, etc.) and multidisciplinary team (MDT) measures (staff levels, sickness rates and training compliance).

Quality improvement projects (QIP) and a continuous drive to improve quality of care for patients should be embedded in team culture.

An example of a well conducted QIP is provided by the forensic violence reduction collaborative of East London NHS Foundation Trust (ELFT) [10]. On five of their seven forensic wards, they managed to achieve a reduction of 46.3%–80.2% in the frequency of incidents of non-physical violence and of 17%–93% in the frequency of incidents of physical violence.

Service User Involvement

Co-production with people with lived experience of services, their families and their carers is one of the common principles of the Five Year Forward View for Mental Health [11].

Involving patients and carers in local meetings (e.g. care quality meetings) can help identify and understand service user needs to transform service delivery and improve overall patient experience.

NICE guidance on service-user experience in mental health services, including quality standards for inpatient contact with staff and inpatient meaningful activity, was updated in July 2019 [12].

Incident Reporting

Staff should have access to established reporting systems (e.g. DATIX) to allow them to log incidents of acute behavioural disturbances and receive timely feedback from managers. All serious incidents should be investigated and accounted for at a senior management level. Those involved in the investigation should establish a detailed understanding of the context of the serious incident, including identifying any predisposing contributing factors using a 'root cause analysis' approach. Inpatient units must have an established process to report, manage and investigate serious incidents, and clear guidance on liaison with external agencies such as local authorities and the police.

'Near miss' or 'no harm' incidents should also be reported and learnt from, and certainly not overlooked.

Factors Contributing to Violence in Mental Health Inpatient Settings

A broad range of factors contribute to violence in mental health inpatient settings, including psychological distress, dysfunctional personality traits or comorbid personality disorder, drug and alcohol use, psychopathological symptoms (e.g. nature of delusions and hallucinations), staff and patient attitudes and restrictions that may limit a service user's freedom (e.g. being denied leave, enforcing ward boundaries, drug treatment given against the patient's wishes). Additional factors that increase the risk of violence in inpatient settings include lack of privacy, poorly kempt wards, overcrowding, lack of structure and routine, authoritarian conditions and no access to fresh air [13].

Environmental Factors

The Department of Health (DoH) has produced guidance to inform the planning and design of inpatient facilities that are fit for purpose. The guidance comprehensively lists service users' needs in relation to the environment, including the need for safety, space, privacy, dignity, access to outside areas, natural light and ventilation and to a variety of activities [14]. NAPICU offer design guidance specifically for Psychiatric Intensive Care Unit (PICU) wards [15].

NICE guidance emphasises the need to address environmental factors in collaboration with service users and carers. Such factors are likely to increase or decrease the need for restrictive interventions and, together with nidotherapy, are discussed further in Chapter 4. Nidotherapy is a relatively new concept that is 'devoted to changing the environment in all its forms so a better fit is established between a person and every aspect of their surroundings' [16].

Staff Factors

Ensuring that patients feel safe requires staff who can work as part of a team and who have a robust knowledge of mental health, good linguistic and communication skills, resilience, empathy, compassion and emotional intelligence. They should be able to remain calm and professional even under stress. This is not easy to do when faced with patients who are abusive or aggressive and acutely mentally unwell. Appropriate supervision is crucial for safe practice, to support staff (clinically and professionally) and in identifying staff who are not coping and may benefit from extra support or training. Proxy measures for the 'health' of an organisation (or team) and how well the organisation (or team) is functioning, include sickness and retention rates, and managers should always be concerned if retention rates fall or sickness absence rises.

Staff Training

Comprehensive staff training is essential to manage acute behavioural disturbance safely. Safe management of violence and aggression is reliant on staff having access to clear guidelines and procedures that they can follow. All staff should receive appropriate training to manage disturbed behaviour, and mental health trusts across the United Kingdom have made it mandatory that all nursing staff working in inpatient settings must receive training in risk assessment and prevention and management of violence and aggression (PMVA).

Staff members with significant experience of working in mental health settings and those who have completed PMVA training have a lower incidence of being assaulted than those who do not [17].

Clinical staff should also receive training on the safe use of pre-rapid and rapid tranquillisation; training that will support them to effectively and with confidence manage aggression using pharmacological interventions.

Staffing Levels and Expertise

As one would expect, staffing levels and expertise influence the safety and quality of care. For example, the increased use of agency staff (often unfamiliar to patients) in ward settings has been shown to be associated with a higher incidence of violent assaults [18].

In the National Audit of Violence (2006–7), respondents were asked whether a range of physical interventions were used 'too quickly' to manage severely challenging behaviour and violent incidents. Responders most frequently mentioned the impact of low ward-staffing levels, meaning that that staff did not have time to de-escalate situations and resorted to using quicker methods instead [1].

Although monitoring and reporting of safe staffing is mandatory on inpatient wards, there are no minimum staffing levels or ratios for mental health wards. NHS England facilitated the production of guidance 'to support the specific requirements of mental health leaders and places the mental health service user at the centre of achieving safe staffing' [19].

Despite the guidance, there remains concern that trusts are managing nursing vacancies by shifting registered nurses to provide cover, by employing more unqualified staff and agency staff and by substituting nurses for allied professionals [20].

Despite nurse vacancies, unit managers should keep in mind CQC guidance for inspections in relation to nurse staffing levels in mental health wards and ensure that:

- The total number of nurses on each shift is sufficient to provide safe care.
- There are enough qualified nurses on each shift.
- There are effective procedures for bringing in additional staff whenever needed.
- All nurses know the service users and are familiar with ward procedures.
- The nurses on duty have the right skills to make the ward safe (e.g. resuscitation, or physical interventions) [21].

Interpersonal Relationships and Communication

An important area in the prevention of violence and skill development amongst mental health staff is the use of 'self' within the context of trusting relationships as a means of de-escalation of disturbance. *Relational security* is the knowledge and understanding staff have of a patient, the environment in which care is provided and the translation of that information into appropriate responses, engagement and care [22]. Relational security is not simply about having 'a good relationship' with a patient. Safe and effective relationships between staff and patients must be professional, therapeutic and purposeful, with clear boundaries.

Effective communication is essential to ensure appropriate care and respect for patients' rights. Staff must communicate in a manner that is straightforward and understandable, and must check that the patient has understood what has been said.

Barriers to effective communication should be identified early, and the patient's care plan should reflect how each barrier will be overcome. Barriers may include the mental state of the patient; racial, cultural, and language differences between staff and patients; difficulty in reading or writing; and hearing or visual impairment.

Health Factors

A number of physical health factors can contribute to acute behavioural disturbances, such as head injury, delirium tremens, encephalopathies, temporal lobe epilepsy, dementia and neoplastic conditions. In such cases, it is essential that the underlying medical condition is treated to reduce the risk of acute behavioural disturbance. Care planning in this group should involve medical specialists, the patient's general practitioner and family members.

Maintaining Ward Safety: Searches

The safety of a ward can be compromised in different ways, such as (a) patients having access to alcohol and drugs, (b) items that may be potentially dangerous going missing from the ward (e.g. cutlery), (c) patients having possession of a prohibited item that might be used as a weapon or to self-harm (e.g. sharp knife, Taser).

Environmental and personal searches are necessary to create and maintain a therapeutic environment and to ensure the security of the unit, the safety of patients, staff and the public. On healthcare premises, appropriately trained members of staff are entitled to undertake lawful searches of patients, visitors and their belongings.

The Mental Health Act 1983 Code of Practice 2015 (Mental Health Act [MHA] Code of Practice) details the legislation regarding conducting searches in the hospital setting for those consenting and those not consenting to searches [23]. The MHA Code of Practice also offers direction on what should be included in an operational policy for searching and all units should have policies in place for both environmental and personal searches.

Search policies should include the actions to be taken if a search uncovers evidence of criminal activity. Protocols should be developed, in liaison with local police, for recording, storing and handing over evidence to the police.

Patients should be informed about environmental searches and verbal consent for a search sought beforehand. Searches should be conducted by at least two members of staff and the patient's dignity should be respected at all times.

Informal patients have the right to refuse a personal search; in such circumstances, the responsible clinician (RC) should assess the patient's risk to self and others and decide whether the patient should continue to be treated on the ward informally.

Nursing staff can ask visitors to undergo a search if there are suspicions about them; however, a search cannot be conducted if the visitor does not consent. Staff can prevent a visitor from entering the ward if they do not adhere to ward rules and regulations.

Healthcare staff are not entitled to undertake intimate body searches. In units where the risks are high, consideration should be given to reporting any evidence of criminal activity, such as illicit drug dealing, to the police. The intrusion needs to be balanced against potential risks and the necessity to protect vulnerable patients and staff from serious harm.

Drug and Alcohol Use

'Dual diagnosis' and 'comorbidity' are terms used to describe coexisting mental health and alcohol and drug misuse problems.

The 2002 Co-morbidity of Substance Misuse and Mental Illness Collaborative study (COSMIC) revealed that dual diagnosis was present in 43% of psychiatric inpatients and 56% of people in secure services [24].

The DoH 2006 guidance on the assessment and management of dual diagnosis in mental health inpatient and day settings identified drug and alcohol use as one of the main triggers for violence in mental health inpatient services [25].

The 2006–7 National Audit of Violence reported that 85% of acute ward nursing staff felt their ward was influenced negatively by alcohol and 88% of acute and 68% of PICU nursing staff identified problems with legal drugs [1]. Large numbers of respondents commented on the problems associated with alcohol, including both a detrimental impact on patient well-being and aggravating the risk of substance misuse and violence.

Staff should have appropriate training in the management of traditional substances of abuse such as alcohol, cannabis, solvents, stimulants, psychedelics and opiates. It is also important that staff receive training in the management of *novel psychoactive substances* [26]. A study that analysed more than 440 admissions to a London NHS Foundation Trust

(Camden and Islington) dramatically demonstrates why [27]. The study showed that the vast majority of admissions of people using 'novel psychoactive substances' were strongly associated with violence. This was both before and during their admission. Specifically, over a six-month period, 13% of admissions to acute psychiatric wards in the study were novel psychoactive substances users (NPSU). Of the 58 NPSU users, around 80% were strongly associated with violence before admission, and a similar percentage during their admission. This compared with 21% and around 16% respectively for non-NPSU. The research also revealed the worrying impact of use on length of hospital admission, with NPSU being admitted for 50 days, compared with 39 days for non-NPSU; NPSU also had a higher readmission rate.

Inpatient admission offers an opportunity to identify or review substance misuse problems, establish appropriate treatment and link patients to services that can help. Substance misuse screening on admission and a high degree of suspicion is required if wards are to maintain a drug-free environment and ensure that patients receive the specialist care they need. If a patient deteriorates, or is slow to improve, especially for no obvious reason, substance misuse should be considered.

Where substance misuse is a factor in the risk of violence, it may be helpful to include drug testing as part of the management plan. Testing may help to elucidate the relationship between intoxication and fluctuations in mental state; it may also provide a therapeutic boundary to help some patients maintain abstinence. Decisions to screen for illicit substances should be taken by the multidisciplinary team in collaboration with the patient and should be documented in a care plan. Arrangements for supervised collection – for example, of urine samples – should give due consideration to the patient's dignity while minimising the opportunities for tampering with or substituting the sample. Test results should be interpreted with due caution in the light of advice from the relevant laboratory.

Environmental random searches by 'sniffer' dogs to detect substances and to dissuade dealers and patients from bringing substances onto the ward may form an important part of an organisational strategy to maintain a therapeutic, drug-free environment [28, 29].

A fuller discussion of dual diagnosis is beyond the scope of this chapter but interested readers should read relevant guidance, including that produced by NICE and the DoH [30, 31].

Sexual Safety

The CQC found that, between April and June 2017, out of a total of nearly 60,000 reports of incidents that took place on wards between April and June 2017, 1,120 were sexual incidents involving patients, staff, or visitors[32]. Although the vast majority were classed as low or no-risk incidents (97%), 24.4% of the total were recorded as 'sexual assault' and 2.6% were allegations of rape. Incidents principally involved patients, and a minority involved staff and visitors.

In response to the CQC report the National Collaborating Centre for Mental Health (NCCMH) was commissioned to develop standards and guidance on improving sexual safety in inpatient environments. A national quality improvement (QI) sexual safety collaborative (SSC) was also developed to support inpatient mental health teams to embed standards and improve ward sexual safety [33].

Any incidents of a sexual nature must be responded to immediately in an appropriate manner by staff. Incidents of a sexual nature in mental health wards include rape, sexual harassment, sexual assault, exposure of genitals, use of sexualised speech to verbally abuse someone and partaking in sexual intercourse (when not having the mental capacity to make an informed decision). All wards must endeavour to facilitate sexual safety by (a) creating a safe space for all patients through adequate supervision and identification of high risk areas within a ward, (b) having separate spaces for men and women within a ward, (c) staff training on safeguarding, clinical risk assessments, sexual safety strategies and management of sexual safety incidents, (d) providing clear guidance on reporting of sexual incidents in clinical care areas (e.g. using posters and leaflets) and (e) reporting sexual safety incidents (e.g. DATIX) and learning from incidents to avoid similar incidents in the future. When a patient reports unwanted sexual behaviour or assault, staff should communicate with the victim in a calm, supportive and compassionate manner in a private space. The incident should be reported to the police. The service user's care plan and risk assessment should be updated and the observation levels reviewed to ensure safety. In the event of a serious sexual assault (e.g. penetrative sexual assault), the victim should be advised not to wash their body or clothes until further medical examination occurs. Following a sexual assault, the incident should be notified to a senior manager, and any disclosures of a sexual nature must be investigated by the hospital regardless of whether the patient wants police involvement or not.

The Role of the Psychiatric Intensive Care Unit (PICU)

PICU's are specialist wards for compulsorily detained patients who can not safely be managed in an acute psychiatric ward. A patient admitted to a PICU is often in an acutely disturbed phase of a serious mental illness and has lost the capacity for self control with a corresponding increase in risk which does not enable their care, therapeutic management and treatment to be in a general adult ward setting [34]. Inpatient mental health teams should refer a patient to PICU if the patient's behaviour, in the context of a mental disorder, is of high risk to self and/or others and cannot safely be managed by conventional treatment in a 'general ward' setting. Behaviour leading to a PICU referral typically consists of one or more of the following: verbal, physical or sexual aggression; property damage; sexual disinhibition; psychomotor overactivity; high absconscion risk and/or significant risk of suicide unresponsive to preventative measures in a general psychiatric ward. Eligible patients can only be accepted under an appropriate MHA section because of the restricted environment of a PICU ward. The use of preventative admission to PICU before an incident has occurred is good practice but is not always achievable given the existing pressure on acute beds.

Principles of Managing Acutely Disturbed Behaviour

Acute behavioural disturbance within inpatient settings should be treated as a clinical emergency requiring urgent intervention to manage risk. Common examples of acute behavioural disturbances include verbal threats, physical aggression, property damage, self-harming behaviour and psychomotor agitation. Prompt use of effective de-escalation techniques and pharmacological interventions can quickly defuse potentially violent behaviour.

A number of fundamental principles should be used by MDT teams in inpatient settings to manage risk in a safe and effective manner. The Joint British Association for Psychopharmacology and NAPICU evidence-based consensus guidelines [35] for the clinical management of acute disturbance recommend the following principles to manage acute behavioural disturbance:

(a) A multidisciplinary approach: The management of acute behavioural disturbance should be carried out using an MDT approach (through psychopharmacological, psychological, environmental and social interventions).

(b) Effective interventions: Interventions used to manage acute disturbance should be based on evidence. Risk should be minimised by prescribing the minimum effective dose of medications and monitoring side effects.

(c) Proportionality of intervention: An intervention should be proportionate to the severity of the risk posed during an episode of acute disturbance. RT should only be used as a last resort once non-pharmacological and oral pharmacological options have been exhausted.

(d) Treatment individualisation and choice: Patient-specific factors should be taken into consideration when an intervention is selected during the decision-making process, such as previous response to specific medications and adverse reactions/allergies.

(e) Treatment optimisation of underlying disorder: Acute disturbances may be partially or wholly caused by an underlying mental illness that should be treated optimally to reduce behavioural disturbances.

(f) The team should continuously monitor and review a patient's (i) mental and physical health, (ii) risk to self and others, (iii) treatment effectiveness or harm, (iv) engagement level.

(g) Consideration of modifiers: Special consideration should be given to sub-populations that require a modified pre-rapid/rapid tranquillisation approach. Special sub-populations in psychiatric inpatient settings include pregnant women, intoxicated patients, medically frail and physically compromised patients, psychotropic naïve patients, patients being treated with regular antipsychotics, patients with learning disability and those at extremes of age [35].

Predicting Violence in Inpatient Settings

Assessing the risk of likelihood of violence should begin from the moment a patient is referred. As part of the provisional risk assessment, all available documentation (historical and current) should be reviewed, with risk assessment documentation being completed after the patient has been seen. The management plan should include the potential risk of violence, including the recommended setting for treatment (e.g. PICU as opposed to a general adult acute ward).

The 2016 Royal College of Psychiatrists College Report (CR201), 'Rethinking risk to others in mental health services' [36], lists a number of factors that should be taken into consideration when conducting a violence risk assessment for mental health patients (see Table 8.1).

Management of Acutely Disturbed Behaviour in Inpatient Settings Observation and Engagement

Background

Observation and engagement is common practice. Bowers found that up to 20% of inpatients had experienced one or more types of enhanced observation [37]. In another of

Table 8.1 Factors to be taken into consideration when conducting a violence risk assessment for mental health patients

History	Environment	Mental State
Previous history of violence	Risk factors may vary by setting and patient group	Evidence of symptoms related to threat or control, delusions of persecution by others, or of mind or body being controlled or interfered with by external forces, or passivity experiences
Relationship of violence to mental state		
Lack of supportive relationships	Risk on release from restricted settings	
Poor concordance with treatment, discontinuation or engagement	Consider protective factors or loss of protective factors	Voicing emotions related to violence or exhibiting emotional arousal (e.g. irritability, anger, hostility, suspiciousness, excitement, enjoyment, notable lack of emotion, cruelty or incongruity)
Impulsivity	Relational security	
Alcohol or substance use	Risks of reduced bed capacity and alternatives to admission	
Early exposure to violence or being part of a violent subculture		Specific threats or ideas of retaliation
Triggers or changes in behaviour or mental state that have occurred prior to previous violence or relapse	Access to potential victims, particularly individuals identified in mental state abnormalities	Grievance thinking
		Thoughts linking violence and suicide (homicide-suicide)
Recent changes in risk factors	Access to weapons, violent means or opportunities	Thoughts of sexual violence
Evidence of recent stressors, losses or threats of loss		Evolving symptoms and unpredictability
	Involvement in radicalisation	Signs of psychopathy
Factors that stopped the person acting violently in the past		Restricted insight and capacity
History of domestic violence		Patient's own narrative and view of risk to others
Lack of empathy		What does the patient think they are capable of? Do they think they could kill?
Relationship of violence to personality factors		Beware of 'invisible' risk factors

his studies, 47% of patients received intermittent observation during the first two weeks of admission, and 16% within reach observation [38].

If implemented and conducted with due care and consideration, observation remains a useful intervention in managing the risk that some patients may pose to themselves and others. However, patients may find observation intrusive, isolative, provocative, humiliating and dehumanising. If conducted poorly, there is potential to do harm (e.g. to damage the therapeutic relationship) and for the risk being managed to increase rather than diminish.

Furthermore, it is a resource-intensive intervention, with estimates of the financial cost to the NHS, of constant observation, ranging from £70,000 per annum per ward to more than £850, 000 per annum on forensic wards and a total estimated national cost of £35 million [39, 40]. As with all restrictive interventions, observation should be proportionate to the risks, only be used after less restrictive measures have failed and only for the minimum time period necessary.

Patients should be informed why they are on observation, be given a clear indication of when observation may cease (what needs to be achieved within a time frame) and have their dignity and rights respected at all times.

'Observation' policies have given way to 'observation and positive engagement' policies in order to emphasise the importance of aligning observation with meaningful therapeutic engagement. NICE guideline NG10 defines positive engagement as an 'intervention that aims to empower service users to actively participate in their care. Rather than 'having things done to' them, service users negotiate the level of engagement that will be most therapeutic' [4].

Observation should be coupled with meaningful interventions, specifically tailored care plans and structured observation reviews [41]. Patients who are actively engaged by empathic individuals have reported that it is potentially therapeutic if staff observing them show an active interest, encourage conversation, listen, and help them feel valued, supported and looked after. In contrast, the perceived attitudes and behaviours of an observer can cause patients distress, which affirms the need for careful supervision of observers [42].

A recent systematic review of interventions to improve constant observation on adult inpatient psychiatric wards suggests that those attempting to improve the quality and safety of constant observations should consider the roles of the team during constant observation, improve teamwork skills, standardise parts of the practice and properly evaluate interventions that may impact constant observations [43].

Observation and Engagement Policies and NG10 (2015)

NG10 states that health and social care provider organisations should have a policy on observation and positive engagement [4], and describes what should be contained in an observation policy, the general principles, the levels of observation and when to use observation.

NG10 suggests three levels of observation:

- Low-level intermittent observation: the baseline level of observation in a specified psychiatric setting. The frequency of observation is once every 30–60 minutes.
- High-level intermittent observation: generally used if a service user is at risk of becoming violent or aggressive but does not represent an immediate risk. The frequency of observation is once every 15–30 minutes.
- Continuous observation: typically used when a service user presents an immediate threat and needs to be kept within eyesight or at arm's length of a designated one-to-one nurse, with immediate access to other members of staff if needed.

In practice, mental health units across the United Kingdom usually use four different observation levels for inpatients. The level of nursing observation for each patient should be determined jointly by the ward's multidisciplinary team.

Level 1: The minimum level of observation for inpatients. A patient does not have to be within eyesight at all times, but staff must be aware of the patient's whereabouts and the patient's location should be checked hourly.

Level 2: Intermittent observations. A patient's whereabouts is checked every 15 minutes by staff. This is the appropriate observation level for a patient at risk of disturbed behaviour who is recovering from the acute phase of his/her mental illness.

Level 3: Eyesight observation. A patient's whereabouts is supervised within eyesight at all times (e.g. 1:1 nursing). This level of observation is appropriate for a patient who poses a high risk of harm to the self or others.

Level 4: Arm's length observation. A patient's whereabouts is supervised at close proximity at all times. This level of observation is reserved for patients who pose the highest risk of harming themselves or others.

For further guidance on observation, please read MHA Code of Practice 2015, NRG10 and your local organisation's policy on observation and engagement.

De-Escalation Techniques

De-escalation is a complex, interactive process in which a patient is redirected towards a calmer personal space. NG10 defines de-escalation as the 'use of techniques (including verbal and non-verbal communication skills) aimed at defusing anger and averting aggression' [4, p. 63]. There is a lack of high-quality research on the effectiveness of individual de-escalation techniques; however, it is widely accepted that de-escalation techniques (see Table 8.2) are effective in reducing aggressive behaviour, and there is widespread advocacy from national bodies for the use of such techniques in mental health settings [44]. For a detailed breakdown of de-escalation components, please also see the NAPICU guidance [35].

The use of effective de-escalation techniques avoids the need for physical restraints and should precede the use of RT and seclusion. Communication is key when de-escalating a potentially aggressive situation: staff should take an attentive, sympathetic and caring attitude towards the patient, using a variety of non-verbal and verbal communication

Table 8.2 De-escalation Techniques

Non-Verbal	Verbal
Maintaining a non-confrontational approach	Speaking in a calm, slow and clear tone
Maintaining appropriate body postures	Speaking in sentences that are short and clear
	Avoiding the use of long sentences
Matching facial expressions to what is being said to the patient	Not retaliating to personal attacks or verbal abuse from patients
Avoiding physical contact with a patient until the situation calms down	Assuring a patient that the team want to help find a solution to the patient's problem
	Explaining to the patient the detrimental effect of the patient's aggressive behaviour on other patients in the ward
Maintaining good eye contact without staring or intimidating the patient	Being an active listener and showing empathy using appropriate verbal clues
	Summarising what the patient says and reflecting on how they may be feeling
	Avoiding arguments, interruptions, sarcasm and blaming
	Helping the patient identify the cause of their anger and setting realistic expectations

techniques. Staff should learn to recognise signs of agitation and escalation, and to present themselves as a calm, caring professional, maintain poise even in the face of a potentially violent patient [45].

Restraint

The MHA Code of Practice (2015) defines physical restraint as 'any direct physical contact where the intention is to prevent, restrict or subdue movement of the body (or part if the body) of another person' [23, p. 295]. Physical restraint should be distinguished from mechanical restraint, which is defined as 'a form of restrictive intervention that refers to the use of a device (e.g. belt or cuff) to prevent, restrict or subdue movement of a person's body, or part of the body, for the primary purpose of behavioural control' [23, p. 296].

The use of restraint is only justified when it is a last recourse measure used to take control of a dangerous situation and to reduce the danger a patient poses to the self or others. The type of restraint and the length of the intervention should be proportionate to the likelihood and seriousness of the harm posed by the patient to themselves or others (see also Chapter 1). The MHA Code of Practice lists five common reasons for restraint of a patient by staff in mental health settings: physical assault; non-compliance with treatment; risk of self-harm or physical injury by accident; prolonged overactivity that is likely to lead to physical exhaustion; and dangerous, threatening or destructive behaviour.

Factors that can increase the risk of injury to a patient during manual restraint include chronic medical conditions (e.g. asthma, cardiac disease), musculoskeletal problems, obesity, substance misuse, pregnancy and the use of psychotropic treatment. Prolonged restraint is associated with a high risk of collapse. NG10 recommends that manual restraint is ceased as quickly as possible and should not be routinely used for more than ten minutes [4]. Restraining a patient in prone position is much riskier than restraining a patient in the supine position, and the MHA Code of Practice states that 'unless there are cogent reasons for doing so, there must be no planned or intentional restraint of a person in a prone position' [23, p. 295]. NG10 states 'taking service users to the floor during manual restraint should be avoided, but that if it is necessary, the supine (face up) position should be used in preference to the prone (face down) position' [4, pp. 57]. Furthermore, 'if the prone (face down) position is necessary' it should be used 'for as short a time as possible' [4, pp. 38]. The exceptional circumstances wherein this advice can be over-ridden are described in Chapter 1. It is recognised that the use of mechanical restraint may be considered to be the least restrictive intervention in some specific cases, and may present less risk to the individual than the alternative of prolonged manual restraint or transfer to a more restrictive setting. This could provide a valid reason for using mechanical restraint in emergency or 'unplanned' interventions as well as planned interventions [46]. However, mechanical restraint should only be used in high secure settings to manage extreme violence directed at others or to limit self-injurious behaviour of 'extremely high frequency and intensity' [4, p. 39].

There is a government directive to reduce all forms of restrictive practices in inpatient mental health units, and all trusts across the United Kingdom are required to reduce the use of restrictive practices and publish data on the use of restrictive interventions. Organisations are encouraged to introduce *restrictive intervention reduction programmes*, which the MHA Code of Practice defines as 'overarching, multi-component action plans which aim to reduce the use of restrictive interventions' [23, p. 281].

Rapid Tranquillisation

Rapid tranquillisation is the use of intramuscular or intravenous medication to sedate a patient urgently if oral medication is not effective or cannot be administered; for further discussion, see Chapter 6.

Seclusion

The MHA Code of Practice defines seclusion as 'the supervised confinement and isolation of a patient, away from other patients, in an area from which the patient is prevented from leaving, where it is of immediate necessity for the purpose of the containment of severe behavioural disturbance which is likely to cause harm to others' [23, p. 300]. Seclusion should always be used as a last resort (and for the shortest time possible) when managing violence, and is to be used only when all other interventions have failed. Prior to placing a patient in seclusion, the multidisciplinary team must attempt de-escalation techniques to manage risk. Seclusion should never be used as a form of punishment or to manage self-harming behaviour. Once seclusion has been instigated, the secluded patient must be within eyesight at all times. The need for ongoing seclusion must be assessed through nursing reviews at least once every two hours. It is recommended that a medical seclusion review is carried out by the patient's RC and ward manager at least once every 24 hours, and further medical reviews at least twice every 24 hours. Once the risk has reduced, following a period of calm, the aim should be to terminate seclusion as soon as possible.

The Extra Care Area

The use of an *extra care area* in which a single patient may receive intensive nursing intervention was advocated in the 2002 Mental Health Policy Implementation Guide as an alternative to seclusion [34].

The principles of the extra care area appear to fulfil much of the function of seclusion by removing a patient who is liable to assault others from the general ward population. It also has the advantage of keeping staff in contact with the patient through the aggressive episode so that they can utilise de-escalation skills. The use of graded observation in the extra care area has been demonstrated to show that seclusion can be completely replaced. However, the extra care area method is not without problems when compared with seclusion. An unintended consequence is that patients receive positive reinforcement of their disturbed behaviour as a result of the special attention they receive from prolonged use of the extra care area. The extra care area can also be difficult for staffing in terms of the numbers needed and the danger of creating 'a ward within a ward'.

In some circumstances, the use of an extra care area may meet the requirements for monitoring of seclusion, and the NAPICU have produced a helpful position statement covering the monitoring, regulation and recording of the extra care area, seclusion and long-term segregation [47].

Leave as a Therapeutic Intervention

Patients under the MHA can be granted leave by their RC. The duration and type of leave should be decided following a consultation between the RC, the ward MDT and the patient.

The therapeutic use of escorted or unescorted leave is a well-accepted strategy for reducing tension and potential escalation towards violence on a ward. Leave should be supported by adequate staffing, risk management and standard operating procedures. Dix et al. [48] suggest a number of procedural steps and measures to facilitate such an approach:

- Prior to commencing escorted leave, staff should check that they have access to an agreed method of communication, such as a two-way radio or mobile telephone. The escorting staff should check the device is working before departure and ensure the shift co-ordinator is aware of their expected time of return.
- If there is a deviation from the stated plan or expected duration of leave, the escort will inform the unit.

Standard operational policy should also recommend the action to take if the service user becomes disturbed or attempts to leave the escort. This includes:

- Attempting verbal negotiation.
- Failing this, contacting the unit and assessing the appropriateness of physical intervention.
- Only attempting physical intervention if safe to do so.
- If physical intervention is inappropriate, following the service user at a safe distance, and contacting the other staff by radio with situation reports at 5-minute intervals.

Nurses must keep accurate records of leave taken by a patient, the destination of their leave and any problems faced during the leave period. Nurses have the right to refuse authorised leave to a patient if the patients mental state deteriorates or the patient is at risk of harming themselves or others.

During the COVID-19 pandemic leave from the ward was in line with government advice and national guidelines. During escorted or unescorted leave, social distancing had to be maintained, the destination of leave agreed beforehand and areas to avoid (e.g crowded places) discussed with the patient. Ethics committees were tasked with considering any restrictive interventions for managing COVID-19 infection risks, including restriction of leave [49].

Therapeutic Activities

Therapeutic activities in inpatient wards play an essential role in reducing acute behavioural disturbances in inpatient settings. Lack of structured activities in psychiatric units identified by the National Audit of Violence 2003–5 found that the resulting boredom increased aggression and violent incidents in the ward and assaults rose during the evenings and weekends (when there are fewer activities available and patients are 'stuck' on wards) [50]. The 2006–7 audit also identified boredom and lack of activities to be an issue: 26% of wards did not have an activity room, 53% of patients thought that there were not enough therapies, 48% thought that there were not enough activities during the day and two thirds did not think there were enough activities available in the evenings and at weekends [1].

NICE defines *meaningful activity* as including any physical, social and leisure activities that are tailored to the person's needs and preferences. Examples range from activities of daily living (such as dressing, eating and washing) to leisure activities (such as reading, gardening, arts and crafts, conversation and singing). NICE quality standard (QS) 14, quality statement 8 discusses meaningful activity [51]:

Staying in hospital for mental health care can be a difficult and worrying experience for some people. Giving people the opportunity to do meaningful activities can help provide a structure to their day and reduce stress, frustration and boredom. It can also help to increase their social interactions, relieve anxiety and improve wellbeing. Being engaged in meaningful activities can help to foster an atmosphere of hope and optimism, which can enhance recovery. Activities can help maximise therapeutic benefits and prevent a ward from being seen as a place of containment.

When suffering an acute mental health crisis, an individual's ability to participate in meaningful activities is diminished; therapeutic activities can help patients maintain and develop the skills required for daily living. Such activities assist in the recovery process, enable distraction from distressing symptoms and help maintain/improve functional skills. Therapeutic activities also give patients the autonomy to choose activities they enjoy and enable engagement with staff and other patients, whilst improving the sense of self-worth and providing a sense of empowerment.

Therapeutic activities within a ward are facilitated by the multidisciplinary team (doctors, nurses, health care assistants, occupational therapists, activity coordinators, physical fitness instructors, volunteers, etc.) and are facilitated within the ward environment, hospital grounds or community.

Individuals suffering from severe mental illness have a significantly reduced life expectancy of 15–20 years, largely due to physical health issues, and thus an inpatient physical exercise programme is of obvious benefit. The National Audit of Violence 2006-7 found that the opportunity to take daily exercise was poor in acute wards and PICUs (49% and 53%, respectively), but was better in forensic and rehabilitation wards (75% and 89%, respectively) [1]. The report noted an 'overwhelming number of requests for access to a gym, organised exercise and walks' (p. 39). The Mental Health Foundation has developed a useful pocket guide to show the positive impact that physical activity can have on mental well-being [52].

At Nile Ward PICU, St Charles Hospital, London, a range of therapeutic activities and a structured physical health programme has reduced violent incidents in the ward by 43% over the course of six months [53].

The Role of Psychology in Reducing Violence

A common complaint from patients, and from staff and carers, is that treatment is focused on medication and the medical model of care as opposed to offering psychosocial interventions, including 'talking therapies'.

The Mental Health Task Force advocated that NHS trusts in England should deliver timely, evidence-based psychological therapies on acute mental health wards. In response, psychologists have proposed how they might support implementation of the NHS's long-term plan pertaining to inpatient services [54].

- Providing wider access to psychological interventions and psychologically informed care during inpatient admission;
- Taking up roles as responsible clinicians to support effective and safe multidisciplinary management of care under the MHA;
- Supporting other professions to deliver trauma-informed care to reduce the potentially traumatising or re-traumatising aspects of inpatient care;
- Contributing to MDT working to support recovery and relapse prevention approaches as part of a personalised approach to case management.

Talk, Understand, Listen for In-Patient Settings (TULIPS) is a research project funded by NICE, with the overall aim of increasing access to psychological therapy on mental health inpatient wards. The pilot study was too small to draw any firm conclusions, but there is evidence to suggest that the level of serious incidents decreased on wards that participated in the scheme. The project proposes that all acute mental health wards should have access to a dedicated ward-based psychologist. The project is ongoing [55, 56].

Psychologists can undoubtedly play an important role in reducing the risk of violence in an inpatient ward and their presence on acute wards is to be welcomed. Patients suffering chronic difficulties in managing and expressing feelings can become aggressive and violent; psychologists can help these patients identify psychological factors and help support and manage their frustrations in a safe, contained manner. Psychological techniques enable patients to manage angry feelings, improve coping skills and develop resilience. Psychologists can also play an important role in providing staff support, such as facilitating formulations to understand patient attitudes and behaviours using a psychological framework (examples include the Reinforce Appropriate, Implode Disruptive 'RAID' programme and trauma-focused case formulations) [57]. Further details on psychological management are given in Chapter 7.

Post-Incident Management

The NICE guidelines support post-incident debriefing and formal review [4]. Every serious incident in a ward must be followed up with a formal debrief facilitated by a manager or senior nurse. The purpose of the debrief is to support staff, patients and carers to address practical and emotional issues around the incident. Staff, patients and/or carers who were directly involved, or witnessed the incident, should all be involved in debriefs. The team can review what went well during the incident, what did not work well, and what action is required to avoid/minimise a similar incident occurring in the future. Post incident management is discussed further in chapter 5.

Criminal Proceedings Against the Perpetrator

Following an assault from a patient, despite a zero-tolerance policy in operation in NHS Trusts, it can be difficult for staff members to decide whether they wish to report the perpetrator to the police. Furthermore, unless the violent act is particularly serious, police officers visiting mental health inpatient units are often reluctant to pursue charges against 'vulnerable' patients with mental health problems; this is one reason to establish robust links with local police.

Assaults may be linked to an individual's condition and some may have little or no insight into their actions or the consequences thereof. However, some assaults may be with intent, and each incident and the appropriateness of sanctions should be investigated on a case-by-case basis.

Factors that influence a staff member's decision to support or encourage police and the CPS to bring charges against a patient include the patient's mental state at the time of the incident, the severity of harm caused, the perceived effect on a patient's mental state if charged and the clinical need for forensic diversion, if this is in the patient's best interests.

COVID-19: Special Considerations

Various professional bodies, including the RCPsych, Royal College of Nursing and NAPICU, provide guidance on COVID-19 and inpatient services [58, 59, 49]. All inpatient mental health units are required to have a protocol in place to minimise the risk of COVID-19 infections, and we briefly describe practice that was in place at the height of the pandemic.

On admission, patients should have a COVID-19 swab test and a comprehensive enquiry should be conducted regarding COVID-19 symptoms. All new patients awaiting COVID-19 swab results (and inpatients showing signs of COVID-19 infection) should be maintained in an isolated ward area consistent with local procedures. Vitals should be monitored daily and patients should have weekly COVID-19 testing. Whilst in isolation, ward staff should make paraphernalia available to patients (e.g. books, puzzles, digital tablets) to reduce isolation and to avoid frustration which may lead to behavioural disturbance. Individual care plans for patients in isolation should be created to maintain cooperation and reduce the need for physical intervention (e.g. restraint) in the event of acutely disturbed behaviour.

In some circumstances, patients that are positive for COVID-19 may refuse to adhere to isolation rules and thereby increase the risk of infection to others. Such patients will require extended segregation in extra care areas, seclusion rooms and other facilities to manage acute behavioural disturbance. Patients may be segregated in bedrooms and in locked-off ward areas if local procedures allow. The need for segregation should be reviewed regularly and should be discontinued in favour of less restrictive isolation methods as soon as the risk has subsided.

If a patient with suspected or diagnosed COVID-19 is acutely disturbed, medication for pre-RT/RT can be used cautiously according to local guidance (if there are no physical health contraindications). As COVID-19 may cause respiratory compromise, psychotropic medications such as benzodiazepines should be used with caution due to the risk of respiratory depression (lorazepam is the preferred benzodiazepine due to its short half-life in such circumstances). Inhaled loxapine is contraindicated in patients with acute respiratory distress or with active airways disease and should be avoided in patients with suspected or confirmed COVID-19 [49].

When restraint is necessary to manage acute behavioural disturbance, staff must wear appropriate personal protective equipment to minimise the risk of infection, which may include face masks, eye/spit guards, aprons (may pose a slip hazard), scrubs, gloves and disposable overalls.

The pandemic was a stressful time for patients, carers and staff. There was a reduction in bed availability with limited community support delivered through remote contact. This may have led to an increase in admissions under the MHA [60]. Extra restrictions were required (e.g. regarding leave, visitors and activities) which are likely to have impacted negatively on patients. The CQC consider that units that managed well during the pandemic focused on the least restrictive principle and meaningfully involved patients and carers in co-producing care plans. The CQC have called for the 'relaxed rules around use of personal technology such as mobile phones' to continue post-pandemic and for services to 'prioritise linked issues such as WIFI connectivity in future estates development' [60].

Conclusion

Violence and aggression commonly occur in inpatient psychiatric units and have a negative impact on patient and carer experience. Providers and clinicians should remain up to date with best-practice evidence-based guidance on the PMVA. Although violence and aggression cannot always be avoided in inpatient settings, this chapter has outlined how to manage violence when it does occur and also how to prevent aggression or a minor violent incident escalating to a severe one.

Furthermore, the chapter encourages organisations to be aware of models of inpatient care that are effective in reducing incidents of violence and consider participation in accredited quality initiatives aimed at delivering high-quality, patient-centred clinical care.

The majority of patients in acute psychiatric inpatient units are detained in hospital against their wishes and are often frightened and distressed. It is of paramount importance that the ward environment is a therapeutic one in which patients, staff and carers feel supported, safe and protected from harm. Patients should be involved in all decisions about their care and treatment, and care and risk management plans should be co-produced. Coercive measures should be avoided if possible, and patients should be made aware that during any restrictive intervention their human rights will be respected and the least restrictive intervention will be used. The patient voice should be empowered, actively listened to and acted upon whenever it is appropriate to do so. Therapeutic wards require good design and sufficient resources, adequate numbers of experienced and appropriately trained empathic staff and meaningful activities for patients to engage in.

Appendix

Table 8.3 Royal College of Psychiatry Areas of Practice for Which Standards have been set for Inpatient Psychiatric Wards

1. Access	12. Patient involvement
2. First 12 hours	13. Carer engagement and support
3. Completing the admission process	14. Compassion, dignity and respect
4. Reviews and care planning	15. Providing information to patients and carers
5. Leave from the ward/unit	16. Patient confidentiality
6. Care and treatment	17. Ward/unit environment
6.1 Therapies and activities	18. Leadership, team-working and culture
6.2 Medication	19. Staffing levels
7. Physical healthcare	20. Staff recruitment, induction and supervision
8. Risk and safeguarding	21. Staff well-being
9. Discharge planning and transfer of care	22. Staff training and development
10. Interface with other services	23. Clinical outcome measurement
11. Capacity and consent	24. The ward/unit learns from feedback, complaints and incidents

The standards are available from www.rcpsych.ac.uk/docs/default-source/improving-care/ccqi/ccqi-resources/rcpsych_standards_in_2019_lr.pdf?sfvrsn=edd5f8d5_2

References

1. Royal College of Psychiatrists. Healthcare Commission National Audit of Violence 2006–7 Final Report – Working Age Adult Services. www.dynamis.training/wp-content/uploads/violence-audit-report.pdf [Accessed 28.4.2022].

2. Royal College of Psychiatrists. Standards for Inpatient Mental Health Services. Third edition. [online 2019]. www.rcpsych.ac.uk/docs/default-source/improving-care/ccqi/ccqi-resources/rcpsych_standards_in_2019_lr.pdf?sfvrsn=edd5f8d5_2 [Accessed 25.4.2022].

3. Care Quality Commission. Key lines of enquiry for healthcare services. 2020. www.cqc.org.uk/guidance-providers/healthcare/key-lines-enquiry-healthcare-services [Accessed 26.4.2022].

4. National Institute of Clinical Excellence. Violence and aggression: short-term management in mental health, health and community settings. NICE guideline NG10 28 May 2015. www.nice.org.uk/guidance/ng10/resources/violence-and-aggression-shortterm-management-in-mental-health-health-and-community-settings-pdf-1837264712389 [Accessed 26.4.2022].

5. National Association of Psychiatric Inpatient Units (NAPICU). National Minimal Standards for Psychiatric Intensive Care in General Adult Services. September 2014. https://napicu.org.uk/publications/national-minimum-standards/ [Accessed 26.4.2022].

6. Safe Wards. www.safewards.net/ [Accessed 26.4.2022].

7. Star Wards. 2004. www.starwards.org.uk/ [Accessed 26.4.2022].

8. The Strategy Unit. Midlands and Lancashire Commissioning Support Unit. November 2019 [online]. www.strategyunitwm.nhs.uk/publications/exploring-mental-health-inpatient-capacity [Accessed 14.4.2022].

9. Royal College of Psychiatrists. Quality Networks and Accreditation. www.rcpsych.ac.uk/improving-care/ccqi/quality-networks-accreditation [Accessed 26.4.2022].

10. O'Sullivan, O. P., Chang, N. H., Njovana, D., Baker, P. and Shah, A. Quality improvement in forensic mental health: The East London forensic violence reduction collaborative. BMJ Open Quality 2020 Sep;9(3):e000803. https://doi.org/10.1136/bmjoq-2019-000803. PMID: 32928782; PMCID: PMC7488843.

11. NHS England. Implementing the Five Year Forward View for Mental Health. www.england.nhs.uk/wp-content/uploads/2016/07/fyfv-mh.pdf [Accessed 26.4.2022]

12. National Institute of Clinical Excellence. Violence and aggression: Service user experience in adult mental health services. Quality standard [QS14] Published: 13 December 2011. Last updated: 31 July 2019. www.nice.org.uk/guidance/qs14 [Accessed 26.4.2022].

13. Beer, M. D., Pereira, S. M. and Paton, C. Psychiatric Intensive Care. 2nd ed. Cambridge, England: Cambridge University Pres, 2008.

14. Department of Health. Health Building Note 03-01: Adult acute mental health units. 2013. https://assets.publishing.service.gov.uk/government/uploads/system/uploads/attachment_data/file/147864/HBN_03-01_Final.pdf [Accessed 26.4.2022].

15. National Association of Psychiatric Inpatient Units (NAPICU). Design Guidance for Psychiatric Intensive Care Units. 2017. https://napicu.org.uk/wp-content/uploads/2017/05/Design-Guidance-for-Psychiatric-Intensive-Care-Units-2017.pdf [Accessed 26.4.2022].

16. NIDUS UK. Nidotherapy. Better Mental Health through Environmental Change. https://nidotherapy.com [Accessed 26.4.2022].

17. Carmel, H. and Hunter, M. Psychiatrists injured by patient attack. Bulletin of the American Academy of Psychiatry and the Law 1991;19(3):309–16. PMID: 1777692.

18. James, D. V., Fineberg, N. A., Shah, A. K. and Priest, R. G. An increase in violence on an acute psychiatric ward: A study of associated factors. *British Journal of Psychiatry* 1990 Jun;156:846–52. https://doi .org/10.1192/bjp.156.6.846. PMID: 2207515.

19. NHS England. Mental Health Staffing Framework. www.england.nhs.uk/6cs/wp-content/uploads/sites/25/2015/06/mh-staffing-v4.pdf [Accessed 26.4.2022].

20. The Kings Fund and Gilburt, H. Securing money to improve mental health care … but no staff to spend it on. October 2019. www.kingsfund.org.uk/blog/2019/10/men tal-health-staff-shortage [Accessed 26.4.2022].

21. Care Quality Commission. Brief guide: staffing levels on mental health wards. htt ps://view.officeapps.live.com/op/view.aspx ?src=https%3A%2F%2Fwww.cqc.org.uk% 2Fsites%2Fdefault%2Ffiles%2FBrief_Guid e_Staffing_levels_on_mental_health_ward s_v4.odt&wdOrigin=BROWSELINK [Accessed 26.4.2022].

22. RCPsych. Your guide to relational security. See Think Act. 2nd ed. [online 2015] www .rcpsych.ac.uk/docs/default-source/improv ing-care/ccqi/quality-networks/secure-forensic/forensic-see-think-act-qnfmhs/st a_hndbk_2nded_web.pdf?sfvrsn=90e1f c26_4 [Accessed 25.04.2022].

23. Department of Health and Social Care. Statutory guidance. Code of Practice: Mental Health Act 1983. [online] Published 2015. Last updated 2017. www .gov.uk/government/publications/code-of-practice-mental-health-act-1983 [Accessed 26.4.2022].

24. Weaver, T., Madden, P., Charles, V. et al. Comorbidity of substance misuse and mental illness in community mental health and substance misuse services. *British Journal of Psychiatry* 2003 Oct;183:304–13. https://doi.org/10.1192/bjp.183.4.304. PMID: 14519608.

25. Department of Health. Dual diagnosis in mental health inpatient and day hospital settings. Guidance on the assessment and management of patients in mental health inpatient and day hospital settings who

have mental ill-health and substance use problems. October 2006. www .drugsandalcohol.ie/17765/1/DOH_Dual_ diagnosis_in_mental_health_inpatien t_and_day_settings.pdf [Accessed 26.4.2022].

26. DrugWise. Promoting Evidence based information on drugs, alcohol and tobacco. www.drugwise.org.uk/new-psychoactive-substances/ [Accessed 26.4.2022].

27. Shafi, A., Gallagher, P., Stewart, N., Martinotti, G. and Corazza, O. The risk of violence associated with novel psychoactive substance misuse in patients presenting to acute mental health services. *Human Psychopharmacology* 2017 May;32(3). https:// doi.org/10.1002/hup.2606. Epub 2017 Jun 19. PMID: 28631373.

28. Smith, M. Barnet, Enfield and Haringey Mental Health Trust to use sniffer dogs in St. Ann's Hospital wards to clamp down on drug use. Tottenham and Wood Green Independent, December 2015. www.thetottenhaminde pendent.co.uk/news/14130697.barnet-enfield-and-haringey-mental-health-trust -to-use-sniffer-dogs-in-st-anns-hospital-wards-to-clamp-down-on-drug-use/ [Accessed 26.4.2022].

29. Nash, M. Who let the dogs in? The use of drug sniffer dogs in mental health settings. *Journal of Psychiatric and Mental Health Nursing* 2005 Dec;12(6):745–9. https://doi .org/10.1111/j.1365-2850.2005.00918.x. PMID: 16336601.

30. Institute of Clinical Excellence. Coexisting severe mental illness and substance misuse: community health and social care services. NICE guideline [NG58]. 30 November 2016. www.nice.org.uk/guidance/NG58 [Accessed 26.4.2022].

31. Department of Health. Health Policy Implementation Guide. Dual Diagnosis Good Practice Guide. www .dualdiagnosis.co.uk/uploads/documents/ originals/Dual_Diagnosis_Good_Practic e_Policy_Implementation_Guide.PDF [Accessed 26.4.2022].

32. Care Quality Commission. Sexual safety on mental health wards. 2017. Last Updated 2018. www.cqc.org.uk/publica

tions/major-report/sexual-safety-mental-health-wards [Accessed 26.4.2022].

33. National Collaborating Centre for Mental Health. Sexual Safety Collaborative. Standards and guidance to improve sexual safety on mental health and learning disabilities inpatient pathways. London: National Collaborating Centre for Mental Health; 2020. www.rcpsych.ac.uk/docs/default-source/improving-care/nccmh/sexual-safety-collaborative/sexual-safety-collaborative--standards-and-guidance.pdf?sfvrsn=1eb6a5b7_2 [Accessed 26.4.2022].

34. Department of Health. Mental health policy implementation guide: National minimum standards for general adult services in psychiatric intensive care units (PICU) and low secure environments. 2002. https://napicu.org.uk/wp-content/uploads/2013/04/2002-NMS.pdf [Accessed 26.4.2022].

35. NAPICU. Joint BAP NAPICU evidence-based consensus guidelines for the clinical management of acute disturbance: De-escalation and rapid tranquillisation. 2018. https://napicu.org.uk/publications/joint-bap-napicu-evidence-based-consensus-guidelines-for-the-clinical-management-of-acute-disturbance-de-escalation-and-rapid-tranquillisation/ [Accessed 26.4.2022].

36. RCPsych. Rethinking risk to others in mental health services. College Report (CR201). [online 2017]. www.rcpsych.ac.uk/docs/default-source/improving-care/better-mh-policy/college-reports/college-report-cr201.pdf?sfvrsn=2b83d227_4 [Accessed 18.4.2022].

37. Bowers, L. and Park, A. Special observation in the care of psychiatric inpatients: A literature review. *Issues in Mental Health Nursing* 2001 Dec;22(8):769–86. https://doi.org/10.1080/01612840152713018. PMID: 11881179.

38. Bowers, L., Simpson, A. and Alexander, J. Patient-staff conflict: results of a survey on acute psychiatric wards. *Social Psychiatry and Psychiatric Epidemiology*. 2003 Jul;38(7):402–8. https://doi.org/10.1007/s00127-003-0648-x. PMID: 12861448.

39. Flood, C., Bowers, L. and Parkin, D. Estimating the costs of conflict and containment on adult acute inpatient psychiatric wards. *Nursing Economics* 2008 Sep-Oct;26(5):325–330, 324. PMID: 18979699.

40. Lambert, K., Chu, S., Duffy, C. et al. The prevalence of constant supportive observations in high, medium and low secure services. *BJPsych Bulletin* 2018 Apr;42(2):54–58. https://doi.org/10.1192/bjb.2017.14. Epub 2018 Feb 6. PMID: 29405902; PMCID: PMC6001855.

41. NHS. The Atlas of Shared Learning. Reducing 'enhanced observations' on a mental health ward. [online]. 2019. www.england.nhs.uk/atlas_case_study/reducing-enhanced-observations-on-a-mental-health-ward/ [Accessed 26.4.2022]

42. Cardell, R. and Pitula, C. R. Suicidal inpatients' perceptions of therapeutic and nontherapeutic aspects of constant observation. *Psychiatric Services* 1999 Aug;50(8):1066–70. https://doi.org/10.1176/ps.50.8.1066. PMID: 10445656.

43. Reen, G. K., Bailey, J., Maughan, D. L. and Vincent, C. Systematic review of interventions to improve constant observation on adult inpatient psychiatric wards. *International Journal of Mental Health Nursing* 2020 Jun;29(3):372–86. https://doi.org/10.1111/inm.12696. Epub 2020 Feb 12. PMID: 32048785.

44. Department of Health. Positive and Proactive Care: Reducing the need for restrictive interventions. [online] 2014. https://assets.publishing.service.gov.uk/government/uploads/system/uploads/attachment_data/file/300293/JRA_DoH_Guidance_on_RP_web_accessible.pdf [Accessed 26.4.2022].

45. Stevenson, S. Heading off violence with verbal de-escalation. *Journal of Psychosocial Nursing and Mental Health Services* 1991 Sep;29(9):6–10. PMID: 1941731.

46. Care Quality Commission. Brief guide: Restraint (physical and mechanical). [online]. www.cqc.org.uk/sites/default/files/20180322_900803_briefguide-restraint_physical_mechanical_v1.pdf [Accessed 26.4.2022].

47. NAPICU. NAPICU position on the monitoring, regulation and recording of the extra care area, seclusion and long-term segregation use in the context of the Mental Health Act 1983: Code of Practice (2015). 2016. https://napicu.org.uk/wp-content/uploads/2016/10/NAPICU-Seclusion-Position-Statement.pdf [Accessed 26.4.2022].

48. Dix, R., Betteridge, C. and Page, M. (2008) Seclusion: Past, present and future. In Psychiatric Intensive Care, 2nd ed., ed. D. Beer, S. M. Pereira and C. Paton. Cambridge: Cambridge University Press, pp. 106–23.

49. National Association of Psychiatric Intensive Care (NAPICU). Managing acute disturbance in the context of COVID-19 [online]. Updated December 2020. https://napicu.org.uk/wp-content/uploads/2020/12/NAPICU-Guidance_rev5_15_Dec.pdf [Accessed 26.4.2022].

50. Royal College of Psychiatrists. The National Audit of violence (2003 – 2005). Final Report. [online]. 2005. www.wales.nhs.uk/documents/FinalReport-violence.pdf [Accessed 26.4.2022].

51. NICE. Service user experience in adult mental health services. Quality standard [QS14]. Quality statement 8: Inpatient meaningful activities. Published: 13 December 2011. Updated July 2019. [online]. www.nice.org.uk/guidance/qs14/chapter/Quality-statement-8-Inpatient-meaningful-activities [Accessed 26.4.2022].

52. Mental Health Foundation. How to look after your mental health using exercise. [online]. www.mentalhealth.org.uk/publications/how-to-using-exercise [Accessed 26.4.2022].

53. Rahman, M., Taylor, C., Abdullahi, R. et al. Nile Ward PICU violence reduction quality improvement project. Published online by Cambridge University Press, 18 June 2021. www.cambridge.org/core/journals/bjpsych-open/article/nile-ward-picu-violence-reduction-quality-improvement-project/18A86956B08923300E523FA803F2C0FD [Accessed 26.4.2022].

54. Psychological Professions Network England. Implementing the NHS Long Term Plan: Maximising the Impact of the Psychological Professions. [online] 2019. www.nwppn.nhs.uk/attachments/article/2578/PPN_Long_Term_Plan_Online_Single_compressed.pdf# [Accessed 26.4.2022].

55. The University of Manchester. Talk, Understand, Listen for In-Patient Settings (TULIPS). [online] https://sites.manchester.ac.uk/tulips/ [Accessed 26.4.2022].

56. Berry, K. Acute inpatient wards: Time to implement psychological therapies. University of Manchester: blog [online]. June 2021. https://blog.policy.manchester.ac.uk/posts/2021/06/acute-inpatient-wards-time-to-implement-psychological-therapies/ [Accessed 26.4.2022].

57. The Association of Psychological Therapies. What does RAID® stand for in mental health? [online]. www.apt.ac/what-does-raid-stand-for-in-mental-health.html [Accessed 26.4.2022].

58. Royal College of Psychiatrists. COVID-19: Guidance for clinicians. www.rcpsych.ac.uk/about-us/responding-to-covid-19/responding-to-covid-19-guidance-for-clinicians [Accessed 6.10.2022].

59. Royal College of Nursing. COVID-19 guidance on mental health care delivery. [online]. Updated June 2021. www.rcn.org.uk/clinical-topics/mental-health/professional-guidance/covid-19-guidance-on-mental-healthcare-delivery [Accessed 21.5.2022].

60. Care Quality Commission. CQC finds mental health inpatient services coped well with coronavirus (COVID-19) but there will have been 'significant unmet need' during lockdown. [online 2020]. Available at: www.cqc.org.uk/news/releases/cqc-finds-mental-health-inpatient-services-coped-well-coronavirus-covid-19-there-will [Accessed 6.10.2022].

Introduction to Section 3

Section 3: Violence in Different Settings

Because violence can manifest anywhere, we all need to be prepared for its impact. The following four chapters describe the main settings outside standard psychiatric inpatient wards where violence is manifest in different ways and how the different environmental circumstances influence management.

In the community, potential victims are much less protected and, as far as is possible, de-escalation (defusion) of violence becomes the primary intervention.

The problem of violence in medical settings has sadly come to the fore in recent years because of an increase in episodes, and its management and prevention need to be developed further. Emergency departments are in the front line here, and paramedics and other ambulance staff are also vulnerable to assault. It is to be expected that when common policies of management are adopted, hospital settings will gain greatly.

The new chapter on forensic psychiatry and adult inpatient secure settings (Chapter 11) offers readers an insight into the historical context behind the existence and development of forensic psychiatric services in England and Wales. Key pieces of legislation are outlined, as is a description of how forensic services are currently configured.

Violence in prisons is unfortunately endemic and illustrates how a combination of overcrowding, boredom and bullying can be a toxic mix (Chapter 12). Until the prison population can be reduced, hope for improvement in this area is limited.

Management of the Risk of Violence in the Community

Dominic Dougall, Sue McDonnell and Masum Khwaja

Introduction

There is broad consensus that public health responses are effective in reducing violence in the general population [1]. Whilst public health measures and addressing social determinants are undoubtedly relevant in reducing violence associated with mental illness, this chapter focuses more on the response of community mental health services, including the modification of clinical risk factors predisposing to violence. Service models that may help promote better risk management are also described, as is the identification and management of domestic violence. Finally, safe working practices, such as lone working, are considered.

Since the 1950s there has been a substantial shift from long-term institutional mental health care to community-based services. Following the closure of large institutions, there has been a further 70% reduction in mental health beds in the United Kingdom since the late 1980s [2]. The introduction of crisis and other specialist community-based teams means people with greater severity of illness and complexity are being treated in the community; one consequence of this is that community mental health teams and other services are more likely to come across violent behaviour in the community.

The National Institute for Health and Care Excellence (NICE) published guidance in 2015 on short-term management of violence and aggression in community settings [3], which recommended that community staff are trained in predicting and de-escalating violence and conducting risk assessments, and that their organisations have policies on both the management of violence and aggression and on lone working. Health and Safety Executive (HSE) guidance reflects that of NICE, in emphasising that violence or aggression in health and social care settings should not be considered as typical, and recommends that employers and employees work collaboratively to prevent or reduce aggressive behaviour [4]. The HSE identifies a range of activities that may place an employee at greater risk: for example, working alone and outside of normal hours, providing or withholding a service and exercising authority, and advises employers to complete risk assessments and implement risk control measures.

The criminal justice system plays an important role in addressing violence, although this is not covered in detail in this chapter (see Chapter 17). Guidance on whether to prosecute suspects with mental illness after a violent episode necessarily has to take into account the circumstances, motivation and mental state of the patient. Of most relevance to the management of violence is public interest. The Code for Crown Prosecutors states that when deciding to prosecute, consideration be given to whether the suspect was affected by mental ill health at the time of the offence, as well as the severity of the offence, likelihood of reoffending and the need to safeguard the public [5]. Multi-agency public protection arrangements (MAPPA) are legislated in the Criminal Justice Act 2003 for England and

Wales [6]. The purpose of these arrangements is to protect the public from serious harm by violent offenders. The essence of MAPPA is that it requires criminal justice and other agencies, such as health and social care, to work together [7]. Collaborative, cross-agency working is a common thread in effective risk management that this chapter seeks to highlight.

Risk Factors for Violence in People With Mental Illness

Increased risk of violence is associated with most mental disorders, although for most conditions violence remains a relatively rare occurrence and the majority of those with mental illness are not violent [8]. The misperception that people with mental illness are inherently dangerous is skewed through reporting in the media, together with the wider potential for stigma [9, 10]. In fact, a person with a mental illness is more likely to be a victim of homicide than the general population [11].

Studies have consistently identified substance misuse and the diagnoses of schizophrenia and/or personality disorder as significant risk factors for violence [8]. The seminal 1990 Epidemiologic Catchment Area survey found that young males of low socio-economic status were more likely to report violent behaviour, and half had one or more mental disorders [12]. Those with drug or alcohol disorders were twice as likely to report violence compared to people with a diagnosis of schizophrenia.

Major mental illness in the absence of other factors does not strongly predict future violence unless there has been past violence, a history of physical abuse, juvenile detention, or parental forensic history [13]. The presence of a comorbid personality disorder in those with an established psychotic illness is a significant and independent predictor of violence [14].

Schizophrenia

In addition to treating comorbid substance misuse and addressing social risk factors, there is a clear role for effective antipsychotic treatment in reducing the risk of violence in schizophrenia [15]. Long-acting injectable antipsychotics help improve adherence and, consequently, effectiveness of treatment. Clozapine, primarily indicated for treatment-resistant schizophrenia, has been shown to have a direct effect on impulsive violence whilst also helping to modify other risk factors such as substance misuse.

Personality Disorder

Underlying the importance of effective treatment of personality disorders is the associated increased risk of violence; those with borderline personality disorder are 3.5 times more likely to be violent compared to people without a personality disorder. This increases to 10 times for those with dissocial personality, and 20 times for those with both borderline and dissocial personality disorder [16]. There is an identified need to improve services involved in treating people with personality disorder – services that predominantly provide treatment in the community. Services need to be able to diagnose and provide effective treatment for people with a diagnosis of personality disorder, and this includes the majority who do not have borderline pathology and generally do not seek treatment [17]. To achieve this, a tiered approach to care is recommended, with services able to provide robust diagnosis, formulation and relational continuity [16]. The focus on complex emotional needs within transformation of community services as part of the NHS Long-Term Plan, and the adoption of structured community treatment, is hoped to provide a less fragmented approach to care and support those with a personality disorder to access treatment [18].

Substance Misuse

The shift to third-sector organisations rather than NHS mental health services delivering substance misuse services has added to the challenge of ensuring the needs of service users with a dual diagnosis are effectively met. Early identification and intervention may help to improve outcomes. Responsibility for the identification of substance misuse falls on all services, be they in primary or secondary health care, social care or housing providers, amongst others. Comprehensive assessment and treatment help to reduce criminal justice contact and potentially devastating outcomes such as homelessness. Services should not exclude someone due to the presence of substance use or major mental illness. Care coordination is recognised to help with engagement and prioritisation of treatment, whilst assertive follow-up after missed appointments also supports engagement [19].

Substance misuse is known to increase the risk of intimate partner violence, increasing the risk of both perpetration and being a victim; this is discussed later in this chapter [20].

Modification and Management of Clinical Risk in the Community

Effective management of risk in the community relies on services that are sufficiently well resourced to be able to respond to the needs of individuals and populations, but also requires staff to have sufficient expertise, training and support to be able to be able to effectively respond to the needs of individuals and their populations. A particular challenge for a service is how to engage an individual who has multiple risk factors, such as personality disorder, comorbid substance misuse and poor housing – essentially, those who are at most risk of falling between gaps in services. An overview of service models which considers this issue is provided in the next section of this chapter. Approaches to risk management of violence should seek to incorporate risk assessment and – arguably, more importantly – focus on addressing and modifying identified risk factors, such as substance misuse, effective management of personality disorders and schizophrenia, as well as addressing social risk factors such as poor housing and lack of social support [21].

Risk Assessment

Risk assessment and management forms one of the cornerstones of what mental health services do. However, the limitations of clinical judgement and structured risk assessment for predicting violence needs to be acknowledged (see also Chapter 4), which is particularly salient for rarer and therefore harder to predict offences such as homicide [22]. There is an inherent challenge in separating those who have identified risk factors for violence and go on to commit a violent act and those who have risk factors for violence but do not become violent. This risk of 'false positives' necessitates a proportionate response by services. Expectations around regular updates to care plans and risk assessments are most clearly defined within the Care Programme Approach (CPA) for those service users with complex needs, risks and multi-agency involvement [23]. Digital patient records have allowed the creation of accessible 'live' risk assessment documents which, together with General Data Protection Regulations (GDPR), allow theoretical greater ease of information sharing.

Multidisciplinary Team Working and Service Models

Until the end of the 1950s, in the United Kingdom a person requiring mental health care would invariably be referred by a general practitioner (GP) to a hospital-based psychiatrist, and consequently receive treatment in an inpatient setting. In the 1960s and 1970s, a GP would have had the option of referring to a psychiatrist-led outpatient clinic. From the early 1980s, multidisciplinary community teams were introduced. The community team model was solidified by the Department of Health introducing the Care Programme Approach in 1990 [24], and in 1999 the Department of Health National Service Framework specified services with specialist teams, such as early intervention and assertive outreach teams.

Community mental health services in the United Kingdom now typically range from more general community mental health teams delivering a wide range of care, to home-treatment teams providing intensive community treatment as an alternative to hospital. Specialist teams may include early intervention in psychosis, forensic community, personality disorder and homeless outreach services, amongst others. Broadly consistent across these teams is the role of the consultant psychiatrist as clinical lead, working alongside health and social care practitioners. The clinical lead, together with the multidisciplinary team, is responsible for the delivery of clinically effective, safe and patient-centred care.

The Department of Health has identified best practice for managing risk in teams, which includes [25]:

- The culture and support systems within the clinical team and wider organisation. A team that fosters openness and transparency, promotes communication, supports reflective practice and seeks to continuously learn will provide a psychologically safe space to allow more effective management of risk.
- Positive risk management, with plans developed collaboratively with service users, families and carers.
- Risk management focused on identifying strengths and the individual's recovery.
- Effective formulation of risk and use of structured clinical judgement rather than relying on risk-assessment tools or, conversely, informal judgement.
- Knowledge of the Mental Health Act.
- Working effectively across organisations.
- Regular risk assessment training.
- Competence in working with diversity.

Effective multidisciplinary working needs to understand and accommodate different professional roles and the values that individuals bring to a team and a particular decision. Promoting the voice of service users may also help to challenge potentially paternalistic practice and build on more collaborative approaches to managing risk [26].

NICE provides guidance on the transition between inpatient mental health settings and community or care home settings. Principles underpinning this guidance are similar to the aforementioned Department of Health guidance, namely that of ensuring collaboration with service users, carers and family, other services and specialists; being recovery focused; offering least restrictive care; and effective communication [27].

The assertive community treatment model (ACT, or assertive outreach in the United Kingdom) emerged in the 1970s as an alternative to standard care for patients who were identified with a higher-level need, such as requiring repeated admissions, difficulty with engaging with services, substance misuse and homelessness [28]. Invariably, this led assertive outreach teams to have caseloads with a high proportion of service users with a history of violence [29].

The assertive outreach model was specified in the 1999 NHS National Service Framework for Mental Health [30]. However, the benefit of this model of care being effective in managing violence was later found to be equivocal. The REACT study did not find a significant difference in outcomes with ACT compared to standard community mental health team (CMHT) care. This included no difference in the number of violent incidents [31]. The closure of assertive outreach teams does not appear to have had a significant impact on outcomes when these teams were integrated into CMHTs employing flexible assertive community treatment (FACT) [32]. However, the need to maintain services caring for people with enduring and serious mental illness has continued to be vociferously advocated [33].

The development in the Netherlands of FACT followed equivocal evidence for dedicated assertive outreach teams. FACT seeks to integrate assertive treatment into generic community mental health teams. However, to date there is no strong evidence, positive or negative, that FACT successfully moderates violence as this has not been specifically evaluated [34, 35].

Another development is that of community forensic services, which aim to treat people who either have offended or are at risk of offending due to their mental illness or personality disorder. These services focus not only on reducing risk of offending or violence, but on overall health and quality of life. Again, the evidence for dedicated community forensic services is debated and good evidence is lacking [36].

Police liaison with health services plays an important role in addressing emerging risk behaviour that could otherwise meet the threshold for formal police and criminal justice involvement, as well as supporting prosecution following a violent incident. Efforts to improve the response of services and police when a member of staff is a victim of violence or a hate crime are underway, such as the adoption of Operation Cavel, which aims to increase convictions when there is violence towards healthcare staff [37]. Assaults on health and social care staff became a specific criminal offence when the Assaults on Emergency Workers (Offences) Act 2018 [38] became law with the intention of delivering longer sentences to act as a deterrent.

The current NHS Long-Term Plan proposes an integrated model of community mental health care, bringing together social and primary care in blended teams within primary care networks. Pilot sites remain in development. The benefits (or otherwise) of this model, and particularly in managing risks such as violence, remain to be seen [18].

The Role of Approved Mental Health Professionals and Mental Health Act Assessments

Statutory criteria for detention in Part II of the Mental Health Act 1983 (MHA) includes detention for the protection of others; consequently, the Mental Health Act has a role in managing risk of violence. Here we discuss the practical aspects of conducting Mental Health Act assessments, whilst Chapter 2 provides an overview of legislation relevant to the management of violence. Also discussed in Chapter 2 is the equivocal evidence for community treatment orders in managing the risk of violence.

As stated earlier, a collaborative approach with service users and others in managing the risk of violence is preferable. However, when engagement and voluntary treatment is not possible, compulsory treatment in hospital may need to be considered. A decision to move to a more coercive approach has the potential to be distressing or divisive for service users and their families, and similarly emotionally demanding and challenging for professionals. Careful preparation, coordination and effective communication helps ensure that when using the Mental Health Act, it is as therapeutic as possible and reduces distress. Before making a referral for a Mental Health Act assessment, a service needs to demonstrate that efforts have been made to engage a service user and provide treatment and support informally. This will typically involve offering clinic-based appointments and home visits, as well as attempts to contact a service user by phone or letter. The Code of Practice sets out other considerations – for example, taking into account factors that might mitigate risk to others through family support [39].

The Code of Practice goes on to set out the role and responsibilities of the approved mental health professional (AMHP) in arranging a Mental Health Act assessment. This includes conducting a risk assessment prior to a Mental Health Act assessment and making arrangements, if required, for the police to attend an assessment. In many areas, police attendance has become the default given the potential for someone detained resisting being conveyed to hospital. The risk assessment will help inform the level of police response in accordance with locally agreed protocols.

For a person to be detained they need to have been assessed by an AMHP, a section-12-approved doctor and another registered medical practitioner who preferably has previous knowledge of the person. The assessment is best done jointly, although it is possible for the first medical recommendation to be done separately as long as there are no more than five clear days between.

The routine option for conveying a person to hospital would be by ambulance. However, if the risk assessment indicated that increased risk secure transport may be required, under section 137 of the Mental Health Act the police are given powers to use force to detain a person to convey them to hospital; this would only be indicated when there is a significant risk to public safety.

Following the completion of an assessment, good practice is for the AMHP to debrief police and others involved to identify concerns or areas for learning resulting from the assessment process.

Once a person is detained in hospital, communication and collaboration between community and inpatient services is vital for longer-term risk management.

Domestic Abuse and Violence

The management and recognition of domestic abuse and violence remains a challenge for services. It is prevalent, is not gender specific and, in the year ending March 2016, 20% of violent crimes in England and Wales were categorised as domestic violence by a partner, ex-partner or family acquaintance [40]. This is thought to be an underestimate as it relies on victims reporting it as such. The Office of National Statistics also reports that one woman in four experiences domestic violence in her lifetime, and two women are killed each week by a current or former partner in England and Wales, as well as 30 men each year through domestic violence.

Stonewall's research shows that one in four lesbian and bisexual women have experienced domestic abuse in a relationship [41]. Two-thirds of those say the perpetrator was a woman, one third a man. Almost half (49%) of all gay and bisexual men have experienced at least one incident of domestic abuse from a family member or partner since the age of 16. There is limited research on how many transgender people experience domestic abuse in the United Kingdom.

The UK government defines domestic abuse as 'any incident or pattern of incidents of controlling, coercive or threatening behaviour, violence or abuse between those aged 16 or over who are or have been intimate partners or family members regardless of gender or sexuality'. The guidance was updated to reflect the impact of the COVID-19 pandemic, for example providing exemptions from self-isolation if a person was a victim of domestic abuse. This temporary guidance has again been updated as mandatory isolation requirements are no longer in place [42]. Types of abuse are not limited to, but can be broadly categorised as including:

- Psychological
- Physical
- Sexual
- Financial
- Emotional

Domestic violence is a major contributory factor to mental ill health across the globe [43]. This impact is found not only in the mental health of the victims of domestic violence but also in the children of these relationships.

Mental health service users have been found to be reluctant to disclose domestic violence for fear of the consequences, and professionals working in mental health find it difficult to enquire about domestic violence as they either feel lacking in the necessary expertise or do not see it as part of their role [44]. Since the Care Act 2014 placed adult safeguarding on a statutory footing equivalent to child safeguarding, clarity around professional obligations to manage adult safeguarding concerns has been settled. This is supported by evidence that service users are in favour of direct enquiry by healthcare professionals [45].

Routine enquiry is also recommended in NICE guidance from 2014 [46], followed in 2016 by the issuing of NICE Quality Standards for Domestic Violence and Abuse [47]. The four quality statements can form the basis of an organisation's policies regarding domestic violence and abuse:

1. People presenting to frontline staff with indicators of possible domestic violence or abuse are asked about their experiences in a private discussion.
2. People experiencing domestic violence and abuse receive a response from level 1 or 2 trained staff.
3. People experiencing domestic violence or abuse are offered referral to specialist support services.
4. People who disclose that they are perpetrating domestic violence or abuse are offered referral to specialist services.

Identification of abuse presents an opportunity to intervene, so all professionals need to be aware of the types and indicators of abuse. The Duluth power and control wheel (theduluthmodel.org) was developed in the USA in 1984 as a way to help victims, perpetrators and professionals to recognise behaviours that could indicate abuse [48].

A disclosing environment where information and advice are clearly displayed in public areas in a range of formats, including areas where service users can pick up information anonymously and staff are aware of specialist agencies and referral pathways to them, will help to facilitate disclosure.

Organisations can offer advice to their staff on how to frame and approach the question as soon as possible in the pathway (i.e. at assessment). Given the sensitive nature of the question it should only be broached when they are alone with the service user and not in the presence of any partner, relative or friends. Curiosity is crucial – an initial negative response does not necessarily indicate the absence of abuse. The service user may not feel ready to disclose, may be frightened or may not recognise their experience as abusive. Specialist websites offer examples of questions (see, for example, http://domesticabuse.stanford.edu/screening/how.html).

Policies should also advise on how to respond to disclosures of domestic abuse. This is likely to have been difficult for the person to speak of and must be met with a non-judgemental and supportive response using validating statements. Where the victim meets the Care Act 2014 criteria, a safeguarding adult referral should be made. Risk assessment procedures should be carried out, leading to an agreed safety plan with the person's views at the centre of all decision-making. Specialist domestic abuse organisations can be contacted as their expertise in this area is invaluable

Domestic violence is associated with many mental disorders, including anxiety, depression, post-traumatic stress disorder, eating disorders and psychosis. There is a high prevalence and increased likelihood of being a victim of domestic violence in men and women across all diagnostic categories, compared to people without mental disorders [49]. These largely refer to affective disorders such as depression, PTSD and anxiety as there are very few comparable studies into domestic violence and psychotic disorders.

The median prevalence of lifetime domestic violence in female mental health outpatients has been estimated at 33% [50]. However, given the reluctance to enquire and also to disclose, this is likely to be an under-representation.

Those with serious mental illness are 2–8 times more likely to experience sexual or domestic violence than others [51]. A report into refuge provision in London for survivors of domestic violence who also have mental health or substance use issues found a lack of tangible data about reasons for refusing access to refuges, but established that services can exclude for reasons such as having a diagnosis of schizophrenia [52]. This poses an extra challenge to community teams seeking to protect their service users.

The obligations placed on local authorities by the Care Act 2014 to safeguard any adult 'who has needs for care and support provide' represents a useful framework for mental health practitioners. Through this act, issues of mental-capacity unwise decision-making and coercive behaviour can be considered. Access to independent domestic violence advocates can be facilitated. Such is the association between domestic violence and adult safeguarding that in 2015 the Directors of Adult social services published a guide to support practitioners and managers [53]. Thus, adult safeguarding policies and procedures, along with links to the local Multi-Agency Risk Assessment Conference (MARAC), are key to supporting this service-user group. A MARAC is a borough-based meeting where information on the highest-risk domestic abuse cases is shared between representatives of local police, health, child protection, housing practitioners, independent domestic violence advisors (IDVAs), probation and other specialists from the statutory and voluntary sectors. The purpose is to discuss options and formulate a plan to safeguard the victim.

Other sources of information and advice can be found here:

www.refuge.org.uk

www.safelives.org.uk

www.womensaid.org.uk

www.hopscotchuk.org.uk

Personal Safety in the Community: Law and Guidance

The Health and Safety Executive (HSE) defines work-related violence as 'any incident in which a person is abused, threatened or assaulted in circumstances relating to their work' [54, p. 1].

There are five main pieces of health and safety law which are relevant to violence at work:

1. **The Health and Safety at Work etc. Act 1974 (HSW Act)**
   Under this, employers have a legal duty to ensure, so far as is reasonably practicable, the health, safety and welfare at work of their employees.
2. **The Management of Health and Safety at Work Regulations 1999**
   These give employers the requirement to assess the risks to employees and make arrangements for their health and safety.
3. **The Reporting of Injuries, Diseases and Dangerous Occurrences Regulations 2013 (RIDDOR)**
   Employers must notify their enforcing authority in the event of an accident at work to any employee resulting in death, major injury or incapacity for normal work for three or more consecutive days.
4. **Safety Representatives and Safety Committees Regulations 1977 (a) and The Health and Safety (Consultation with Employees) Regulations 1996 (b)**
   Employers must inform, and consult with, employees in good time on matters relating to their health and safety.
5. **The Corporate Manslaughter and Corporate Homicide Act 2007**
   An organisation can be prosecuted and receive an unlimited fine, particularly if it is found to be in gross breach of health and safety standards and the duty of care owed to the deceased.

The HSE has published several guidance documents for employers, including *Violence at Work: A Guide for Employers* [54], *Lone Working* [55], and *Preventing Workplace Harassment and Violence* [56], the latter being jointly published by employer and employee representative organisations.

Lone Working in the Community

Community-based work invariably involves individuals working alone or in situations where they may not have the immediate support of others. The HSE describes lone working as 'someone who works by themselves without close or direct supervision' [55]. Safety measures need to be proportionate to the type of work, and should be guided by risk assessment.

The Health, Safety and Wellbeing Partnership Group (HSWPG) part of NHS Employers has providing the following advice [57]:

- Staff should be trained in de-escalation and breakaway techniques.
- Staff skilled in dynamically assessing risk and, when identified, recording and sharing of clinical risk
- Availability of personal safety equipment such as lone working alarm devices.
- A system to ensure that the whereabouts of community staff is always known.
- Awareness of safety precautions when using public transport or walking between visits
- Awareness on how to assess the environment and act during community visits.
- Post-incident support, reporting and review.

Further advice on precautions and information about lone working safety devices and apps can be found at www.suzylamplugh.org.

Conclusion

Successful management of violence in the community is predicated on a wide range of factors which have been described briefly in this chapter. The need for collaboration not just between different services, but also with service users and their networks, forms a vital component of good risk management. This has to be allied with services that are well resourced, with trained staff who work in a supportive and open culture where they are able to identify, assess and manage risk. This remains an evolving challenge.

References

1. Dahlberg, L. L. and Mercy, J. A. History of violence as a public health issue. *AMA Virtual Mentor*, February 2009 (11)2:167–72. http://wiki.preventconnect.org/wp-content/uploads/2018/08/History-of-Violence-as-a-Public-Health-Issue.pdf [Accessed 7.9.2021].

2. The Strategy Unit. Exploring Mental Health Inpatient Capacity across Sustainability and Transformation Partnerships in England. [online]. November 2019. www.strategyunitwm.nhs.uk/publications/exploring-mental-health-inpatient-capacity [Accessed 7.9.2021].

3. National Institute for Health and Care Excellence. Violence and aggression: Short-term management in mental health, health and community settings [online]. [London]: NICE; 2015. (Clinical guideline [NG10]). www.nice.org.uk/guidance/ng10 [Accessed 7.9.2021].

4. Health and Safety Executive. Violence at Work: A Guide for Employers. HSE, INDG69. [online]. 1996. www.hse.gov.uk/pubns/indg69.pdf [Accessed 7.9.2021].

5. Crown Prosecution Service. Mental Health: Suspects and Defendants with Mental Health Conditions or Disorders. [online]. 2019. www.cps.gov.uk/legal-guidance/mental-health-suspects-and-defendants-mental-health-conditions-or-disorders [Accessed 7.9.2021].

6. Criminal Justice Act 2003, c. 44. www.legislation.gov.uk/ukpga/2003/44/contents [Accessed 7.9.2021].

7. College of Policing. Major investigation and public protection: Managing sexual offenders and violent offenders: Multi-agency public protection arrangements (MAPPA). [online]. 2017. www.app.college.police.uk/app-content/major-investigation-and-public-protection/managing-sexual-offenders-and-violent-offenders/mappa/ [Accessed 7.9.2021].

8. Whiting, D., Lichtenstein, P. and Fazel, S. Violence and mental disorders: A structured review of associations by individual diagnoses, risk factors, and risk assessment. *Lancet Psychiatry* 2021; 8:150–61.

9. Chan, S. K. W., Li, O. W. T., Hui, C. L. M. et al. The effect of media reporting of a homicide committed by a patient with schizophrenia on the public stigma and knowledge of psychosis among the general

population of Hong Kong. *Social Psychiatry and Psychiatric Epidemiology* 2019. 54:43–50.

10. McGinty, E. E., Goldman, H. H., Pescosolido, B. A. et al. Communicating about mental illness and violence: Balancing stigma and increased support for services. *Journal of Health Politics, Policy and Law* 2018; 43:185–228.

11. Rodway, C., Flynn, S., While, D. et al. Patients with mental illness as victims of homicide: A national consecutive case series. *Lancet Psychiatry* 2014; 1:129–34.

12. Swanson, J. Holzer, C. E., Ganju, V. K. et al. Violence and psychiatric disorders in the community: Evidence from the Epidemiologic Catchment Area surveys. *Hospital and Community Psychiatry* 1990; 41:761–70.

13. Elbogen, E. B. and Johnson, S. C. The intricate link between violence and mental disorder. Results From the National Epidemiologic Survey on Alcohol and Related Conditions. *Archives of General Psychiatry* 2009; 66:152–61.

14. Moran, P., Walsh, E., Tyrer, P. et al. Impact of comorbid personality disorder on violence in psychosis. *British Journal of Psychiatry* 2003; 182:129–34.

15. Strassnig, M. T., Nascimento, V. N., Deckler, E. et al. Pharmacological treatment of violence in schizophrenia. *CNS Spectrums* 2020; 20:207–15.

16. Royal College of Psychiatrists. Services for people diagnosable with personality disorder PS01/20. [online]. 2020. www.rcpsych.ac.uk/docs/default-source/improving-care/better-mh-policy/position-statements/ps01_20.pdf?sfvrsn=85af7fbc_2 [Accessed 7.9.2021]

17. Duggan, C. and Tyrer P. (2022). Specialist teams as constituted are unsatisfactory for treating people with personality disorders. *BJPsych Bulletin* 46, 100–102.

18. Bell, A. NHS England's new framework for community mental health services. 8 Nov. 2019. www.nationalelfservice.net/populations-and-settings/community-settings/nhs-england-framework-community-mental-health-services/ [Accessed 7.9.2021].

19. National Institute for Health and Care Excellence. Coexisting severe mental illness and substance misuse qs188. [online]. 2019. www.nice.org.uk/guidance/qs188/resources/coexisting-severe-mental-illness-and-substance-misuse-pdf-75545728091845 [Accessed 7.9.2021].

20. Department of Health. Drug misuse and dependence. [online]. 2017. https://assets.publishing.service.gov.uk/government/uploads/system/uploads/attachment_data/file/673978/clinical_guidelines_2017.pdf [Accessed 7.9.2021].

21. Coid, J. W., Ullrich, S., Kallis, C. et al. Improving risk management for violence in mental health services: A multimethods approach. Programme Grants for Applied Research NIHR, 2016.

22. Large, M. and Nielssen, O. The limitations of future of violence risk assessment. *World Psychiatry* 2017; 16:25–6.

23. Department of Health. Refocusing the Care Programme Approach: Policy and positive practice guidance. [online]. 2008. https://webarchive.nationalarchives.gov.uk/20130105012529/http://www.dh.gov.uk/en/PublicationsandstatisticsPublications/PublicationsPolicyAndGuidance/DH_083647 [Accessed 7.9.2021].

24. Turner, J., Hayward, R., Angel, K. et al. The history of mental health services in modern England: Practitioner memories and the direction of future research. *Medical History* 2015; 59:599–624.

25. Department of Health. Best Practice in Managing Risk. [online]. 2009. https://assets.publishing.service.gov.uk/government/uploads/system/uploads/attachment_data/file/478595/best-practice-managing-risk-cover-webtagged.pdf [Accessed 7.9.2021].

26. Haines, A., Perkins, E., Evans, E. A. et al. Multidisciplinary team functioning and decision making within forensic mental health. *Mental Health Review (Brighton)* 2018; 23:185–96.

27. National Institute for Health and Care Excellence. Transition between inpatient mental health settings and community or care home settings. [online]. 2016. www

.nice.org.uk/guidance/ng53/resources/transition-between-inpatient-mental-health-settings-and-community-or-care-home-settings-pdf-1837511615941 [Accessed 7.9.2021].

28. Stein, L. I. and Test, M. A. Alternative to mental hospital treatment. Conceptual model, treatment program, and clinical evaluation. *Arch Gen Psychiatry* 1980; 37:392–7.

29. Priebe, S., Fakhoury, W., Watts, J. et al. Assertive outreach teams in London: Patient characteristics and outcomes. *British Journal of Psychiatry* 2003; 183:148–54.

30. Department of Health and Social Care. National service framework: Mental health. [online] 1999. www.gov.uk/government/publications/quality-standards-for-mental-health-services [Accessed 10.10.2022].

31. Killaspy, H., Bebbington, P., Blizard, R. et al. The REACT study: Randomised evaluation of assertive community treatment in north London. *BMJ* 2006; 332:815–20.

32. Firn, M. Hindhaugh, K. Hubbeling D. et al. A dismantling study of assertive outreach services: Comparing activity and outcomes following replacement with the FACT model. *Social Psychiatry and Psychiatric Epidemiology* 2013; 48:997–1003.

33. Dissanayaka, N. Meet my patients who've been left out of the mental health conversation. The Guardian [online], 2019. https://www.theguardian.com/society/2019/feb/28/meet-patients-left-out-mental-health-conversation [Accessed 06.01.2023].

34. Norden, T. and Norlander, T. Absence of positive results for flexible assertive community treatment. What is the next approach? *Clinical Practice in Epidemiology and Mental Health* 2014; 10:87–91.

35. Sood, L., Owen, A., Onyon, R. et al. Flexible assertive community treatment (FACT) model in specialist psychosis teams: An evaluation. *BJPsych Bulletin* 2017; 41:192–6.

36. Latham, R. and Williams, H. K. Community forensic psychiatric services in England and Wales. *CNS Spectrums* 2020; 25:604–17.

37. Crown Prosecution Service. London-wide launch of operation to convict those who assault NHS staff. [online] 2021. www.cps.gov.uk/cps-london-north-london-south/news/london-wide-launch-operation-convict-those-who-assault-nhs-staff [Accessed 7.9.2021].

38. Assaults on Emergency Workers (Offences) Act 2018. Gov.uk [online]. www.legislation.gov.uk/ukpga/2018/23/contents/enacted [Accessed 29.4.2022].

39. Department of Health and Social Care. Code of Practice: Mental Health Act 1983. [online] 2015. www.gov.uk/government/publications/code-of-practice-mental-health-act-1983 [Accessed 7.9.2021].

40. Office of National Statistics. Overview of violent crime and sexual offences. [online] 2017. www.ons.gov.uk/peoplepopulationandcommunity/crimeandjustice/compendium/focusonviolentcrimeandsexualoffences/yearendingmarch2016/overviewofviolentcrimeandsexualoffences [Accessed 7.9.2021].

41. Stonewall. Domestic Abuse: Stonewall Health Briefing (2012) [online] 2015. www.stonewall.org.uk/resources/domestic-abuse-%E2%80%93-stonewall-health-briefing-2012 [Accessed 7.9.2021].

42. Home Office. Domestic abuse: How to get help [online] 2021. www.gov.uk/guidance/domestic-abuse-how-to-get-help [Accessed 12.10.2022b].

43. Hegarty, K. Domestic violence: The hidden epidemic associated with mental illness. *BJPsych* 2011; 198:169–70.

44. Rose, D., Trevillion, K., Woodall, A. et al. Barriers and facilitators of disclosures of domestic violence by mental health service users: Qualitative study. *BJPsych* 2011; 198:189–94.

45. Trevillion, K., Hughes, B., Feder, G. et al. Disclosure of domestic violence in mental health settings: A qualitative meta-synthesis. *International Journal of Psychiatry* 2014; 26:430–44.

46. National Institute for Health and Care Excellence. Domestic violence and abuse: Multi-agency working PH50. [online]

2014. www.nice.org.uk/guidance/ph50 [Accessed 7.9.2021].

47. National Institute for Health and Care Excellence. Domestic Violence and Abuse: Quality Standard QS116. [online] 2016. www.nice.org.uk/guidance/qs116 [Accessed 7.9.2021].

48. Domestic Abuse Intervention Programmes. [online] 2021. www .theduluthmodel.org [Accessed 7.9.2021].

49. Trevillion, K., Oram, S., Feder, G. et al. Experiences of domestic violence and mental disorders: A systematic review and meta-analysis. *PLOS One* 2012; 7:e51740.

50. Oram, S. Trevillion, K., Feder, G. et al. Prevalence of experiences of domestic violence among psychiatric patients: systematic review. *BJPsych* 2013; 202:94–9.

51. Khalifeh, H., Moran, P., Borschmann, R. et al. Domestic and sexual violence against patients with severe mental illness. *Psychological Medicine* 2015; 45:875–86.

52. Harvey, S., Mandair, S., Holly, J. Case by Case: Refuge provision in London for survivors of domestic violence who use alcohol and other drugs or have mental health problems. Solace Women's Aid, Stella Project. [online] 2014. https://ava project.org.uk/wp-content/uploads/2016/0

3/Case-by-Case-London-refuge-provision-Full-Report.pdf [Accessed 7.9.2021].

53. Local Government Association. Adult Safeguarding and Domestic Abuse: A guide to support practitioners and managers. [online] 2015. www .local.gov.uk/publications/adult-safeguarding-and-domestic-abuse-guide-support-practitioners-and-managers-second [Accessed 7.9.2021].

54. Health and Safety Executive. Violence at Work: A Guide for Employers. [online] 1996. www.hse.gov.uk/pubns/indg69.pdf [Accessed 7.9.2021].

55. Health and Safety Executive. Protecting lone workers: How to manage the risks of working alone. [online] 2020. www .hse.gov.uk/pubns/indg73.htm [Accessed 7.9.2021].

56. Health and Safety Executive. Preventing Workplace Harassment and Violence. [online] 2010. www.hse.gov.uk/violence/p reventing-workplace-harassment.pdf [Accessed 7.9.2021].

57. NHS Employers. Improving the personal safety for lone workers. [online] 2018. www .nhsemployers.org/system/files/media/HS WPG-Lone-Workers-staff-guide-210218-FINAL_0.pdf [Accessed 12.10.2021].

Chapter 1

Management of Violence in Acute Medical Hospital Settings

Sachin Patel, Emma Valentine and Eric Baskind

Introduction

Violence is unfortunately a hazard encountered across all health and social care settings to some degree. This chapter aims to provide a framework for non-mental health care workers to approach the issue through understanding why violence occurs in the medical setting, where the risk areas are and how to develop a workforce that can prevent, assess and manage situations they are likely to encounter. There are particular considerations for the acute medical setting; this includes the physical healthcare needs of the patient population, staffing mix, their training, environmental factors and the applicability of legal frameworks.

Violence in the medical hospital setting is common. A special report by the HSJ and Unison estimated that in 2018 there were approximately 75,000 reported assaults on NHS staff equating to approximately 200 per day (1). In reality, this figure is likely much greater as not all assaults are reported. Rates of self-reported violence are higher in the Ambulance and Mental Health sectors and across all groups appear to be slowly reducing over recent years (see Table 10.1; data compiled from annual NHS staff surveys). Amongst acute sector staff, there are similar patterns of self-reporting as seen in the mental health sector of being the victim of violence on repeated occasions. This suggests that this is as much of an embedded hazard as it is in the mental health sector.

Despite high gross numbers of incidents reported in the acute healthcare setting, violence is still relatively rare when compared to the rates seen in mental healthcare settings. Training in the assessment and management of violence and formal guidance in acute sectors varies between hospitals but is generally not on a par with that provided in mental healthcare settings. Nevertheless, the principles and practices in violence reduction are equally valid across all healthcare settings and can be readily transferred for use across organisations.

Aetiology, Perpetrators and Victim Profile

Violence, either physical or non-physical, can arise in many parts of the hospital in different patient groups. One of the most common drivers of violence is substance misuse and intoxication. Patients presenting with acute psychiatric crises can also present to the emergency department (ED) and risks arise of the same nature as those seen in mental health settings. Other causes include cognitive impairment leading to attempts to leave the hospital, acute confusional states, patient discomfort, the use of restraints and transitions in patient care. An analysis of the age and sex profile of perpetrators of violence in NHS settings between 2010–15 identified that males aged 75–95 were the most likely to commit acts of violence [2]. This suggest strongly that dementia, confusional states and delirium

Table 10.1 NHS Staff Survey data on violence experienced by NHS staff from patients, relatives or other members of the public

YEAR OF NHS Staff Survey	Percentage of Ambulance NHS Trust staff who experienced any violence in the past 12 months	Percentage of Mental Health NHS Trust staff who experienced any violence in the past 12 months	Percentage of Acute NHS Trust staff who experienced any violence in the past 12 months	Percentage of Community NHS Trust staff who experienced any violence in the past 12 months
2017	35%	18%	15%	9%
2018	34%	16%	14%	8%
2019	33%	17%	14%	8%
2020	33%	15%	14%	7%
2021	31%	14%	14%	7%

Source: NHS annual staff survey: https://public.tableau.com/app/profile/piescc/viz/ST21_national_data_2022-03-30_PIEFH25/Aboutthissurvey

are the most likely drivers of violence. Acute behavioural disturbance (ABD) or excited delirium (ExD) can be associated with 'hyper-aggression'. It is a controversial term that divides the medical community [3]. Cases of ABD and ExD frequently occur outside of medical units and present in a variety of settings, including in the EDs of acute hospitals. The College of Paramedics has recommended that pathways and guidance are developed with police and emergency departments to support early recognition as well as the appropriate management of suspected cases, and that training takes places in partnership with police, particularly in relation to restraint and de-escalation techniques [4]. Eric Baskind, who has appeared as an expert in a number of court cases and inquests/fatal accident inquiries, in the United Kingdom and overseas, discusses this topical issue later in the chapter.

Particular staff groups are more prone to become victims of violence. These include nursing staff, those working in the ED, staff working in complaints management roles and security staff. In addition, violence and abuse tends to be perpetrated more outside of core working hours and towards younger, male staff [5].

Acute Behavioural Disturbance and Excited Delirium

ABD is often cited in cases of deaths in custody, especially where restraint has been used. It describes a constellation of symptoms that may indicate an acute medical crisis. ExD, first described in the mid-1800s, is a form of ABD and has subsequently been referred to by other names, including Bell's mania, lethal catatonia, acute exhaustive mania and agitated delirium [6]. Of all the forms of ABD, ExD has been described as 'the most extreme and potentially life threatening' [7, p. 1]. Faculty of Forensic and Legal Medicine of the Royal College of Physicians original guidelines on management of ABD in police custody, from which this quote was taken have recently been updated [8]. It is said to exist where the subject displays constant or near constant physical activity, pain tolerance, superhuman strength, sweating, rapid breathing, tactile hyperthermia and, where police are involved, a failure to respond to police presence [9]. It remains a controversial term because it is not currently a recognised medical or psychiatric diagnosis according to either the International Classification of Diseases of the World Health Organisation or the Diagnostic and Statistical Manual of Mental Disorders of the American Psychiatric Association. Further controversy arose following a statement issued on 16 July 2021 by the Royal College of Psychiatrists (RCPsych) withdrawing its 23 June 2021 statement on ExD and ABD on the grounds that the terms ExD and ABD had 'no empirical evidential basis' [10]. This further divided the opinion of doctors and restraint experts/practitioners. It also received condemnation from the Police Federation of England and Wales, who described it as 'hugely damaging'. In its scathing criticism, the Federation pointed out that

> [T]he current version of the *College of Policing* guidelines emphasises the early recognition of ABD, as well de-escalation as the first approach, and that restraint should be minimised. Officers are not required to diagnose the cause of ABD but to treat it as a medical emergency so that the emergency department is the right place for the person and not as a s136 or psychiatric referral. It is about the recognition of ABD, and treating individuals presenting with these symptoms as patients not prisoners. ABD is a term used for police, ambulance trust and emergency physicians, and psychiatrists are not involved in these cases until all medical causes are ruled out and the person is in a safe and stable condition. Therefore, the management of ABD is out of scope for a psychiatrist. [11]

Such controversies are unfortunate because, notwithstanding the debate as to the existence of these conditions, the symptoms are widely recognised and included in the majority of prevention and management of violence and aggression [PMVA] training programmes, wherein they are noted as a medical emergency. The question should not, therefore, centre on whether the conditions exist on the WHO database, but what ABD/ExD involves, how it can lead to death, and what can be done to improve the safety of restraint to prevent these deaths from occurring. There is, of course, no diagnostic test for ABD/ExD; diagnosis depends on the recognition of clinical features and on the exclusion of differential diagnoses. It is therefore important for investigations to be undertaken to exclude other causes of altered mental behaviour and to assess for the complications of psychomotor overactivity, such as acidosis, cardiac arrhythmias, hyperkalaemia, hyperthermia and rhabdomyolysis.

Ruttenber et al. [12] point to the many known causes of ABD, such as brain tumours, infection, heat exhaustion, thyroid disease, illegal drugs and psychiatric medications, although they assert that ExD is a largely unknown medical condition. Accordingly, some of those who die from a restraint-related ExD syndrome are victims of their own, usually long-term, cocaine and amphetamine abuse, which causes heart disease and can trigger this fatal syndrome [12, 13]. Costello [14] notes that those who take large quantities of antipsychotic medications and who are susceptible to ExD may also have the same effects as those taking stimulants. These individuals can suddenly become extremely agitated and aggressive, resulting in death during or shortly after being restrained. Gillings et al. [15] describe patients typically presenting with tachycardia, tachypnoea, hyperthermia (often with undressing), excessive physical strength with apparent lack of fatigue, insensitivity to pain (including that associated with irritant sprays) and acute psychosis often accompanied by paranoia. Common causes include use of stimulant drugs, such as cocaine, and exacerbation of underlying mental health disorder. Karch [16] discusses the role of sudden cardiac death, noting that its cause is not fully understood in the context of restraint-related deaths. What is known, however, is that death can occur during or following restraint, although the infrequency and complex circumstances of these events hamper scientific investigation in the real world [17].

The College of Paramedics issued a Position Statement on ABD and ExD in October 2018, describing them as 'medical emergencies' [4]. Noting that there is no consensus on definition, the College recognises the definition set out by the Royal College of Emergency Medicine as a 'sudden onset of aggressive and violent behaviour and autonomic dysfunction'.

Differentiating between a service user who is in a state of ExD and someone who is simply otherwise violent/aggressive is often difficult. The following may indicate the presence of ExD:

- Exhibition of unexpected physical strength or endurance
- Exhibition of abnormal tolerance to pain
- Feeling hot to touch and profuse sweating
- Extreme agitation or hostility
- Acute paranoia
- Bizarre behaviour and speech
- Disorientation and impaired thinking
- Hallucinations
- Sudden tranquillity following a period of frenzied activity

It is because these symptoms are often difficult to detect and/or distinguish from episodes of non-medical-emergency violence that clear guidelines must be provided and incorporated into PMVA training. Unfortunately, many current guidelines lack consistency and best cross-sector expertise, which can create 'a risk of death through ignorance of a potentially life-threatening condition' [18, p. 7].

Excellent guidance in dealing with suspected cases of ABD has been provided by the College of Policing [19]:

> Prolonged restraint and struggling can result in exhaustion, reduced breathing leading to build up of toxic metabolites. This, with underlying medical conditions such as cardiac conditions, drugs use or use of certain antipsychotics, can result in sudden death with little warning. The best management is de-escalation, avoiding prone restraint, restraining for the minimum amount of time, lying the detainee on their side and constant monitoring of vital signs . . . Officers should note that the effects of a violent struggle or restraint and build-up of lactic acid can exacerbate the effects of drugs, alcohol or medication.

In many cases, it is only apparent that a service user is suffering with ABD/ExD when they suddenly collapse. It is for this reason that staff should be alert to a service user's sudden tranquillity following a period of frenzied activity. This may be due to severe exhaustion, asphyxia or cardiorespiratory compromise. Training must emphasise that a person suffering with ABD/ExD is at risk of sudden death and should be treated as a medical and psychiatric emergency.

Special Considerations in the Acute Hospital Setting

Staff Training and Skills

There is a notable difference in staffing skill mix and risk awareness between physical and mental health settings. This is naturally the case given that their respective care delivery focuses on different aspects of health. It is recognised that there are drivers to integrate healthcare and incorporate better mental health and physical health training for staff working across settings. Training on PMVA is not yet mandatory for staff working in physical healthcare settings as it is in psychiatric settings. The general awareness of the drivers for disturbed behaviour, exposure to violence and vigilance levels are lower than those seen in staff working in psychiatric settings. A National Confidential Enquiry into Patient Outcome and Death (NCEPOD) survey of NHS staff working in the acute hospital setting found that 41.4% had no training on risk assessment and 19.1% had no training on the management of violence and aggression [20].

Specialist registered mental health nurse (RMN) input in acute medical settings is available when needed, often via bank or agency deployment, and this is usually used on an ad hoc, case-by-case basis. There can be delays in getting such input at short notice when the need for specialist nursing and implementation is identified. The ED, on the other hand, is a special case in that this cohort of frontline staff is often experienced in de-escalating and managing violence and many have access to some training. It is also commonly the case that RMNs are embedded routinely in the nursing complement of EDs given that their need can be anticipated on a daily basis.

In contrast to acute mental health settings, the majority of medical hospitals do not have a dedicated 'control and restraint team' which can respond to escalating aggression or incidents of violence. The initial responders are often staff in the vicinity of the perpetrator, and escalation in high-risk scenarios is usually to hospital security staff who are trained in control and restraint.

Risk Assessment

Risk assessment in the acute setting invariably falls to one based on clinical judgement rather than actuarial tools or a structured approach. This is likely due to a combination of the absence of embedded structured risk assessment tools, training factors and also system factors. The latter include recording systems which are not designed to flag and record historical risk factors.

The likelihood of specific incidents of violence and aggression can to some extent be assessed through the process of risk assessment. In practice, certain service areas are more adept in assessing risk through clinical experience and formal training on the process. As expected, these areas include the ED and acute medical admissions units, wherein incidents of violence are most common. Nevertheless, risk assessment and management is often overlooked in the acute hospital, as highlighted in the NCEPOD report, Treat as One [20]. This study assessed the quality of care provided to those with serious mental illness admitted to acute hospital settings and found that only 33.8% of patients had their risk assessed at any stage in their admission; of these, risk management plans were put in place in 47.3% of patients. Structured risk assessment tools can be useful, in particular when integrated into broader psychiatric assessment tools with clear, linked, risk-based actions. The Royal College of Emergency Medicine provide a useful toolkit for individual EDs in how to prepare a pro forma which prompt areas of inquiry and observations which are vital in determining specific risks [21].

Environmental and Systemic Considerations

When assessing and mitigating risk in the acute hospital, the structural environment and function of the hospital contrasts with psychiatric settings and represents an important consideration. The hospital has general access to the public, with barriers into wards often

1. Clash of people in over-crowded area
2. Lack of progression/waiting times
3. Inhospitable environments
4. Dehumanising environments
5. Intense emotions in a restricted space
6. Unsafe environments
7. Perceived inefficiency
8. Inconsistent response to 'undesirable' behaviour
9. Staff fatigue

Figure 10.1 Triggers of Violence in Emergency Departments

being simple and easily negotiated. Patients are usually cared for based on physical health need rather than any other particular psychological need or vulnerability factor. The ward furniture, access to medical instruments, high demand for side rooms and a less restrictive capability leads to challenges in the prevention and management of violence.

The ED environment can also be a bewildering and frustrating environment for patients and visitors, and this goes beyond specific characteristics that may make an individual more or less likely to be violent or aggressive. Research has identified specific triggers to violence in the ED which are typically experienced in combination (Figure 10.1 [22]). The Design Council has developed a useful, evidence-based toolkit setting out principles in spatial design, information design and service design which can lessen the chances of violence and lower the level of frustration for both patients and visitors [22]. The RCPsych affiliated Psychiatric Liaison Accreditation Network (PLAN) sets standards for psychiatric assessment rooms in EDs which are designed to be safe yet dignified, and are a core requirement for meeting the needs of patients who present with a mental health crisis and who may pose an associated risk of violence [23].

Legal Frameworks

The application of legal frameworks in the acute setting can be challenging due to a number of factors, including the interplay between physical health and mental health needs, overlap between the Mental Capacity Act (MCA) and Mental Health Act (MHA), and the level of staff training. In practice, awareness of the MCA and its informed application is generally of a higher standard in the medical setting when compared to that of the MHA. Confusion over which Act to follow can arise when the underlying aetiology of challenging behaviour in medical settings is still unsure. This often arises in situations when there is an acute need for organic intervention, when the MCA is often used; subsequently, the MHA could also be invoked to manage the consequent or associated mental disorder. Specialist guidance is often required when managing cases such as these, when violence is persistent and restrictive practice is necessary.

Consent and Standards of Behaviour

In contrast to mental health admissions, admissions to physical healthcare settings are almost exclusively on a voluntary basis or in patients' best interests in those who are incapacitated. Information provision and consenting is often fluidly approached over the course of admissions when these are unplanned. The opportunity to more fully inform patients of the specifics of care delivery can occur when arranging elective admissions. However, when codes of conduct for patients' behaviour are considered, there is little formalised contract or relaying of the expectations of a medically admitted patient when compared to psychiatric admissions. It often follows that a divergence in expectations between patient and care providers is a trigger for frustration and violence. In the case of violence and aggression, NHS organisations tend to revert to legislation which safeguards staff and so have a duty 'so far as it is reasonably practical' to protect the health, safety and welfare of staff members under the 1974 Health and Safety at Work Act [24]. NHS employers provide standards aimed at NHS organisations for ensuring the health and safety of their employees [25]. In addition to employee rights, patients causing a nuisance or disturbance on NHS property are ultimately liable to removal from NHS premises under section 120 of the Criminal Justice and Immigration Act 2008 [26]. It is understandable that there will be ethical considerations in certain scenarios when delivery of patient care conflicts with the need to protect staff and the general public.

Rapid Tranquillisation

The use of rapid tranquillisation (RT) in the chemical restraint of acutely disturbed patients needs special consideration in the acute hospital setting. RT is relatively rare in the hospital setting and individual members of staff involved are often exposed to these situations for the first time. Many of the incidents requiring RT will involve patients with physical health comorbidities, and the safe use of potentially harmful medication should take into account all aspects of pathology, particularly those involving interaction between drugs. The use of RT in the management of violence involves quick clinical decision-making, and for the inexperienced there is a risk of deviation from safe and effective practices, particularly regarding the dosage of medication. In contrast to psychiatric settings, the combination of unfamiliarity with local RT guidance and the presence of emergency medical response teams can lead to error and less stringent monitoring. ABD and ExD have already been discussed, and these presentations in combination with poorly considered or monitored RT can lead to potentially fatal consequences.

There has been growing concern regarding the controversial practice in some hospitals for anaesthetists to be routinely involved in RT [27]. Both the Royal College of Psychiatrists and the Royal College of Anaesthetists provide guidance on the role of anaesthetists in managing highly disturbed behaviour, with a particular focus on multidisciplinary working and training. It is also vital for acute hospitals to produce local guidance on RT, and there is opportunity for sharing and adaptation of well-established protocols such as those included in the Maudsley Guidelines [28].

Post-incident Support and Reporting

Staff support after each violent incident is vital for an organisation to ensure the emotional well-being of staff, and to learn from and improve future care delivery. Policies and provision of post-incident support, debriefing and a system for learning from incidents is key in the overall governance of risk management. Given the uncommon frequency of such risk events occurring in any particular service, gold standard guidance may not always be followed.

The NHS Staff Survey results highlight the level of under-reporting of incidents of physical violence in acute medical trusts. Of those staff responding, 27% of acute trust staff who had been involved in an incident of workplace-based physical violence did not report the incident [29]. This compares to just 6% of respondents in the same survey working in mental health trusts. The reasons for under-reporting are likely to be multifactorial and similar to those in found in a 2015 survey of US ED nurses [30]. This suggested that many of the reasons involve a level of desensitisation or acceptance of workplace violence.

The lack of a national agency or national guidelines (see Chapter 1) that focus on the safety of staff and allow for standardised reporting of incidents of violence across the NHS has led to challenges in governance [1]. In the absence of national structures, local governance plays a crucial role in identifying areas of need and where to focus limited resources.

Emergency Department Specific Challenges

The ED in the acute setting plays a central role in the emergency psychiatry pathway, receiving the ambulatory and emergency conveyances of mentally and physically unwell patients. There is also a disproportionately high number of intoxicated patients in a highly stimulating and claustrophobic environment. The staff working in this area often have more experience and are more vigilant in the assessment of risk and management of violence. Risk assessment as a core component in the triage of all presentations to EDs is crucial in the early identification and avoidance of risk of the violence [30]. The Royal College of Emergency Medicine provides guidance on how departments can design local risk assessment tools which meet the needs of their patients [21].

Particular challenges exist in the ED because of growing pressure in the mental healthcare system, and this is illustrated by an alarming increase in section 136 Mental Health Act (s136) conveyances to the ED. Prior to recent legislation change, s136 conveyances to the ED were in practice only accepted if there was a demonstrable physical healthcare need. The 2017 changes to the Code of Practice opened the ED to conveyances of those without a medical need if no other health-based place of safety (HBPoS) is practically accessible by the police [31]. The staffing and environmental risk management arrangements in a mental-healthcare-based PoS are rarely replicable in the acute medical setting. This increases the potential for aggression and violence, especially when overstretched police and hospital services attempt to deflect what they perceive as inappropriate pressures on their services.

Role of Liaison Psychiatry

Liaison psychiatry services can play a central role in the prevention and management of violence in the acute hospital setting. There is value in sharing knowledge and skills from working across mental and physical healthcare settings and being able to undertake, shape and model good practice. The responsive provision of mental healthcare with early identification of high-risk patients and mitigation in parallel to the delivery of physical health care is recommended. A core function of many liaison psychiatry services is also to provide training and education to the staff of the acute hospital, and this can promote a safer culture across the acute hospital.

Recommendations

- Training in risk assessment and the management of violence should be provided to all acute hospital staff.
- Acute hospitals are advised to develop local policies on control and restraint procedure and on RT.
- Emergency departments should specifically consider the management of violence. This should include training and staffing needs in order to maintain a safe environment.
- Acute hospital staff should be encouraged to report incidents of violence, allowing organisations to learn and adapt.
- Comprehensive liaison psychiatry services may have a positive impact on violence reduction across acute hospitals and should be approached for assistance.

Conclusion

Violence is commonplace in the acute hospital setting, with some services and patient groups at increased risk of being perpetrators and victims. The attention on robust risk assessment, management and prevention seen in other areas of healthcare is not always applied in acute hospitals, and this is due to a variety of particular challenges and barriers. Some of the most potentially challenging cases of ABD and ExD may enter the acute hospital setting, and the early identification and potential morbidity related to these conditions can be overlooked. We advocate the promotion of safer healthcare environments for patients and staff of the acute hospital settings through a process of training and education. This will ideally involve cross-organisational partnership work and a process of shared learning under robust localised governance systems.

References

1. HSJ Guides. Violence against NHS staff: A special report by HSJ and Unison, 2017; https://guides.hsj.co.uk/5713.guide [Accessed 29.4.2022].

2. Harwood RH. How to deal with violent and aggressive patients in acute medical settings. *Journal of the Royal College of Physicians of Edinburgh* 2017;47(2):94–101.

3. Rimmer, A. Excited delirium: What's the evidence for its use in medicine? *BMJ* 2021 May 5;373:n1156. https://doi.org/10.1136/bmj.n1156. PMID: 33952574.

4. College of Paramedics. Position Statement on Acute Behavioural Disturbance. [online]. 2018. www.collegeofparamedics.co.uk/COP/News/Statements%20and%20Consultations/COP/News/Statements_and_consultations.aspx?hkey=58e66fcf-4996-4b0a-b599-b3d52fc19348 [Accessed 29.4.2022].

5. Arnetz, J. E., Hamblin, L., Essenmacher, L. et al. Understanding patient-to-worker violence in hospitals: A qualitative analysis of documented incident reports. *Journal of Advanced Nursing* 2015;71(2):338–48.

6. Sztajnkrycer, M. D. and Baezz, A. A. Cocaine, excited delirium and sudden unexpected death. *Emergency Medical Services* 2005; 34(4):77–81.

7. Faculty of Forensic and Legal Medicine of the Royal College of Physicians. Acute behavioural disturbance (ABD): Guidelines on management in police custody. 2016.

8. Faculty of Forensic and Legal Medicine of the Royal College of Physicians. Acute behavioural disturbance (ABD): Guidelines on management in police custody. 2022. [online]. https://fflm.ac.uk/wp-content/uploads/2022/10/ABD-Guidelines-on-Management-in-Police-Custody-Oct-2022.pdf [Accessed 14.10.2022].

9. American College of Emergency Physicians. White Paper Report on Excited Delirium

Syndrome. [online]. 2009. www.prisonle galnews.org/media/publications/acep_re port_on_excited_delirium_syndrome_ sept_2009.pdf [Accessed 29.4.2022].

10. RCPsych. Follow-up on our statement regarding Acute Behavioural Disturbance (ABD); July 2021. [online]. www.rcpsych .ac.uk/news-and-features/latest-news/detai l/2021/07/16/follow-up-on-our-statement-regarding-acute-behavioural-disturbance-(abd) [Accessed 23. 4.22].

11. Police Federation of England & Wales (PFEW). PFEW totally refute statement on ABD by The Royal College of Psychiatrists; June 2021. [online]. www.polfed.org/news/ latest-news/2021/pfew-totally-refute-state ment-on-abd-by-the-royal-college-of-psy chiatrists/ [Accessed 23. 4.22].

12. Ruttenber, A. J., McAnally, H. B. and Wetli, C. V. Cocaine-associated rhabdomyolysis and excited delirium: Different stages of the same syndrome. *American Journal of Forensic Medicine and Pathology* 1999 Jun;20(2):120–7https://doi.org/10.1097/00 000433-199906000-00003. PMID:10414649.

13. Paquette, M. Excited delirium: Does it exist? *Perspectives in Psychiatric Care* 2003 Jul-Sep;39(3):93–4. https://doi.org/10.1111/j.17 44-6163.2003.00093.x. PMID: 14606228.

14. Costello, D., 'Excited delirium' as a cause of death, Los Angeles Times, April 21, 2003. https://www.latimes.com/archives/la-xpm-2003-apr-21-he-delirium21-story.html [Accessed 05.01.2023].

15. Gillings, M., Grundlingh, J. and Aw-Yong, M., Guidelines for the Management of Excited Delirium/Acute Behavioural Disturbance (ABD). Royal College of Emergency Medicine. 2016. See also RCEM Best Practice Guideline. Acute Behavioural Disturbance in Emergency Departments 2022.

16. Karch, S. B. The problem of police-related cardiac arrest. *Journal of Forensic and Legal Medicine* 2016 Jul;41:36–41. https://doi.or g/10.1016/j.jflm.2016.04.008. Epub 2016 Apr 9. PMID: 27126838.

17. Sethi, F., Parkes, J., Baskind, E., Paterson, B. and O'Brien, A. Restraint in mental health settings: is it time to declare a position? *British Journal of Psychiatry* 2018 Mar;212(3):137–141. https://doi.org/10.11 92/bjp.2017.31. PMID: 30071907.

18. Sheriffdom of Lothian and Borders at Edinburgh. Fatal Accident Inquiry into the Death of Allan Marshall. Sheriff Gordon Liddle. FAI 35, para 2. [online]. 2018. https:// scotcourts.gov.uk/docs/default-source/cos-g eneral-docs/pdf-docs-for-opinions/2019fa i35.pdf?sfvrsn=0 [Accessed 29.4.2022].

19. College of Policing. Authorised Professional Practice on Detention and Custody (control, restraint and searches). [online] 2016. www.app.college.police.uk/ app-content/detention-and-custody-2/con trol-restraint-and-searches/ [Accessed 28.4.2022].

20. NCEPOD. Treat as One: Bridging the gap between mental and physical healthcare in general hospitals, 2017. www.ncepod .org.uk/2017report1/downloads/TreatAsO ne_FullReport.pdf [Accessed 29.4.2022].

21. The Royal College of Emergency Medicine. Mental health in emergency departments: A toolkit for improving care. Revised April 2021. https://rcem.ac.uk/wp-content/uplo ads/2021/10/Mental_Health_Toolkit_Jun e21.pdf [Accessed 28.4.2022].

22. Department of Health. Reducing violence and aggression in A&E through a better experience. www.designcouncil.org.uk/site s/default/files/asset/document/ReducingVi olenceAndAggressionInAandE.pdf [Accessed 28.4.2022].

23. Royal College of Psychiatrists. Psychiatric Liaison Accreditation Network (PLAN) Quality Standards for Liaison Psychiatry Services, 6th ed., January 2020. www.rcpsych .ac.uk/improving-care/ccqi/quality-net works-accreditation/psychiatric-liaison-accre ditation-network-plan [Accessed 29.4.2022].

24. Health and Safety at Work Act 1974. www.legislation.gov.uk/ukpga/1974/37/ contents [Accessed 28.4.2022].

25. NHS Staff Council. Workplace health and safety standards, Revised 2013. www.csp .org.uk/system/files/documents/2019-07/ nhs_workplace_health_safety_stds_2013 .pdf [Accessed 29.4.2022].

26. HM Government. Criminal Justice and Immigration Act 2008. www.legislation.gov.uk/ukpga/2008/4/contents [Accessed 29.4.2022].

27. Royal College of Psychiatrists. Position statement on anaesthetics in restraint teams. www.rcpsych.ac.uk/docs/default-source/members/faculties/liaison-psychiatry/rcoa_rcpsych-restraint-statement.pdf?sfvrsn=61b12951_2 [Accessed 29.4.2022].

28. Taylor, D. M. , Barnes, T. R. E. , Young, A. H. *The Maudsley Prescribing Guidelines in Psychiatry*. 13th ed. 2018. London: Wiley-Blackwell.

29. HM Government. Official statistics NHS Staff Survey 2016. www.gov.uk/government/statistics/nhs-staff-survey-2016 [Accessed 29.4.2022].

30. Stene, J., Larson, E., Levy, M. and Dohlman, M. Workplace violence in the emergency department: Giving staff the tools and support to report. *The Permanente Journal* 2015 Spring;19(2):e113–7. https://doi.org/10.7812/TPP/14-187. PMID: 25902352; PMCID: PMC4403590.

31. Department of Health and Social Care. Code of Practice: Mental Health Act 1983: Published January 2015. Last updated October 2017. www.gov.uk/government/publications/code-of-practice-mental-health-act-1983 [Accessed 27.4.2022].

Forensic Psychiatry and Adult Inpatient Secure Settings

Elliott Carthy and Bradley Hillier

Introduction

Forensic psychiatry is a relatively new medical discipline that focuses on the assessment and treatment of mental disorders that appear to be associated, though not necessarily causally so, with offending behaviour. It is a multidisciplinary speciality that requires a close relationship with the legal system; one that is not always harmonious, but one that is necessary to balance the welfare of the individual with the duty to protect the public. The specific roles of a forensic psychiatrist include:

- the exploration, investigation and understanding of the relationship between mental disorder, violence and serious offending behaviour(s);
- the identification, assessment and treatment of mentally disordered offenders (MDOs) interfacing with the criminal justice system at various stages. This requires an in-depth knowledge of mental health and criminal legal (medico-legal) frameworks;
- the specialised management of severely disturbed, violent and aggressive behaviour occurring in the context of mental disorders in various settings;
- the use of therapeutic security within the secure psychiatric system to assess, treat and rehabilitate MDOs and/or those with significant risks of violence to others, thereby reducing recidivism.

To fully appreciate the current provision of forensic inpatient services, it is necessary to understand the historical context which has brought about their existence and distribution. This chapter will therefore be divided into two parts: we will first set the context within which forensic services in England and Wales (E&W) have developed through a brief description of the history of forensic psychiatry and how this influenced the development of secure psychiatric services. In the second part we will outline the current structure of inpatient secure psychiatric settings, including the current challenges in managing this complex cohort of individuals.

A Brief History of Forensic Psychiatry in England and Wales

The existence and development of forensic psychiatric services in E&W are best understood within their historical context, since there are a number of key events, cases, incidents and inquiries which have shaped it, rather than through strategically planned service development.

Like most mental health inpatient settings in E&W, the origins of forensic services can be found in the 'asylum' system. At the end of the sixteenth century, there was only one public asylum for the 'insane' in England: Bethlehem Hospital in London (also known as

'Bethlem' and, notoriously, as 'Bedlam'). By the end of the seventeenth century, there were several others in cities such as Liverpool, Manchester, York and Norwich [1]. However, places were limited, and there was an expansion of privately owned 'madhouses' operating for profit. Understandably, concerns arose about a conflict of interest, with unjust admissions for the sake of commercial gain. This led to the first major attempts to formalise the detention of people with mental illnesses in statute through the Act for Regulating Madhouses (1774) (otherwise known as the 1774 Madhouses Act; Table 11.1) [2]. This was the first time that private 'madhouses' became subject to state regulation and responsibility.

Although there has been recognition of mental disorders playing a role in offending since at least the seventh or eighth centuries, the Prerogativa Regis (1322) formally defined the role of the King in scenarios where an individual could not be tried, or was mentally ill and could not be held responsible [3]. In this circumstance, the individual was usually released to their family or held in prison pending a Royal Pardon, even for capital offences such as murder or treason. The prevailing legal concept was (by modern standards, stigmatising and pejorative) the 'wild beast test' [4].

The awareness of mental illness increased significantly during the reign of George III (1760–1820), not least owing to the king's own mental health problems, as he suffered from porphyria (although other severe and enduring mental illness has also been proposed) [5]. There were also significant developments at the start of the nineteenth century within the criminal justice system. These arose from several notorious, high-profile cases which required the state to enact legislation to account for these scenarios – a process which has become familiar in forensic psychiatric service development in general. These were the cases of James Hadfield, Pritchard and Daniel M'Naghten.

James Hadfield and the Criminal Lunatics Act 1800

James Hadfield [1, 6, 7] was a British soldier who sustained a traumatic brain injury at the Battle of Lincelles in Flanders in 1794 and suffered from 'violent episodes of madness' thereafter. He was discharged from the Army on the grounds of insanity. In May 1800, he attempted to assassinate King George III by firing a pistol towards the Royal Box in the Drury Lane Theatre in London as the king entered. Hadfield believed that God had decreed that he needed to die to save the world but that he must not die by his own hand and therefore sought to commit treason, an offence he knew was punishable by death. However, his mental illness was identified at trial and, ultimately, Lord Kenyon, Lord Chief Justice and the judge in the case of such gravity, directed the jury to find him 'Not guilty: he being under the influence of insanity at the time the act was committed'. Although acquitted, his dangerousness rendered it unsafe for him to be released into the community, with His Lordship adding that the verdict 'was clearly an acquittal . . . but . . . the prisoner, for his own sake, and for the sake of society at large, must not be discharged' [7, p. 508].

Owing to the very specific circumstances of the case – involving the king and being heard by the Lord Chief Justice – urgent provisions were made for the detention of those found to be insane, though acquitted of treason, murder or certain other capital offences at 'His Majesty's Pleasure', this being in the form of the rapidly progressed Criminal Lunatics Act 1800 which gained Royal Assent on 28 July 1800 [4]. It did not state where individuals should be detained or any details regarding treatment for a mental disorder. The Act for the Better Care and Maintenance of Pauper and Criminal Lunatics 1808 then specified provisions to permit admission of these individuals to asylums providing funding was available [4]. The Amendment Act 1816 permitted transfer of sentenced prisoners to asylums for those with mental illness while serving a penal sentence, whilst later acts also considered those on remand awaiting trial, the transfer of those with intellectual disabilities and extended the jurisdiction to cases of lesser offending in due course.

R v. *Pritchard* (1836) and Fitness to Plead and Stand Trial

The next major development in clinic-legal frameworks relating to MDOs was the case of Pritchard, who was deaf and mute; he was accused of bestiality, which was a capital offence. Through having been educated in an institution for individuals with such disabilities, Pritchard was able to indicate a sign that he was 'not guilty', meaning that a jury considered that he was able to plead. The judge, Baron Alderson, did not consider that being able to indicate a plea was the same as being fit to plead and proposed a state and functionally based test for a jury to consider [8] (as was the case at that time, as opposed to now where it is a single judge). This invited them to consider first whether the defendant was sane or not, and, if not, to consider three elements:

> First, whether the prisoner is mute of malice or not; secondly, whether he can plead to the indictment or not; thirdly, whether he is of sufficient intellect to comprehend the course of proceedings on the trial, so as to make a proper defence – to know that he might challenge any of you to whom he may object – and to comprehend the details of the evidence.

These principles have been further developed through case law and informed by expert evidence, though they remain under constant debate as to their suitability for the modern legal system and understanding of mental disorders, which is beyond the scope of this chapter (however, this is discussed by Brown [9], and the Law Commission Discussion Paper on Unfitness to Plead [10] for those who are interested). Box 11.1 details the current Pritchard Criteria, and their most recent interpretation, and a helpful review of their historical development, including case law, is found in *Marcantonio* v. *R* (2016) [11]. It could be reasonably said that it is a highly subjective test (on the part of the assessor) and does not infrequently lead to contested opinion in court, the issue ultimately being decided by a single judge on the strength of the arguments.

Daniel M'Naghten and the M'Naghten Rules (1843)

The third significant case in further establishing the role of mental disorder in considerations of criminal responsibility is that of Daniel M'Naghten. In January 1943,

---

Box 11.1 Pritchard Criteria

To be fit to plead and stand trial, the defendant must be able to:
1. Understand the charges and evidence
2. Understand the difference between a guilty and not guilty plea
3. Instruct a defence counsel
4. Challenge a juror
5. Follow proceedings
6. Give evidence in their own defence

M'Naghten shot Edward Drummond, Prime Minister Sir Robert Peel's private secretary, in the back in the mistaken belief that he was shooting the prime minister. Drummond died five days later and M'Naghten was placed on trial for the 'wilful murder of Mr Drummond' [12].

M'Naghten harboured delusional beliefs of a conspiracy against him, led by the Tory party (the precursor of the Conservative political party in the United Kingdom), and at his trial said:

> The Tories in my native city have compelled me to do this. They follow, persecute me wherever I go, and have entirely destroyed my peace of mind … It can be proved by evidence. That is all I have to say. [13, 14]

Medical evidence and other witnesses in court highlighted that 'M'Naghten's delusions had deprived him of "all restraint over his actions"', leading to him being found 'not guilty by reason of insanity' (NGRI). He spent the rest of his life in an asylum.

This outcome, and subsequent debate, led to the referral of the issues identified in the case to the House of Lords (the highest criminal court at that time) in the form of a series of hypothetical questions. Subsequently, a formalised set of more specific principles to limit the circumstances in which such a verdict could be reached were developed. The outcome of this was the M'Naghten Rules 1843 [15], which form the ongoing basis of insanity defences in common law jurisdictions as follows:

> the jurors ought to be told in all cases that **every man is to be presumed to be sane**, and to possess a sufficient degree of reason to be **responsible** for his crimes, until the contrary be proved to their satisfaction; and that **to establish a defence on the ground of insanity**, it must be **clearly proved** that, **at the time** of the committing of the act, the party accused was labouring under such a **defect of reason**, from **disease of the mind**, as **not to know the nature and quality of the act he was doing**; or, **if he did know it, that he did not know he was doing what was wrong**.

These principles have been subject to ongoing legal interpretation, including clarifications on what constitutes 'disease of the mind', and the meaning of 'wrong' as legally wrong. It is broadly recognised that there are challenges in the use of a 170-year-old set of legal rules in conjunction with the advances that have occurred in modern neuroscience and psychiatry; nonetheless, they form the current position, and this is discussed in a recent Law Commission Discussion Paper on Insanity and Automatism [16]. It is somewhat paradoxical that the eponymous rules would have led to M'Naghten himself being found guilty, rather than NGRI which, perhaps, indicates their intention.

Development of the Secure Psychiatric Estate

When James Hadfield was detained, the only appropriate setting was Bethlem Royal Hospital, where he subsequently escaped before being returned to prison, then later back to hospital, where he was then detained for the rest of his life. The Hadfield case therefore not only highlighted a gap in legislation about the disposal options for such individuals but also the risks associated with admitting 'dangerous' individuals to county asylums. This consequently led to the development of purpose-built institutions for MDOs, either in purpose-built wings within larger asylums or entirely separate buildings. Two 'criminal' blocks were built as part of the new Bethlem Hospital that opened in 1816 [1], whereby the discharge of patients from these settings would be at the discretion of the Home Secretary.

They quickly filled to capacity, and debates continued about the most suitable setting to manage such patients – bearing in mind that 'care' at this time primarily constituted physical and mechanical restraint.

In 1850, the Dundrum Central Criminal Asylum was built outside Dublin (at that time part of the United Kingdom) as the first wave of the developing philosophy to separate MDOs from prison settings. This was the first secure psychiatric hospital in the world and preceded the construction of Broadmoor Criminal Lunatic Asylum in Berkshire in 1863, with subsequent additional secure hospitals being established owing to increasing capacity requirements: these included Rampton Criminal Lunatic Asylum (as a Broadmoor 'branch') in Nottinghamshire in 1913, and two hospitals in Liverpool called Moss Side and Park Lane, which later merged to become Ashworth Hospital in the 1970s. In Scotland, the State Hospital at Carstairs served a similar function.

The E&W institutions remained under the supervision of the Board of Control for Lunacy and Mental Deficiency, including following the foundation of the National Health Service in 1948, although on the introduction of the Mental Health Act (MHA) 1959 [17], the ownership and responsibility for the institutions in E&W were transferred to the Ministry of Health and later become known as the Special Hospitals, with their own administrative arrangements. A detailed history of the administration and oversight until approximately 1999 is contained in the Fallon Report into Ashworth Hospital Personality Disorder Unit [18].

Now, the management of these hospitals is by three separate NHS trusts in the form of the High Secure Psychiatric Estate. For many years these institutions formed the only type of secure psychiatric inpatient setting, meaning that there was a significant step in both security and expertise when a patient reached the point of discharge.

Table 11.1 outlines key pieces of legislation which have impacted on the interface between secure psychiatric services and the criminal justice system (CJS). At the time of writing, the current MHA is under consultation and may introduce further changes to the way MDOs are diverted from the CJS [19].

The Creation of Stepped Secure Services: The Butler Review

In the latter part of the twentieth century, the combination of overcrowding and change in the focus of mental health care away from inpatient provisions to the community meant that the model of secure care needed to adapt. There was a clear need for secure beds outside of specialist hospitals that balanced the need for protection of the public with least restrictive practice. The specialised, maximum-security hospitals were full, leading to many mentally ill patients being sent to prison as an alternative and struggling to access appropriate treatment and support. In 1961, the Working Party on Special Hospitals recommended that regional hospital boards provide a variety of types of hospital units, including secure units, though these recommendations were never implemented [20, 21]. It was the case of Graham Young (see Box 11.2) that accelerated reforms of secure mental health care and risk management following public outcry, leading to the commissioning of the Butler Review into procedures for releasing offenders for psychiatric hospitals and supervision of released patients [22]. This recommended the creation of regional secure units (RSUs), which forms the basis of the forensic inpatient system that exists today. Later events (e.g. the killing of Jonathan Zito by Christopher Clunis and the subsequent Ritchie Enquiry) [23] led to the development of community forensic services, which are

Table 11.1 Key pieces of legislation in the development of forensic psychiatry

Legislation	What did it do?
Madhouses Act 1774	Set limits on the number of admissions Created licences and regular inspections for madhouse proprietors Medical certification became necessary for the incarceration of lunatics
The Criminal Lunatics Act 1800	Provisions for the detention of those found to be insane, though acquitted of treason, murder or felony at His Majesty's Pleasure
The County Asylums Act 1808	Specified provisions to permit admission of pauper lunatics to asylums, including from workhouses and prisons
The Madhouse Act 1828	Increased the number of Commissioners and extend their role to include inquiry of behaviour of attendants and investigate patient complaints. Appointment of lay members as well as the medically qualified Commissioners given powers to revoke a proprietor's licence if the conditions were inadequate
The Lunatics Act 1845	Empowered Commissioners (by now called Lunacy Commissioners) to inspect asylums throughout the country and workhouses and gaols
Trial of Lunatics Act 1883	Prompted by Queen Victoria to remove NGRI to a verdict of 'guilty but insane'; later repealed by the Criminal Procedure and Insanity Act 1964
The Lunacy Act 1890	Private asylums permitted to receive both voluntary and involuntary admissions Public asylums limited to admissions under an order of the Act or following inquisition
The Mental Treatment Act 1930	Temporary admission orders for up to six months to allow for shorter admissions Allowed voluntary admissions to public mental hospitals
Homicide Act 1957	Inclusion of diminished responsibility in English law as a partial defence to murder of manslaughter, in context of a death penalty existing at that time for murder
The Mental Health Act 1959	Compulsory civil admissions became medical rather than judicial matters Criminal admissions and transfers from prison remained the concern of the judiciary and the Home Office
Criminal Procedure and Insanity Act 1964	Introduced the formal legal procedure and outcomes for individuals considered unfit to plead and stand trial, and found to be NGRI; some procedural amendments in 1991 and 2004
Mental Health Act 1983	Primary legislative framework defining the legal rights and powers concerning those with a mental disorder
The Mental Health Act 1983 (amended 2007)	Updated version of the MHA that included consent to treatment, Community Treatment Orders (CTOs) and broadened definition of 'Mental Disorder'
Coroners and Justice Act 2009	Amended the criteria for Diminished Responsibility to a test with narrower interpretation and with a capacity-based component

---

Box 11.2 Graham Young and regional secure units

Graham Young, otherwise known as the 'Teacup Poisoner' or 'St Albans Poisoner', was detained at Broadmoor Hospital in 1962 at the age of 14 [24]. He was convicted of administering a poison to his father, sister and school friend, although his step-mother also died but he was not charged with her murder since poisoning was not noted as her cause of death. He was assessed as suffering from a psychopathic disorder and admitted to Broadmoor, although he was discharged in 1971. However, he was able to obtain work on the tea trolley in a factory making lenses in 1972 and, although he was known to probation services, details of his index offences were not shared. Whilst he worked at the factory, multiple mysterious 'outbreaks' of illness attracted the attention of public health professionals who were investigating an infective source of unknown origin. Young's inability to refrain from demonstrating his knowledge of poisons being associated with the symptoms described drew attention to him, and further investigations on the victims, including two deaths, demonstrated the presence of antimony and thallium. He was convicted of two murders and two attempted murders and spent the rest of his life in prison.

---

described in Chapter 17. We will now describe the current structure and function of forensic inpatient services.

Current Structure and Function of Forensic Inpatient Services

Secure inpatient services provide assessment and treatment of adults with complex mental disorders linked to behaviours that are seriously harmful to others and/or associated with offending. Inpatients in forensic services are invariably detained under the MHA, and their risk of harm to others and risks associated with escape from hospital cannot be contained within non-secure settings. In E&W, these services are commissioned by NHS England, which provides the service specifications for all three levels of secure psychiatric settings: high, medium and low secure [25–27]. The key concepts when understanding how forensic inpatient services work relate to:

- Therapeutic security and how it is defined;
- Levels of security and how security needs for patients are assessed;
- Interfaces with other settings and pathways through secure services to discharge;
- Services for women and other specialist need groups.

Domains of Therapeutic Security

Therapeutic security in forensic settings is conceptualised within three broad domains: physical, procedural and relational security. These are summarised in Box 11.3 and have been developed progressively as secure services have developed. Kennedy [28] provides a comprehensive overview of these different security concepts and the ways in which they may flex and predominate in differing levels of secure setting, although clear service specifications whereby these were formally operationalised did not occur until the mid-2000s [29].

Since that time, there have been significant developments in characterising and measuring the more conceptually challenging relational security, which can be more

Box 11.3 Types of Therapeutic Security

Physical security: the specifications of the secure environment (e.g. height of perimeter fences, number of airlocks, design to impede or prevent escape).

Procedural security: timely, correct and consistent application of effective operational procedures and policies (e.g. sign out process for keys, appropriate use of alarm equipment).

Relational security: understanding and use of knowledge about individual patients, the environment and population dynamics to inform risk assessment, management and therapeutic interventions accordingly (e.g. as elaborated in 'See Think Act' [30, 31]).

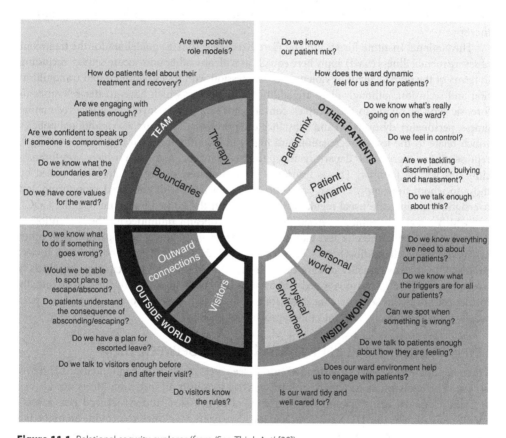

Figure 11.1 Relational security explorer (from 'See Think Act' [30])

readily identified by clinicians as the basis of the therapeutic practice and principles guiding treatment in secure settings. The practical policy guide 'See Think Act' was developed in 2010 in conjunction with the Quality Network for Forensic Mental Health Services (QNFMHS) at the Royal College of Psychiatrists' (RCPsych) College Centre for Quality Improvement (CCQI); it provides a core framework for approaching relational security and has been used to develop tools to measure this [31, 32]. Figure 11.1 shows the 'Relational Security Explorer' and the key domains that inpatient teams should be considering when approaching the care and treatment of MDOs in forensic settings [33].

Secure services do not differ from non-secure services in terms of the types of staff working within them. However, unlike non-forensic services, there has been significantly less pressure to reduce the number of beds, with approximately 50% of the current number of psychiatric beds in E&W being in secure settings [2]. As in non-secure settings, the team works in a multidisciplinary way, although the focus of any admission is significantly influenced by the risk assessment, particularly of violence to others, using structured risk assessment tools (such as the HCR-20) [34], the legal circumstances within which the individual finds themselves, occupational therapy, psychology and nursing assessment, and the way in which the individual engages and responds to therapy.

The National Institute for Health and Care Excellence (NICE) guidelines for the treatment of severe mental illness (SMI) apply here equally as with any other non-secure setting, including in terms of the management of violence and aggression with de-escalation, rapid tranquillisation and seclusion, although there are additional guidelines which have greater relevance in forensic services owing to the complex comorbidities frequently involving a triad of mental illness, personality dysfunction and substance use problems. There are also additional policies which relate to the use of segregation and night-time confinement (in high secure settings), representing a significant departure from the standard practice with which non-forensic clinicians will be familiar. This is informed proportionately by the risk to others posed by those to whom they apply. These procedures are associated with enhanced monitoring and oversight, including the usual regulatory bodies within the United Kingdom (e.g. the CQC), and which can also be subject to inspection by the European Committee for the Prevention of Torture (CPT) [35]. There is also increasing and beneficial regional collaboration with other services to ensure that idiosyncratic practice does not arise, as well as supportive peer review processes to improve quality of care through the QNFMHS [32], participation in which is a requirement of being commissioned. Importantly (and not without controversy when initially introduced owing to security concerns), former forensic inpatients form a part of the peer review team and directly feed into the improvement process.

Levels of Security and Pathways Within and Between Them

Forensic inpatient services are divided into three levels of security: high, medium and low secure. The decision as to which level of security to admit an individual to is not always a straightforward decision and, beyond clinical impression and structured risk assessment, tools such as the 'DUNDRUM Quartet' have been developed to provide an objective evidence-based assessment of this [36], as well as the use of independent admission panels and appeals processes (in particular with regard to high secure services). However, these are used by services on an individual basis rather than forming any part of a service specification. Table 11.2 outlines the approximate numbers and cost for each of the levels of security.

High Secure Services

There are three hospitals in the United Kingdom that provide dedicated high-security services for males with severe and enduring mental illness and/or personality disorder:

Table 11.2 Demographics of secure services [25, 37, 38]

Conditions	Number of units	Number of beds	Average length of stay	Approximate cost per person per annum (£)
High security	3 (Broadmoor, Rampton and Ashworth)	630	5–6 years	250–350,000
Medium security	60 (approximately)	2800	2–4 years	175–200,000
Low security	Not known	2500	Not known	Up to 150,000

Broadmoor Hospital in Berkshire, Rampton Hospital in Nottinghamshire and Ashworth Hospital in Merseyside; these hospitals cover London and the South, the Midlands and the North of England, respectively. Rampton Hospital also provides national specialist high secure services for women, people who are deaf and males with learning disabilities [25]. The physical security arrangements within high secure services are equivalent to that of a Category B prison, though they can treat those who would have otherwise required a Category A prison environment. High secure hospitals are subject to the High Security Psychiatric Services (Arrangements for Safety and Security) Directions 2019 [39], which outline requirements concerning safety, security and the management of patients. The high secure hospitals must adhere to the Clinical Security Framework and will engage with the Clinical Secure Practice Forum (CSPF) and the National Oversight Group (NOG), which provides line of sight for the Secretary of State for Health. They also actively participate in the Offender Personality Disorder (OPD) pathway [40] and continue to provide specific forensic personality disorder inpatient services in contrast to the shift to prison-based PD services at lower levels of security. The acceptance criteria for admission to high secure services is summarised in Box 11.4.

High secure services provide care to those deemed a 'grave and imminent risk to the others that cannot be managed in lower levels of security' [25 p.4]. Crucially, these services are for individuals who **must not** be able to escape from hospital. All patients are detained under the MHA. Patients may be admitted directly from the CJS, including prisons, or as an escalation from medium security. Further assessment and treatment then aims for patients to be stepped-down to lower levels of security, usually on a 'trial leave' basis for six months, although return to prison remains a discharge pathway. It is exceptionally rare for patients to be discharged from high secure settings directly to the community.

There are some forms of investigation and treatment which tend to be only considered in high secure settings for reasons of proportionality and coercion, as well as most other standard treatments having been exhausted by the time a high secure admission occurs. Although high secure admission is not a requirement to do so, these may include:

- Nasogastric administration of Clozapine [41];
- Electroconvulsive therapy in highly refractory treatment-resistant SMI [42];
- Use of depot anti-libidinal medication [43], often guided with penile plethysmography (PPG) assessment.

Box 11.4 High Secure Service Acceptance and Exclusion Criteria

Acceptance Criteria

- The patient must be suffering from a mental disorder (including mental illness, neuro-developmental disorder and personality disorder), as defined within the Mental Health Act 1983, which is of a nature and/or degree warranting detention in hospital for medical treatment and that appropriate treatment is available.
- The patient must be assessed as presenting a grave risk of harm to others; appropriate management of the risk requires inpatient care, specialist risk management procedures and treatment interventions that cannot be provided safely in lower levels of security.
- Patients suitable for transfer from prisons under the Mental Health Act will generally be charged with or have been convicted of a specified violent or sexual offence as defined in Schedule 15 of the Criminal Justice Act 2003, or another serious offence such as murder or arson with intent to endanger life.
- On occasion, patients will be accepted without criminal charges pending where there is clear evidence of grave risk of harm to others. In such cases, there will generally be a pattern of assaults and escalating threats which may, in the light of an access assessment, constitute grounds for admission.
- Patients directed to conditions of high security by the Ministry of Justice even if they have not been assessed to be a grave risk of harm to others by the individual hospital.

Exclusion Criteria

- People who do not present a grave risk of harm to others should not be admitted to high secure services and should be referred to medium or low secure services.
- People with a severe learning disability and who present with dangerous behaviours will in most cases require bespoke packages of care in non-high secure settings.
- People who present with severe self-harm should only be admitted to high secure services if their risk to others clearly necessitates it.

Medium Secure Services

Medium secure services are provided by both the NHS and the independent sector, with the latter providing approximately 35% of medium secure care nationally [26, 44]. Medium secure services care for those presenting a 'serious risk of harm to others and whose escape from hospital must be prevented' [26 p.2]. As noted in Table 11.2, there are approximately 2,800 medium secure beds in E&W, with average length of stay being 2–4 years. The primary routes of admission are mainly from the courts and prisons (either remand or sentenced prisoners), and occasionally from lower levels of security where the risks require higher therapeutic security. Step-down from high security also constitutes an admission route through a trial leave and full transfer process, as does urgent recall from the community for conditionally discharged patients.

There are various models of care within medium secure services, which can be determined by the size of the unit (some services have only two or three wards) and collaboration with other services (both NHS and independent); for example, some services operate on the basis of a specified admission ward which carries out a (usually) twelve-week initial assessment by members of the multidisciplinary team, at which point the information is reviewed in a Care Programme Approach (CPA) meeting to identify further treatment needs and pathways. Larger services, or those with a collaborative relationship with partner organisations, may have wards specifically focused on medium or higher dependency needs for more complex cases. A similar arrangement is often made for patients with treatment-resistant illness or greater risks, in addition to the provision of rehabilitation wards. Smaller services may collaborate with forensic providers within their region to specialise within the catchment area, although large services may also benefit from such collaborations where more specialised services are needed (e.g. medium secure LD settings, women's services or where there are exclusion zone issues relating to victims that prevent leave from being granted).

Low Secure Services

Low secure services provide care and treatment who present a 'significant risk of harm to others and whose escape from hospital must be impeded' [27 p.2]. However, low security is a more ill-defined concept, comprising dedicated low secure units, but also long-stay secure wards, locked rehabilitation wards and psychiatric intensive care units. It is therefore unclear how many low secure services are available nationally and the length of stay. In 2013, the independent charity, the Centre for Mental Health, estimated that there were 2,500 low secure beds available, with an annual cost of approximately £150,000 per bed [38], and the National Association of Psychiatric Intensive Care and Low Secure services (NAPICU) [45] has collaborated with the RCPsych QNFMHS to provide clearer service specifications and requirements in conjunction with the national low secure specification from NHS England [27]. However, commissioning arrangements can vary depending on the region and historical context. The transfer between medium and low secure services can often be a bottleneck and can lead to patients remaining at an inappropriate (and more expensive) level of security. The development of specialist Community Forensic Teams (CFTs) that provide more assertive 'in-reaching' to both medium and low secure wards has recently been introduced as a partial solution to this challenge, as well as partnership between provider organisations to use these expensive resources as effectively as possible across a wider geographical area. CFTs are discussed further in Chapter 17.

Although beyond the scope of this chapter, and discussed further in Chapter 17, it should be acknowledged that there remain gaps in provision of the secure pathway, primarily arising from the way that it is currently commissioned. These include, for example: the lack of a clear pathway to CFTs for prisoners with mental disorder who do not meet the threshold for a secure admission during their sentence, or who may have to be returned to prison before release; and the pathway for individuals who may be in non-forensic services, but may benefit from forensic community management. For this group, specialised CFT input is not commissioned, and local arrangements may be required. These gaps highlight ongoing challenges with integration of this complex group with healthcare services.

Women's Secure Services

Women comprise only 6% of the prison population and are responsible for 6% of murders, 1.5% of attempted murders, 16% of manslaughters and 1.3% of sexual crimes [46]. Most women detained in conditions of security have convictions for arson [47] and are admitted to high and medium security due to self-harm, suicidal acts, aggression towards staff and damage to property [48]. Most have a primary diagnosis of emotionally unstable personality disorder [49, 50].

Rampton Hospital provides the national high secure service for women from England and Wales (and, with commissioner approval, referrals from Scotland and Northern Ireland) and works closely with the women's OPD pathway [25]. Prior to this, women could be detained in all three high secure hospitals. In 2007, three Women's Enhanced Medium Secure Services (WEMSS) were developed to provide care for those women who no longer needed high security, but whose risk to others required conditions of enhanced relational security. Subsequently, the number of women in high secure settings dropped from 345 in 1991 to 50 in 2008, with Rampton then becoming the sole provider of women's high secure care [46]. At present the provision of WEMSS beds occurs at three sites in London, Manchester and Leicestershire, all having national catchment and amounting to approximately 40 beds. In 2009, there were 27 standard women's medium secure units (18 within the NHS and 9 in the independent sector), amounting to a total of 543 beds.

Deaf Secure Services

Rampton Hospital provides a designated National High Secure Deaf Service, which includes specialist deaf staff, access to sign language interpreters and communication support workers [25]. Therapeutic interventions can also be delivered using British Sign Language where necessary. This unit can accommodate up to ten male patients irrespective of diagnosis. Rampton also provides a deaf prison in-reach service. At lower levels of security, there has been development of deaf services to meet the needs of this group, provided primarily within the independent sector, although support is provided on an ad hoc basis by the National Deaf Service at South West London and St George's NHS Trust on request [51].

Learning Disability and Neurodevelopmental Secure Services

Rampton Hospital provides a national service for men with learning disability from England and Wales. This dedicated unit comprising 54 beds across four wards supports all male patients with a learning disability requiring conditions of high security, irrespective of diagnosis. There are also services within medium and low security (and increasingly specialist community forensic neurodevelopmental teams), although access to these is strictly assessed owing to the 'Transforming Care' agenda in response to the Winterbourne View Hospital scandal [52]. There are also services available for autistic individuals without a learning disability where this is related to their offending.

Pathways Through Secure Services and Part III of the MHA

While some patients may be escalated to secure services under a civil section of the MHA, most are detained under Part III of the Act, which is indicative of the stage of their legal proceedings, their status as a sentenced or unsentenced prisoner and the nature of any

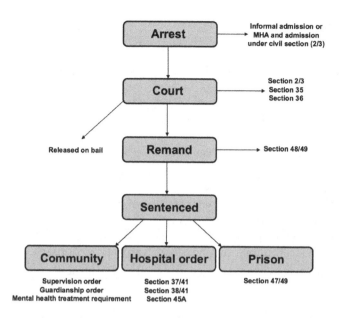

Figure 11.2 Criminal justice pathway for offenders with a mental disorder, highlighting the stages at which the role of the MHA may be considered and the relevant Section depending on whether the individual has been arrested, charged and held or remand or sentenced.

restrictions to which they are subject. As shown in Figure 11.2, forensic practitioners and frameworks can play a role before, during and after court proceedings for patients with known or suspected mental disorders. Diversion from the CJS is covered in Chapter 17.

Table 11.3 summarises the commonly used sections for MDOs and the clinico-legal implications that these may indicate for an individual's pathway. The primary difference between forensic and non-forensic services is the volume of individuals who are under special restrictions with either Section 41 or 49 of the MHA applying, owing to their status as restricted patients or prisoners. Although individual factors will determine the rate at which individuals pass along the forensic pathway to obtain escorted and unescorted leave, and ultimately discharge, there is a significant difference between those who are restricted and those who are not. The management of patients who are subject to restrictions with regards to obligations clinicians and services have for reporting, risk management and victim liaison is detailed in recent guidance from the Ministry of Justice [53].

Discharge from Inpatient Forensic Services

It is the aim for all individuals admitted to forensic services to progress along a care pathway towards discharge through rehabilitation and recovery, reduction of risk through biopsychosocial interventions, and a period of gradual but proportionate testing in settings of least restriction. It is important to recognise that for some individuals this may be a challenging process, and there is evidence that a significant proportion of individuals may be regarded as 'long-term'. Based on recent studies, this comprises approximately 24% of high secure patients and 17% of those in medium secure units [44]. There have been calls for a strategy to address this, and it may be that the specialised CFTs in combination with a potential expansion of low secure services may provide this. However, for the majority who do progress to discharge to live in the

Table 11.3 Forensic Sections under Part III of the Mental Health Act with practical considerations

Section	Details
Section 35	Purpose: Remand to hospital for report on accused's mental condition Available at any stage of the court case Duration: 28 days (extended to a maximum of 12 weeks) Recommended by: Magistrates or Crown Court Appeal: No grounds to appeal Leave: Emergency only, usually requiring handcuffs and multi-staff escort.
Section 36	Remand to hospital for treatment of the accused's mental condition Available at any stage of the court case Duration: 28 days (extended to a maximum of 12 weeks) Recommended by: Magistrates or Crown Court Appeal: No grounds to appeal Leave: Emergency only, usually requiring handcuffs and multi-staff escort.
Section 48/49	Section 48: Transfer direction from prison to hospital for **unsentenced** prisoners Section 49: Restriction direction Duration: Until statutory criteria for detention no longer met, or disposed in some other way (including other MHA orders) Recommended by: Two medical recommendations and agreement from the Ministry of Justice Appeal: Once during the first 6 months, once during the next 6 months, and once in every year after that, although 'discharge' is back to prison. Leave: Emergency only, usually requiring handcuffs and multi-staff escort.
Section 38	Section 38: Interim hospital order (convicted and detained for further assessment before sentencing) Duration: Initially 3 months and thereafter renewable for 28 days at a time up to 12 months Recommended by: Two medical recommendations (at least one Section 12 approved) and agreement from the Crown Court Appeal: No grounds to appeal Leave: Emergency only, usually requiring handcuffs and multi-staff escort.
Section 37/41	Section 37: Hospital order (disposal) Section 41: Restriction order – leading to supervision by Secretary of State for Justice Duration: Section 37: Until nature and degree no longer satisfied Section 41: Without limit of time and until nature and degree and risks to public no longer satisfied Recommended by: Two medical recommendations (at least one Section 12 approved and for Section 41 oral evidence from one) at the Crown Court Appeal: May not apply during the 6 months starting with the day the court made the hospital order. After that, may apply once during the next 6 months and then once in every year after that. In Section 41 cases discharge can only occur by the tribunal or at the discretion of the Secretary of State for Justice

Table 11.3 (cont.)

Section	Details
	(rarely exercised) and is almost always subject to 'conditions' being a 'Conditional Discharge' under Section 42, with burden of proof on patient to satisfy tribunal statutory criteria no longer met. Leave: Section 37: At discretion of responsible clinician. Section 37/41: Only with express permission from the Ministry of Justice on application.
Section 45A	Hospital direction and limitation direction ('Hybrid order' – a prison sentence is given but starts in hospital; transfer back to prison can occur at any point prior to earliest release date). These are controversial within forensic and legal circles. Duration: Dependent on tariff/sentence and/or until statutory criteria for admission no longer met. Recommended by: Two medical recommendations (at least one Section 12 approved and on oral evidence from one) and agreement from the Crown Court Appeal: May not apply during the 6 months starting with the day the court made the order. After that, may apply once during the next 6 months and then once in every year after that, although if within tariff 'discharge' is to prison. Leave: At discretion of the Ministry of Justice and likely to be informed by stage in care pathway.
Section 47/49	Section 47: Transfer direction from prison to hospital (sentenced prisoner) Section 49: Restriction direction Duration: Until statutory criteria no longer met or sentence has ended (converted to notional s37 if ongoing treatment in hospital is required) Recommended by: Two medical recommendations and agreement from the Ministry of Justice Appeal: Once during the first 6 months, once during the next 6 months, and once in every year after that; 'discharge' within tariff is back to prison. Leave: At discretion of the Ministry of Justice and likely to be informed by progress/individual factors given status as sentenced prisoner.

community, there are specific services available to provide support and supervision to facilitate recovery and greater independence, whilst aiming to prevent recidivism, relapse and readmission or imprisonment. The role of community forensic services is discussed in Chapter 17.

Impact of COVID19 on Secure Psychiatric Settings

Inpatient forensic mental health services have not been immune to the impact of the COVID-19 pandemic. A recent systematic review and meta-analysis found that the presence of a pre-existing mental disorder and exposure to antipsychotics, antidepressants and anxiolytics were associated with increased odds of hospitalisation and mortality from COVID-19 [54]. For those detained in secure hospitals, the pandemic was associated with an overall increase in long-term segregation and, in some cases, violence and self-harm [55]. There have also been some anecdotal reports of reduced adherence to public health measures, such as social distancing and wearing masks. The risks are accentuated further by the longer length of stay in secure hospitals, pre-existing physical health comorbidities and greater socio-economic deprivation, and high rates of metabolic side effects of psychotropic medication. Those who recover from COVID-19 may also be at increased risk of future mental disorders [56]. Ross et al. [57] have produced a helpful guide to assist decision-making on issues around the COVID-19 vaccination for those with SMI.

The Role of the Inpatient Psychiatrist as Professional and Expert Witness

Forensic (and non-forensic) psychiatrists will often be asked to provide expert assistance on medico-legal matters, particularly in the criminal courts, and often for their own or other inpatients, including in response to incidents within their own wards between patients or towards staff. These requests may include (but not be limited to):

- The state of mind of defendants in criminal cases;
- Sentencing of offenders with mental disorders;
- Psychiatric defences such as diminished responsibility and NGRI;
- Fitness to plead and stand trial;
- The mental capacity of people making legal decisions.

It is important that those accepting instructions to provide independent expert evidence are familiar with an expert's duties, have undertaken appropriate training and comply with the relevant practice directions of the criminal or civil justice system.

It is also important to consider whether what is being asked from any agency, be it solicitor, police or court, is information that places the doctor in the role of a *professional* or *expert* witness. The primary distinction is that the former provides evidence of fact, whereas the expert can give specialist opinion within their area of expertise. An example might be the distinction between advising a court of a diagnosis that a patient has (professional) as opposed to providing an opinion on that person's 'capacity to form intent' (expert).

This is a complex area and there are frequent requests of all clinicians to share information and potentially give opinions that may inadvertently lead to a clinician stepping across the dividing line between professional and expert witness, which can have serious legal implications for both the clinician and the subject individual concerned. Clinicians should also remain mindful of the potential conflict of interest that may arise from giving 'independent' expert evidence on one's own patients. There are arguments both for and against this, and ultimately the decision as to who the most appropriate expert is lies with the court, although a responsible clinician may be required to provide evidence under certain circumstances – for example, to make recommendations regarding the availability of a bed in hospital order disposals.

The RCPsych has produced a helpful guide on the responsibilities of both professional and expert witnesses, and the clinic-legal and ethical considerations that may arise [58]. There are also entire textbooks written and conferences held on this highly specialised aspect of practice, which any practitioner would be wise to explore to ensure they are informed of the requirements and implications of doing this.

Conclusion

In this chapter we have provided an overview of the development of forensic psychiatry as a specialty and the forensic psychiatric system both structurally and functionally. It can be seen that the development of forensic services has not consistently been subject to careful planning and evidence, but rather as a response to tragic incidents with political ramifications, broadly leading to the structures in place today.

Nonetheless, policy and practice concerning forensic services is continuously developing to address complex clinical needs and legal pathways. It is anticipated that there will be a greater emphasis on community forensic services and least restrictive practice, which may include a reduction in high secure patient populations even further. The overall structure of services may change with the formation of Integrated Care Systems in accordance with the NHS Long-Term Plan, with greater regional integration across larger areas to make most efficient use of services, as well as with attempts to utilise NHS services as opposed to independent providers.

'Forensic' patients have often undergone major adversity in their lives and it is the role of all services, forensic or otherwise, to work across security and professional boundaries to eliminate the stigma associated with being a forensic patient and support the individual to recover and eventually seamlessly integrate into non-forensic services allowing for the negative aspect of risk and the positive one of recovery.

References

1. Forshaw, D. *The Origins and Early Development of Forensic Mental Health. Handbook of Forensic Mental Health.* London: Routledge; 2008.

2. Crane, J. *1774 Madhouses Act:* Warwick University; 2013 https://warwick.ac.uk/fac/arts/history/chm/outreach/trade_in_lunacy/research/1774madhousesact/.

3. Crotty, H. D. The history of insanity as a defence to crime in English criminal law. *California Law Review* 1924;12(2):105–23.

4. Hamilton, J. R. Insanity legislation. *Journal of Medical Ethics* 1986;12(1):13–17.

5. Peters, T. King George III, bipolar disorder, porphyria and lessons for historians. *Clinical Medicine (London)* 2011;11(3):261–4.

6. Gutheil, T. G. The history of forensic psychiatry. *Journal of the American Academy of Psychiatry and the Law Online* 2005;33(2):259.

7. Moran, R. The origin of insanity as a special verdict: The trial for treason of James Hadfield (1800). *Law & Society Review.* 1985;19(3):487–519.

8. Pritchard Rv. 7 Car & P 303, 7 Car and P 304, 173 ER 135, [1836] EWHC KB 1, 7 Car & P 303 1836. www.bailii.org/ew/cases/EWHC/KB/1836/1.html. Accessed 01.05.2022].

9. Brown, P. Unfitness to plead in England and Wales: Historical development and contemporary dilemmas. *Medicine, Science and the Law* 2019;59(3):187–96.

10. Law Commission. Unfitness to Plead: Law Commission; 2016. www.lawcom.gov.uk/project/unfitness-to-plead/. Accessed 01.05.2022.

11. Marcantonio v R. (Rev 1) [2016] EWCA Crim 14. www.bailii.org/ew/cases/EWCA/Crim/2016/14.html. Accessed 01.05.2022.

12. West, D. J. and Walk, A. *Daniel McNaughton His Trial and the Aftermath*. London: Gaskell; 1977.

13. Ellison, D. R. and Hass, H. E. A recent judicial interpretation of the M'Naghten Rules. *The British Journal of Delinquency* 1953;4(2):128–33.

14. Moran, R. *Knowing Right from Wrong. The Insanity Defense of Daniel McNaughtan*. New York: The Free Press; 1981.

15. Daniel M'Naghten's Case UKHL J16, 8 ER 718 1843. www.bailii.org/uk/cases/UKHL/1843/J16.html. Accessed 01.05.2022.

16. Law Commission. *Insanity and Automatism*: Law Commission; 2013. www.lawcom.gov.uk/project/insanity-and-automatism/. Accessed 01.05.2022.

17. HM Government. Mental Health Act 1959. London: HMSO; 1959. www.legislation.gov.uk/ukpga/Eliz2/7-8/72. Accessed 01.05.2022.

18. HM Government. Report of the Committee of Inquiry into the Personality Disorder Unit, Ashworth Special Hospital. London: HMSO; 1999. https://assets.publishing.service.gov.uk/government/uploads/system/uploads/attachment_data/file/265696/4194.pdf. Accessed 01.05.2022.

19. HM Government. *Reforming the Mental Health Act: Summary*, Department of Health and Social Care. London: HMSO; 2021. www.gov.uk/government/consultations/reforming-the-mental-health-act/reforming-the-mental-health-act. Accessed 01.05.2022.

20. Pollitt, J. D. Management of the mentally abnormal offender. *Proceedings of the Royal Society of Medicine* 1977;70:877–80.

21. HM Government. Special Hospitals. Ministry of Health. London: HMSO; 1961.

22. Ewins, D. The Butler Report. *British Journal of Law and Society* 1976;3(1):101–9.

23. Coid, J. W. The Christopher Clunis enquiry. *Psychiatric Bulletin* 1994;18(8):449–52.

24. Bowden, P. Graham Young (1947–90); the St Albans poisoner: his life and times. *Criminal Behaviour and Mental Health* 1996;6(S1):17–24.

25. NHS England, Services specification: High secure mental health services (Adult). London: NHS England 2021. www.england.nhs.uk/publication/service-specification-high-secure-mental-health-services-adult/. Accessed 04.01.2023.

26. NHS England. Service specification: Medium secure mental health services (Adult). London: NHS England; 2018. www.england.nhs.uk/publication/service-specification-medium-secure-mental-health-services-adult/. Accessed 01.05.2022.

27. NHS England. Service specification: Low secure mental health services (Adult). London: NHS England; 2018. www.england.nhs.uk/publication/service-specification-low-secure-mental-health-services-adult/. Accessed 01.05.2022.

28. Kennedy HG. Therapeutic uses of security: Mapping forensic mental health services by stratifying risk. *Advances in Psychiatric Treatment* 2002;8(6):433–43.

29. HM Government. Best practice guidance: Specification for adult medium-secure services. Department of Health. London: HMSO; 2007. http://data.parliament.uk/DepositedPapers/Files/DEP2007-0001/DEP2007-0001.pdf. Accessed 02.05.2022.

30. Quality Network for Forensic Mental Health Services. Physical Security in Secure Care London: RCPsych. www.rcpsych.ac.uk/docs/default-source/improving-care/ccqi/quality-networks/secure-forensic/qnfmhs-physical-security-in-secure-care.pdf?sfvrsn=9a67ef6d_2. Accessed 01.05.2022.

31. Quality Network for Forensic Mental Health Services. *See Think Act*. London: RCPsych. www.rcpsych.ac.uk/improving-care/ccqi/quality-networks-accreditation/forensic-mental-health-services/see-think-act. Accessed 01.05.2022.

32. Royal College of Psychiatrists. *Quality Network for Forensic Mental Health Services* London: RCPsych. www.rcpsych.ac.uk/im

proving-care/ccqi/quality-networks-accreditation/forensic-mental-health-services. Accessed 02.05.2022.

33. Quality Network for Forensic Mental Health Services. Relational Security Explorer. London: RCPsych. www.rcpsych.ac.uk/docs/default-source/improving-care/ccqi/quality-networks/secure-forensic/forensic-see-think-act-qnfmhs/sta_hndbk_2nded_web.pdf?sfvrsn=90e1fc26_4. Accessed 01.05.2022.

34. Douglas, K. S., Hart, S. D., Webster, C. D. et al. Historical-Clinical-Risk Management-20, Version 3 (HCR-20V3): Development and Overview. *International Journal of Forensic Mental Health* 2014;13 (2):93–108.

35. Council of Europe. *European Committee for the Prevention of Torture and Inhuman or Degrading Treatment or Punishment (CPT)*. Strasbourg: Council of Europe. www.coe.int/en/web/cpt. Accessed 02.05.2022.

36. Kennedy H. G., O'Neill, C., Flynn, G., Gill, P. and Davoren, M. The DUNDRUM Toolkit V1.0.30. Dublin: Trinity's Access to Research Archive; 2016. www.tara.tcd.ie/handle/2262/76545. Accessed 01.05.2022.

37. Institute of Mental Health. Secure hospital care: Information for carers 2018. https://institutemh.org.uk/images/research/7778_Secure_Hospital_Care_Brochure_A5_Online.pdf. Accessed 04.01.2023.

38. Centre for Mental Health. Briefing Note: Secure Care Services 2013. www.centreformentalhealth.org.uk/sites/default/files/2018-09/securecare.pdf. Accessed 04.01.2023.

39. HM Government. High security psychiatric services directions 2019: Arrangements for safety and security. London: HMSO; 2019.

40. NHS England. The offender personality disorder pathway strategy 2015. London. www.england.nhs.uk/commissioning/wp-content/uploads/sites/12/2016/02/opd-strategy-nov-15.pdf. Accessed 17.04.2022.

41. Till, A., Selwood, J. and Silva, E. The assertive approach to clozapine: Nasogastric administration. *BJPsych Bulletin* 2019;43(1):21–6.

42. Blott, H., Bhattacherjee, S. and Harris, E. An evaluation of the use of electroconvulsive therapy in a United Kingdom high secure psychiatric hospital. *European Psychiatry* 2017;41 (S1):S373-S.

43. Saleem, R., Kaitiff, D., Treasaden, I. and Vermeulen, J. Clinical experience of the use of triptorelin as an antilibidinal medication in a high-security hospital. *Journal of Forensic Psychiatry & Psychology* 2011;22 (2):243–51.

44. Hare Duke, L., Furtado, V., Guo, B. and Völlm, B. A. Long-stay in forensic-psychiatric care in the UK. *Social Psychiatry and Psychiatric Epidemiology* 2018;53(3):313–21.

45. National Association of Psychiatric Intensive Care & Low Secure Units 2022. https://napicu.org.uk/. Accessed 17.04.2022.

46. Sarkar, J. and di Lustro, M. Evolution of secure services for women in England. *Advances in Psychiatric Treatment* 2011;17 (5):323–31.

47. Sahota, S., Davies, S., Duggan, C. et al. Women admitted to medium secure care: Their admission characteristics and outcome as compared with men. *International Journal of Forensic Mental Health* 2010;9(2):110–17.

48. Bartlett, A. and Hassell, Y. Do women need special secure services? *Advances in Psychiatric Treatment* 2001;7(4):302–9.

49. Milne, S., Barron, P., Fraser, K. and Whitfield, E. Sex differences in patients admitted to a regional secure unit. *Medicine, Science and the Law* 1995;35 (1):57–60.

50. Coid, J., Kahtan, N., Gault, S. and Jarman, B. Women admitted to secure forensic psychiatry services: Comparison of women and men. *Journal of Forensic Psychiatry* 2000;11(2):275–95.

51. National Health Service. National Deaf Services: South West London and St George's Mental Health NHS Trust. www.swlstg.nhs.uk/our-services/specialist-services/national-deaf-services. Accessed 01.05.2022.

52. HM Government. Transforming care: A national response to Winterbourne View Hospital. Department of Health. London: HMSO; 2012.

53. HM Government. Mentally disordered offenders – the restricted patient system. Ministry of Justice. London: HMSO; 2020.

54. Vai, B., Mazza, M. G., Delli Colli, C. et al. Mental disorders and risk of COVID-19-related mortality, hospitalisation, and intensive care unit admission: A systematic review and meta-analysis. *Lancet Psychiatry* 2021;8(9):797–812.

55. Puzzo, I., Aldridge-Waddon, L., Stokes, N., Rainbird, J. and Kumari, V. The impact of the COVID-19 pandemic on forensic mental health services and clinical outcomes: A longitudinal study. *Frontiers in Psychiatry* 2022;12:1–12.

56. Taquet, M., Luciano, S., Geddes, J. R. and Harrison, P. J. Bidirectional associations between COVID-19 and psychiatric disorder: retrospective cohort studies of 62,354 COVID-19 cases in the USA. *The Lancet Psychiatry* 2021;8(2):130–40.

57. Ross, C., Brown, P., Brown, C. et al. COVID-19 Vaccination in those with mental health difficulties: A guide to assist decision-making in England, Scotland, and Wales. *Medicine, Science and the Law* 258024221086054. 11 Mar. 2022, https://doi.org/10.1177/00258024221086054.

58. Rix, K., Eastman, N. and Adshead, G. [on behalf of the Special Committee for Professional Practice and Ethics]. Responsibilities of psychiatrists who provide expert opinion to courts and tribunals. London: RCPsych; 2015.

Chapter 2

Management of Violence in Prisons

Louise Robinson and Andrew Forrester

Introduction

More than 11 million people are thought to be held in prisons across the world, this population having increased in size by 24% since 2020. The median global rate of imprisonment is 145 per 100,000 people; however, there are considerable variations in rates of imprisonment across the world, with the highest rates appearing in the USA (655/100k), El Salvador (604/100k), Turkmenistan (552/100k) and Thailand (526/100k). Between them, five countries – the USA, China, Brazil, Russia and India – account for just under half of the world's imprisoned people [1].

Rates of imprisonment also vary between the nations of the United Kingdom, with 143/100k being held in Scotland, 140/100k in England and Wales and 76/100k in Northern Ireland. In England and Wales, almost 80,000 people are currently detained, of whom around 4% are female [2]. Men and women are held in different situations (on remand or pre-trial, while convicted but unsentenced, or after being sentenced) and in institutions with four different security categories (A = high security; B and C = medium security; D = open conditions). Progress through these security levels, to less secure and then open conditions, is dependent upon assessments of risk (of both escape and violence) over time.

In England and Wales, people of Black, Asian and minority ethnicities are over-represented and make up 27% of the prison population. Sentence lengths are growing; 48% of prisoners are serving a sentence of at least four years, while 28% of prisoners are in custody for offences of violence against the person, with sexual offences being the second most common offence category [3]. Many prisoners return to prison soon after they are released. The overall proven reoffending rate is 28% in England and Wales, while for those serving sentences of less than 12 months it is 61%, raising serious questions about the effectiveness of the management in these institutions in preventing further crime [4]. Other countries are more successful (see Chapter 3).

His Majesty's Inspectorate of Prisons (HMIP), an independent organisation that inspects prisons and provides reports which are made available publicly on their website, has described significant problems with drugs, violence, living conditions and lack of access to meaningful activity [5]. Meanwhile, 44% of prisons in England and Wales were recorded as over-crowded in 2021 [3]. In 2020, the Council of Europe's Committee for the Prevention of Torture (CPT) described the present crisis in the prison system in England, with continued deterioration of conditions since 2012. Many prisoners were spending up to 23 hours per day in their cells, incidents of self-harm had increased by 63% (to more than 60,000 per annum), assaults had increased by 53% and episodes of prisoner on staff violence had increased by 70% [6, 7].

The prevalence of all mental disorders is higher in prisoners than in the general population [8]. This is particularly the case for major depression and psychosis, which are said to affect one in seven prisoners [9]. Estimates of rates of neurodevelopmental disorder are highly variable and reflect methodological challenges in this environment [9]. Rates of mental illness comorbid with substance misuse are high, and rates of mental disorder are even higher amongst female prisoners. Rates of suicide and self-harm are higher than in the community and increasing [10]; additionally, prisoners have high rates of physical ill-health [11].

In 1982, the United Nations General Assembly adopted the principle of equivalence, meaning that 'Health personnel, particularly physicians, charged with the medical care of prisoners and detainees, have a duty to provide them with protection of their physical and mental health and treatment of disease of the same quality and standard as is afforded to those who are not imprisoned or detained' [12; 13, p. 3]. Thus, according to the United Nations Basic Principles for the Treatment of Prisoners, 'prisoners shall have access to the health services available in the country without discrimination on the grounds of their legal situation' [14].

In the nations of the United Kingdom, prison healthcare, including primary and secondary mental healthcare, is provided by the National Health Service and is meant to observe both the principle of equivalence and the associated right to health [15]. In England and Wales, these services are monitored and reported on by HMIP and the Care Quality Commission in accordance with a number of core domains, including whether establishments are safe, effective, caring, responsive and well-led, and the international principles of equivalent care and right to health are central to this approach.

Violence in Prisons

Violence is more common in prisons than in the community [8] and can take a number of different forms, including physical violence amongst prisoners, sexual assaults, violence towards staff, riots, the destruction of property and excessive violence from staff towards prisoners. Incidents of violence are thought to be significantly under-reported due to concerns around reprisals. However, in one Australian study, 34% of male and 24% of female prisoners reported having experienced physical assault in prison [16], and rates of physical assault are estimated to be between 13 and 27 times higher in US prisons than in the community [8]. Meanwhile, estimates of sexual assault victimisation have varied between 1% and 41% of the prison population [17].

In England and Wales, in the 12 months ending March 2020, there were 31,568 reported assaults (i.e., 380 per 1,000 adult prisoners), of which 9,784 were on staff. This represented a reduction in rates which had increased steeply over the preceding decade and reached a record high in 2019 [18]. Rates of violence fell still further from March to June 2020 (to 336 incidents per 1,000 prisoners), coinciding with restriction of prison regimes due to the COVID-19 pandemic [10]. Homicides are much rarer, with three having taken place in the prison population of England and Wales in 2019 [18]. In their most recent report, HM Inspectorate of Prisons noted similar concerns to those described by the CPT, prison safety remaining 'a major problem in men's prisons' [5].

What Does Prison Violence Look Like?

Prisons are establishments that have some unique characteristics associated with violence. There are gangs: groups of prisoners within prisons with distinct identities, and who are responsible for a great deal of violence [19]. Prisons also have a large illicit economy relating to the use of alternative currencies and trade, which is forbidden [20]. Traded items include toiletries, tobacco, mobile telephones and drugs, and this illicit economic system is strongly associated with debt and violence [21]. As prisoners have moved away from so-called 'hard drugs' and towards the use of novel psychoactive substances (NPS), these newer drugs, and the systems involved in their finance and supply, are thought to be more strongly associated with violence in UK prisons [22]. This appears to relate to their role in the illicit economy, but it has also been suggested that they can cause violence during intoxication [23]. They may be administered to other prisoners without consent (known as 'spiking') as a form of bullying. Bullying is assumed to be common but it is difficult to measure because of probable under-reporting [24]. However, its use as a term can minimise serious offences. It can include assault, verbal abuse and humiliation, and it often relates to the illicit economy. Hidden weapons may be used in prison violence – either obtained illicitly or created by, for example, attaching a razor blade to a toothbrush (a 'shank').

Reasons given by prisoners for violence often include demonstrating toughness ('projecting an image'), managing conflict or punishing behaviour (particularly in women) [25]. Causes of prison violence are often considered and categorised as either individual (i.e., imported), a consequence of the prison environment or the result of an interaction between the two [21]. However, there is no single identifiable cause of prison violence. According to His Majesty's Prison and Probation Service (HMPPS), 'it is too simplistic to say prison violence is caused by drugs or bullying or debt, or imported vulnerabilities or poor relationships with staff'; instead, 'prison violence is caused by multiple or related factors' [26]. According to HMPPS, these factors include:

- Individuals who have a tendency to violence;
- Unkempt environments that leave people feeling uncared for;
- Cultural norms that accept violence as a solution to difficulties or a way of establishing respect;
- A lack of activity so people feel bored and frustrated, and turn to illicit drugs to help pass the time;
- Interactions with staff where prisoners feel neither treated kindly nor have decisions explained [26]

There is a large research literature on predictors of violence, much of which has been conducted in the USA. The strongest individual risk factor is youth [21, 27]. Others include a history of violence in prison and/or violent convictions, short sentences, gang membership, impulsiveness, anger, antisocial attitudes, educational attainment and mental disorder [21, 27, 28]. In the USA there are higher rates of violence in African American, Hispanic and Native American than white prisoners, but these studies are difficult to interpret [21]. Prison factors include high security levels, prison gang activity [28] and poor conditions [29, 30]. Unevenly applied rules, perceived unfairness and feeling unsafe also increase risk [21]. Prison visits can both increase and reduce risk: Siennick, Mears and Bales showed that rates reduce before, and increase after, visits [31]. Meanwhile, the impact of overcrowding is often discussed but is not straightforward and appears to relate to the additional impact upon staff resources [21, 28].

Mental disorders are associated with both increased risk of perpetuating violence and risk of becoming a victim of violence in prison [8]. Amongst male prisoners, mental illness is associated with increased risk of violence if there is a history of perpetrating violence. Risk is higher where there is comorbid substance misuse with mental illness in both sexes [32, 33].

Holding the belief that thoughts are being controlled is a particularly pertinent symptom relating to risk of perpetrating violence in prison [34]. But there are also associations between antisocial, narcissistic and paranoid personality disorders and violence against other prisoners [35, 36].

Perpetrators of violence are also more likely to also be victims of violence [33]. Sexual victimisation is higher in women and those with mental disorder [37]. Being in debt and borrowing in prison also increases risk of victimisation [38].

Managing Violence in Prisons

Prisoners have a right to protection against violence. Principle 5 of the United Nations Basic Principles for the Treatment of Prisoners states that 'except for those limitations that are demonstrably necessitated by the fact of incarceration, all prisoners shall retain the human rights and fundamental freedoms set out in the Universal Declaration of Human Rights' [3]. The State is therefore obliged to protect prisoners from violence, this also being essential to meet the stated aims of His Majesty's Prison Service – namely, to 'keep those sentenced to prison in custody, helping them to lead law-abiding and useful lives, both while they are in prison and after they are released'. [39]. In keeping with these aims, the Ministry of Justice and HMPPS have a policy of zero tolerance towards violence, their stated objective being to ensure its overall reduction [26].

Prevention

Prison violence is likely to be multifactorial; some prisoners bring an increased risk of violence into prison with them when they enter, and the prison environment is also one that can promote violence. In practice, there is unlikely to be a single response which can be used effectively alone. Each prison requires an individual violence reduction strategy, and many have a dedicated violence reduction co-ordinator. In some places, specific initiatives have been developed: for example, in London, the Mayor's Office of Policing and Crime (MOPAC) has implemented a violence reduction programme which aims to provide a trauma-informed model for gang interventions, while improving relationships and employment skills, and also providing an increased police presence inside prisons [40]. Although this is one example, its multi-faceted approach does reflect thinking in this area, in which violence is understood to have multiple, inter-related underlying causations.

In keeping with this, HM Inspectorate of Prisons [5] described finding that 'peer support and a collaborative approach to addressing violence' were features of the safer prisons they reviewed, while 'a combination of poor living conditions and lack of purposeful regime contributed to continued drug misuse and violence' (p. 22).

HM Inspectorate of Prisons has set out expectations which have led to criteria for assessing the treatment for individual prisoners and conditions in prison [41]. Those relevant to evidence of a whole-prison approach to ensuring prisoners are safe from violence include:

- An effective multidisciplinary strategy to reduce violence and antisocial behaviour
- Staff to promote positive relationships, identify and challenge problematic behaviour and model pro-social behaviour
- Use of mediation where appropriate to resolve disputes
- Investigate allegations of violence promptly and take action where required

- Protect vulnerable prisoners
- Support perpetrators of violence to change behaviour
- Encourage meaningful occupation

At the level of the prison, incident monitoring and the use of intelligence, reporting and information sharing are all vital to understand patterns and causes of violence. Investment in security to reduce the supply of contraband is also required, given that supply routes may include visitors, staff, prisoners, postal deliveries and the passage of objects over walls or via drones [42]. It is vital to ensure that aspects of daily life in prisons are understood to be reasonable and fair, in order to maintain order, and given the potential for strong feelings of perceived injustice. Therefore, it is important to take prisoners' perspectives into account, via mechanisms such as focus groups or questionnaires.

Many prisons hold vulnerable offenders separately in specific wings – often known as vulnerable prisoners' (VP) wings. These wings usually aim to provide cellular accommodation and enhanced safety for those who are thought to be at a higher risk of potential victimisation, often because of their original offences (e.g. sex offenders).

Generally, staff training should include skills in de-escalating conflict; use of force should be a last resort, and recording of all violent incidents should be both made and reviewed regularly. Staff must be properly supervised and supported, and at adequate levels.

Opportunities for structured and purposeful activities must also be provided: there are significantly fewer violent incidents in areas such as workshops and education [21] and lower rates of violence associated with prison employment [28]. There is little evidence at present that any psychological treatments aiming to reduce prison violence are effective [43, 44]. Readers are also referred to the initiatives mentioned in Chapter 4, such as prison councils and greater prisoner involvement in their environment and regime.

A substance misuse strategy must include accurate, relevant and accessible information tailored to the specific groups it is aimed at, as well as attempts to reduce drugs entering prison [42], in combination with appropriate treatments provided by healthcare services.

While there are no evidence-based interventions which address gang activity [45], it may be reduced by promoting alternative social groups and activities, monitoring gang membership and providing support to prisoners who may wish to leave gangs, as well as identifying those recruiting into gangs [46].

An important intervention focused on the individual is the cell-sharing risk assessment (CSRA). A review of homicides in prison found that half of the prisoners died in this way when locked in with a cellmate [47]. This risk assessment should be completed for all prisoners to assess the likelihood of harming or killing a cellmate, as currently most prisoners share cells. However, to be effective they must be properly completed with all relevant information.

Segregation can be used to separate individual prisoners at high risk of immediate harm to others, or those in need of protection, from the rest of the prison population. However, there is little evidence of its impact on violence [48].

The UK government reports several current strategies for violence reduction [49]. The national Prison Safety Framework (5 Ps) is based around the five principles of people, physical, population, partnerships and procedural to address violence, self-harm and self-inflicted deaths. They report prioritising investment in prison security to reduce contraband in prison and thereby improving safety and expanding intelligence and counter-corruption. They also recognise the role of loss of staff in increasing violence and report plans to increase numbers. They have introduced the CSIP model (Challenge Support and Intervention Plan). This is a multidisciplinary case management approach to managing prisoners at increased risk of violence mandated across prisons in England and Wales in 2018. To protect staff they have introduced use of PAVA, a synthetic pepper spray, in men's prisons as part of a package for staff to de-escalate incidents. Body-worn video cameras have also been introduced to prevent ill-treatment by staff and allow investigation of incidents.

The Crime in Prison Referral Agreement, published in 2019 [50], sets out which crimes in England and Wales should be reported to police rather than managed via internal adjudication procedures.

Mental Health Clinicians in Prisons

Different jurisdictions take different approaches to the provision of mental health assessment and treatment in prisons. In many places, there are very serious problems arising in prisons that can contribute to the development of mental disorders (e.g. physical or sexual assaults, unchecked violence, insufficient medical care, or the use of corporal punishment or the death penalty) [51]. In England and Wales, the agreed national approach has been to provide mental health teams that are meant to be similar in design and function to teams that are provided in the community – that is, community mental health teams [52]. The most recent national service specification confirms the primacy of the principle of equivalence, and specifies the necessity for mental health services that can provide a broad range of interventions, including crisis intervention, recovery-focused models and treatments for, amongst other things, personality disorder, substance misuse, dementia and learning disabilities. Teams are also meant to provide care and treatment for both those with common mental disorders and those who require specialist interventions, through the provision of an integrated model that is based on a stepped model of care [53]. However, despite advances in service specifications, there are concerns that prison healthcare remains underfunded, that many are not receiving the treatment they should be and that many teams remain inadequately resourced [54–57]. Some prisons provide healthcare wings, usually for prisoners who present with serious physical and/or mental health problems such that they cannot be managed on ordinary prison wings [58]. Many such prisoners await transfer to secure hospitals for further care and treatment. This wait has historically been excessive [59, 60].

Multidisciplinary teams play a role in assessing prisoners at all stages of their imprisonment, starting at prison reception and continuing subsequently. They have a duty to work together with prison governors and operational staff to ensure appropriate access to healthcare services [61]. This includes a necessity to document and raise concerns where vulnerability is detected, including those who may be vulnerable to violence because of their own mental disorder [62]. There is also a need for environmental awareness, such as ensuring sufficient space and staff presence for assessments to take place safely, and gathering information from a range of sources before going to assess a prisoner on a wing or in segregation. Additionally, clinicians have a clear role in identifying and reporting security issues when they arise (e.g. witnessing violence or hearing threats of serious harm or death).

Risk Assessment and Risk Management

Assessing and managing risk of violence is a core activity of prisons, and clinicians working in prisons have various levels of access to this information. The main vehicle used to identify and manage risk in England and Wales is the Offender Assessment System (OASys), which is used to examine both the risk that reoffending will occur and the risk of serious harm. This system has been in place since 2001 and it is designed to recognise the multiple factors that can contribute to offending behaviour, including individual, social and environmental factors [63, 64]. It identifies risk according to four main categories (low, medium, high or very high) as well as specifying who will be at risk (e.g. the general public, a named individual, other prisoners, vulnerable adults, an ethnic minority group, children or staff).

Clinical teams may also use additional internationally validated and effective risk assessment instruments, such as the HCR-20 or the PCL-R [65]; however, many unfortunately have insufficient resources to undertake potentially lengthy risk assessments and instead must be focused on the various urgent clinical issues that tend to arise within any given day. For this to work as effectively as it can, greater emphasis on the provision of clinical psychology services and improved liaison with forensic psychologists who already work in the prison estate but are not employed by healthcare providers are likely to be required.

Violence Related to Mental Disorder

Violence occurring in prisons can be related to underlying mental disorder [66], and can be linked to the use of substances, including new psychoactive substances [23]. For many prisoners who present with serious or recurrent violence, segregation units with relatively high staffing ratios are used to remove them from other prisoners and thereby attempt to manage the risk they present. However, although people with acute mental health needs or serious vulnerabilities are not meant to be managed in these units, in reality segregation units often contain a mixed group of people with complex needs. These presentations may include unmet mental health needs, learning disabilities, protection needs arising from threats from other prisoners and serious risks to self and/or others [67].

The correct pathway for those who present with acute mental illness, including those in whom there is an association with violence, is admission to the prison's healthcare wing in the first instance. This admission should also, depending on the specific circumstances, be accompanied by an urgent referral to the relevant local secure mental health service (in the United Kingdom, these being provided at a range of security levels – high, medium, low and psychiatric intensive care – depending upon the needs of the particular prisoner being referred). However, there are substantial limitations within this process, meaning that morbidity within these healthcare wings is often extreme and untreated [58]. Firstly, in many jurisdictions, including England and Wales, it is not possible to invoke compulsory treatment in prisons using mental health legislation. There are important reasons for this, not least the concern that abuses may arise through pharmacological attempts to manage difficult behaviour under the guise of treatment. For this reason, the World Health Organisation has clearly stated that 'there must be a clear acceptance that penal institutions are seldom, if ever, able to treat and care for seriously and acutely mentally ill prisoners' [68; 69, p. 6]. Secondly, although acutely mentally ill people should be transferred to hospital quickly, in reality this process is often considerably delayed, meaning that the clinical team in the prison must continue to manage in challenging clinical circumstances [60].

With regard to the pharmacological management of mental disorders in prisons, practice is intended to be no different from that in the general community. In England and Wales, this means it is guided by the evidence that is assimilated by the National Institute for Health and Care Excellence (nice.org.uk), which provides guidelines for the assessment and management of a wide range of physical and mental health disorders.

Treatment can be provided on a voluntary basis in prisons. Some mood-altering medications have a trading value and can be sought for this purpose, quickly entering the prison's illicit economy following prescription. Sometimes, prisoners may act under the coercion of others to seek medication – for example, for the payment of a debt. Although this should not interfere with treatments that should be provided when appropriate and necessary, this aspect of imprisonment does need to be borne in mind lest the unwitting clinician inadvertently contributes to the wider climate of prison coercion and violence by enhancing the supply of particular drugs within the illicit economy. Various drugs have entered into this economy at different times, including sedative drugs such as benzodiazepines, drugs used for anxiety and pain such as pregabalin, and even antipsychotics such as quetiapine.

Other forms of management may include non-pharmacological techniques. HMPPS uses the principles of risk, needs and responsivity to match prisoners to accredited offending behaviour programmes [70], aiming to encourage attitudes that are pro-social and meant to assist them in developing new skills [71]. Additionally, for people who present with personality disorders, the Offender Personality Disorder Pathway is in place to focus on the management of risk of reoffending and violence through a focus on early intervention, sentence planning and building relationships [72].

Clinicians working in prisons must also take time to review the environment in which risk is presented, and keep in mind the common co-occurrence of violence and self-harm [73, 74]. Several questions need to be asked continually. Does the individual require transfer to a single cell because of the risk they present to their cellmate? Are regular observations by staff required to ensure safety? Are immediate cellular adaptations required (e.g. the removal of a weapon or obvious ligature point)? Should the individual be moved to another part of the prison? Regular reviews by nursing or psychology staff can assist in defusing crisis-type situations [75] and continued appraisal of historical clinical and risk information can help ensure that teams can anticipate the risk and threat of violence.

COVID-19 and Prisons

Particular concerns have arisen in prisons throughout the world since the onset of the COVID-19 pandemic in early 2020. Reasons for this include the concentration of people who are already vulnerable to infection, the necessity for close contact in over-crowded conditions, problems with ventilation and sanitation, and difficulties with healthcare access [76]. This has led to the conclusion that prisons are 'in no way equipped' to deal with COVID-19, with UK prisons operating at 107% of capacity and many other countries providing conditions that are ripe for the spread of the virus [77]. Measures taken to manage COVID-19 in prisons include a technique known as compartmentalisation, with associated reductions in activities such as education and gym, increased time in the cell (potentially amounting to solitary confinement for many), and the cancellation of prison visits. All of this can have adverse mental health consequences [78]. However, in these abnormal and highly restrictive times, some things can still be done to mitigate adverse mental health effects and the challenges that are presented may nonetheless offer some opportunities for growth [79, 80]. The most recent safety in custody statistics for prisons in England and Wales show a substantial reduction in assaults by 37%, to 4,550 incidents between March and June 2020 [18]. This trend is continuing, and the data obtained will be useful in planning future strategies. Whilst we are still in the midst of the pandemic we cannot predict successfully, and the longer-term effects of COVID-19 have yet to be fully understood.

Conclusion

Violence is common in prisons and is associated with the unique characteristics of prison environments and culture. There is no single cause of prison violence and strategies to reduce prison violence must operate at both the individual and the prison levels. Mental health clinicians working in prisons will encounter perpetrators and victims of violence in their day-to-day practice. Clinicians have a role in managing prison violence through individual risk assessment and subsequent environmental management, and treatment of acute mental disorder. They should also report prison-level risks when they are encountered. However, much prison violence stems from factors unrelated to mental disorder. It is crucial that the clinician has an understanding of these individual and cultural factors in order to work effectively with this population, provide risk assessments for individuals, and contribute to the future reduction of prison violence. While the severe restrictions associated with COVID-19 have significantly affected the quality of life and, it is likely, mental health, of prisoners, it is hoped that some of the lessons learnt during this period will help to reduce future prison violence in a less restrictive context.

References

1. Walmsley, R. *World Prison Population List.* London: Institute for Criminal Policy Research; 2018.

2. Ministry of Justice. Population and Capacity Briefing for Friday 4th December 2020 [online]. 2020. www.gov.uk/govern ment/statistics/prison-population-figures-2020 [Accessed 28.4.2022].

3. Sturge, G. House of Commons Library Research Briefing UK Population Statistics [online] 29 October 2021 Available from https://researchbriefings.files.parliament.u k/documents/SN04334/SN04334.pdf [Accessed 1.5.2022].

4. Ministry of Justice. Proven reoffending statistics quarterly bulletin, October 2018 to December 2018. [online]. 29 October 2020. www.gov.uk/government/statistics/p roven-reoffending-statistics-october-to-de cember-2018 [Accessed 28.4.2022].

5. HM Inspectorate of Prisons for England and Wales Annual Report 2018-19 9 July 2019. The annual report of HM Chief Inspector of Prisons from 1 April 2018 to 31 March 2019. [online]. July 2019. www .justiceinspectorates.gov.uk/hmiprisons/ wp-content/uploads/sites/4/2019/07/6.556 3_HMI-Prisons-AR_2018-19_WEB_FINA L_040719.pdf [Accessed 28.4.2022].

6. Council of Europe. Report to the United Kingdom government on the visit to the United Kingdom carried out by the European Committee for the Prevention of Torture and Inhuman or Degrading Treatment or Punishment (CPT) from 13 to 23 May 2019. Council of Europe; [online]. 2020. https://rm.coe.int/16809e4404 [Accessed 28.4.2022].

7. Ismail, N. and Forrester, A. The state of English prisons and the urgent need for reform. *Lancet Public Health* 2020 Jun. 5(7): e368–e369.

8. Fazel, S., Hayes, A. J., Bartellas, K., Clerici, M. and Trestman, R. Mental health of prisoners: Prevalence, adverse outcomes, and interventions. *The Lancet Psychiatry* 2016 Sep 1;3(9):871–81.

9. Fazel, S. and Seewald, K. Severe mental illness in 33 588 prisoners worldwide: Systematic review and meta-regression analysis. *The British Journal of Psychiatry* 2012 May;200(5):364–73.

10. Ministry of Justice Safety in Custody Statistics, England and Wales, [internet] 30 July 2020. https://assets.publishing.ser vice.gov.uk/government/uploads/ system/uploads/attachment_data/file/905 064/safety-in-custody-q1-2020.pdf [Accessed 28.4.2022].

11. Fazel, S. and Baillargeon, J. The health of prisoners. *The Lancet* 2011 Mar 12;377 (9769):956–65.

12. Till, A., Forrester, A. and Exworthy, T. The development of equivalence as a mechanism to improve prison healthcare. *Journal of the Royal Society of Medicine* 2014 Feb. 107(5):179–182.

13. United Nations. Principle of Medical Ethics. 1982. A/RES/37/194. [online]. http://britishjustice.org/docs/UNResolution .pdf [Accessed 28.4.2022].

14. United Nations. Basic principles for the Treatment of Prisoners: adopted by the United Nations General Assembly, 14 December 1990. [online]. A/RES/45/111. www.ohchr.org/EN/ProfessionalInterest/P ages/BasicPrinciplesTreatmentOfPrisoner s.aspx [Accessed 28.4.2022].

15. Exworthy, T., Samele, C., Urquía, N. and Forrester, A. Asserting prisoners' right to health: Progressing beyond equivalence. *Psychiatric Services* 2012 Mar;63(3):270–5.

16. Schneider, K., Richters, J., Butler, T. et al. Psychological distress and experience of sexual and physical assault among Australian prisoners. *Criminal Behaviour and Mental Health* 2011, 21(5):333.

17. Wolff, N. and Shi, J. Patterns of victimization and feelings of safety inside prison: The experience of male and female inmates. *Crime & Delinquency* 2011 Jan;57 (1):29–55.

18. Ministry of Justice. Safety in custody statistics England and Wales: deaths in prison custody to September 2020, assaults and self-harm to June 2020 [online]. Oct. 2020. https://assets.publishing.service.gov .uk/government/uploads/system/uploads/ attachment_data/file/930458/safety-in-cus tody-q2-2020.pdf [Accessed 28.4.2022].

19. Gundur RV. Prison Gangs. In *Oxford Research Encyclopedia of Criminology and Criminal Justice* [online]. 2020. https://doi .org/10.1093/acrefore/9780190264079.013 .397 [Accessed 28.4.2022].

20. Gooch, K. and Treadwell, J. Prisoner society in an era of psychoactive substances, organized crime, new drug markets and austerity. *The British Journal of Criminology* 2020;60(5):1260–81.

21. McGuire, J. Understanding prison violence: A rapid evidence assessment HM

Prison and Probation Service Analytical Summary 2018, [online] 2018. https://asse ts.publishing.service.gov.uk/government/u ploads/system/uploads/attachment_data/fi le/737956/understanding-prison-violence. pdf [Accessed 28.4.2022].

22. HM Inspectorate of Prisons. Changing patterns of substance misuse in adult prisons and service responses. December 2015. [online]. www.justiceinspectorates.g ov.uk/hmiprisons/wp-content/uploads/sit es/4/2015/12/Substance-misuse-web-2015 .pdf [Accessed 28.4.2022].

23. Mason R, Smith M, Onwuegbusi T, Roberts A. New Psychoactive Substances and Violence within a UK Prison Setting. Subst Use Misuse. 2022; 57(14): 2146–2150. doi: 10.1080/10826084.2022.21299 99. Epub 2022 Oct 21. PMID: 36269768.

24. Gooch, K., Treadwell, J. and Trent, R. Preventing and reducing prison bullying. *Prison Service Journal* 2015 Sep 30; 25–9.

25. Edgar, K. Conflicts in prison. *Prison Service Journal* 2015 Sep 30; 20–4. www.crimeand justice.org.uk/sites/crimeandjustice.org.u k/files/PSJ%20221%2C%20Conflicts%20in %20prison.pdf.

26. Her Majesty's Prison and Probation Service. Violence reduction in prisons. 2019.

27. Schenk, A. M. and Fremouw, W. J. Individual characteristics related to prison violence: A critical review of the literature. *Aggression and Violent Behavior* 2012 Sep 1;17(5):430–42.

28. Gonçalves, L. C., Gonçalves, R. A., Martins, C. and Dirkzwager, A. J. Predicting infractions and health care utilization in prison: A meta-analysis. *Criminal Justice and Behavior* 2014 Aug;41(8):921–42.

29. Bierie, D. M. Is tougher better? The impact of physical prison conditions on inmate violence. *International Journal of Offender Therapy and Comparative Criminology* 2012 May;56(3):338–55. https://doi.org/10 .1177/0306624X11405157. Epub 2011 Apr 13. PMID: 21489998.

30. Rocheleau, A. M. An empirical exploration of the 'pains of imprisonment' and the level

of prison misconduct and violence. *Criminal Justice Review* 2013; 38, 354–74.

31. Siennick, S. E., Mears, D. P. and Bales, W. D. Here and gone: Anticipation and separation effects of prison visits on inmate infractions. *Journal of Research in Crime and Delinquency* 2013; 50, 417–44.

32. Houser, K. A. and Welsh, W. Examining the association between co-occurring disorders and seriousness of misconduct by female prison inmates. *Criminal Justice and Behavior* 2014; 41:650–66.

33. Wood, S. R. and Buttaro, Jr A. Co-occurring severe mental illnesses and substance abuse disorders as predictors of state prison inmate assaults. *Crime & Delinquency* 2013 Jun;59 (4):510–35.

34. Friedmann, P. D., Melnick, G., Jiang, L. and Hamilton, Z. Violent and disruptive behavior among drug-involved prisoners: Relationship with psychiatric symptoms. *Behavioral Sciences & the Law* 2008 Jul;26 (4):389–401.

35. Coid, J. W. Personality disorders in prisoners and their motivation for dangerous and disruptive behaviour. *Criminal Behaviour and Mental Health* 2002 Sep;12(3):209–26.

36. Newberry, M. and Shuker, R. Personality Assessment Inventory (PAI) profiles of offenders and their relationship to institutional misconduct and risk of reconviction. *Journal of Personality Assessment* 2012 Nov 1;94 (6):586–92.

37. Wolff, N., Blitz, C. L. and Shi, J. Rates of sexual victimization in prison for inmates with and without mental disorders. *Psychiatric Services* 2007 Aug;58 (8):1087–94.

38. Copes, H., Higgins, G. E., Tewksbury, R. and Dabney, D. A. Participation in the prison economy and likelihood of physical victimization. *Victims & Offenders* 2010, 6 (1):1–18.

39. Her Majesty's Prison Service. About us [online]. 2020. www.gov.uk/government/organisations/hm-prison-service/about [Accessed 28.4.2022].

40. Mayor of London. Reducing violence in prisons [online]. 2019. www.london.gov.uk/city-hall-blog/reducing-violence-prisons [Accessed 28.4.2022].

41. HM Inspectorate of Prisons. Expectations Criteria for Assessing the treatment of prisoners and conditions in prisons Version 5. [online]. 2017. www.justiceinspectorates.gov.uk/hmiprisons/wp-content/uploads/sites/4/2020/04/Expectations-for-publication-FINAL-Dec-2019.pdf [Accessed 28.4.2022].

42. Wheatley, M., Stephens, M. and Clarke,M. Violence, aggression and agitation: What part do new psychoactive substances play? *Prison Service Journal* 2015 Sep 30;36–41.

43. Byrne, G. and Ní Ghráda, A. The application and adoption of four 'third wave' psychotherapies for mental health difficulties and aggression within correctional and forensic settings: A systematic review. *Aggression and Violent Behavior* 46, 2019:45–55. https://doi.org/10.1016/j.avb.2019.01.001.

44. Auty, K. M., Cope, A. and Liebling, A. Psychoeducational programs for reducing prison violence: A systematic review. *Aggression and Violent Behavior* 2017 Mar 1;33:126–43.

45. Home Office. Early Intervention Foundation. What works to prevent gang involvement, youth violence and crime. A rapid review of interventions delivered in the UK and abroad. London. [online] 2015. www.eif.org.uk/files/pdf/preventing-gang-and-youth-violence-rapid-review.pdf [Accessed 28.4.2022].

46. Horan, R., Dean, C. and Sutcliffe, P. Reducing gang-related prison violence. *Prison Service Journal* 2015 Sep 30, 42–6.

47. Prisons and Probation Ombudsman for England and Wales. Learning lessons bulletin: Fatal incident investigations. Issue 5, December 2013.

48. Labrecque, R. M., Mears, D. P. and Smith, P., Gender and the effect of disciplinary segregation on prison misconduct. *Criminal Justice Policy Review* 2020 31(8):1193–216.

49. Council of Europe. Response of the United Kingdom Government to the report of the

European Committee for the Prevention of Torture and Inhuman or Degrading Treatment or Punishment (CPT) on its visit to the United Kingdom from 13 to 23 May 2019 Strasbourg, 30 April 2020. https://rm.coe.int/16809e4406 [Accessed 28.4.2022].

50. HM Prison and Probation Service, National Police Chief's Council, Crown Prosecution Service. Crime in Prison Referral Agreement 7 May 2019. https://assets.publishing.service.gov.uk/government/uploads/system/uploads/attachment_data/file/800040/Crime_in_Prison_Referral_Agreement_-_7_May_19.pdf [Accessed 28.4.2022].

51. Forrester, A. and Piper, M. The WPA's prison health position statement and curriculum. *World Psychiatry* 2020 Feb;19(1):125.

52. Steel, J., Thornicroft, G., Birmingham, L. et al. Prison mental health inreach services. *The British Journal of Psychiatry* 2007 May;190(5):373–4.

53. NHS England. Service specification – integrated mental health services for prisons in England. 2018. www.england.nhs.uk/wp-content/uploads/2018/10/service-specification-mental-health-for-prisons-in-england-2.pdf [Accessed 28.4.2022].

54. Ismail, N. The politics of austerity imprisonment and ignorance: A case study of English prisons. *Medicine, Science and the Law* 2020 Apr; 60(2):89–92.

55. Piper, M., Forrester, A. and Shaw, J. Prison healthcare services: The need for political courage. *The British Journal of Psychiatry* 2019 Oct;215(4):579–81.

56. Patel, R., Harvey, J. and Forrester, A. Systemic limitations in the delivery of mental health care in prisons in England. *International Journal of Law and Psychiatry* 2018 Sep 1;60:17–25.

57. Forrester, A., Exworthy, T., Olumoroti, O. et al. Variations in prison mental health services in England and Wales. *International Journal of Law and Psychiatry* 2013 May 1; 36(3–4):326–32.

58. Forrester, A., Chiu, K., Dove, S. and Parrott, J. Prison health-care wings:

Psychiatry's forgotten frontier? *Criminal Behaviour and Mental Health* 2010 Feb;20(1):51–61.

59. Hopkin, G., Samele, C., Singh, K. and Forrester, A. Letter to the editor: Transferring London's acutely mentally ill prisoners to hospital. *Criminal Behaviour and Mental Health* 2016;26:76.

60. Woods, L., Craster, L. and Forrester, A. Mental Health Act transfers from prison to psychiatric hospital over a six-year period in a region of England. *Journal of Criminal Psychology* 2020;10(3):219–31.

61. Forrester, A., Till, A., Simpson, A. and Shaw, J. Mental illness and the provision of mental health services in prisons. *British Medical Bulletin* 2018;127(1):101–9.

62. Stevens, E. Safeguarding vulnerable adults: Exploring the challenges to best practice across multi-agency settings. *Journal of Adult Protection* 2013;15(2):85.

63. National Offender Management Service. A compendium of research and analysis on the Offender Assessment System (OASys), 2009–2013 (publishing.service.gov.uk). [online]. 2015. https://assets.publishing.service.gov.uk/government/uploads/system/uploads/attachment_data/file/449357/research-analysis-offender-assessment-system.pdf [Accessed 21.10.2022].

64. Howard, P. D. and Dixon, L. The construction and validation of the OASys Violence Predictor: Advancing violence risk assessment in the English and Welsh correctional services. *Criminal Justice and Behavior* 2012 Mar;39(3):287–307.

65. Nicholls, T. L., Ogloff, J. R. and Douglas, K. S. Assessing risk for violence among male and female civil psychiatric patients: The HCR-20, PCL: SV, and VSC. *Behavioral Sciences & the Law* 2004 Jan;22(1):127–58.

66. Felson, R. B., Silver, E. and Remster, B. Mental disorder and offending in prison. *Criminal Justice and Behavior* 2012 Feb;39(2):125–43.

67. Shalev, S. and Edgar, K. Deep custody: Segregation units and close supervision centres in England and Wales. Prison Reform Trust. 2010. www.prisonreformtrust.org.uk/wp-content/uploads/old_files/

Documents/deep_custody_111215.pdf [Accessed 28.4.2022].

68. Carroll, A., Ellis, A., Aboud, A., Scott, R. and Pillai, K. No involuntary treatment of mental illness in Australian and New Zealand prisons. *Journal of Forensic Psychiatry & Psychology*. 2020 Sep 27:1–28.

69. World Health Organization. Trencin statement on prisons and mental health. 2007. https://apps.who.int/iris/bitstream/h andle/10665/108575/E91402.pdf [Accessed 28.4.2022].

70. Ministry of Justice. Correctional services accreditation and advice panel – currently accredited programmes. [online]. February 2021. https://assets.publishing.s ervice.gov.uk/government/uploads/sys tem/uploads/attachment_data/file/96009 7/Descriptions_of_Accredited_Program mes_-_Final_-_210209.pdf [Accessed 28.4.2022].

71. Ministry of Justice. Offending behaviour programmes and interventions. [online]. 2018. www.gov.uk/guidance/offending-be haviour-programmes-and-interventions [Accessed 28.4.2022].

72. Skett, S. and Lewis, C. Development of the Offender Personality Disorder Pathway: A summary of the underpinning evidence. *Probation Journal* 2019 Jun;66(2):167–80.

73. Slade, K. Dual harm: The importance of recognising the duality of self-harm and violence in forensic populations. *Medicine, Science and the Law* 2019 Apr; 59(2);75–7.

74. Slade, K., Forrester, A. and Baguley, T. Coexisting violence and self-harm: Dual harm in an early-stage male prison population. *Legal and Criminological Psychology* 2020 Apr 7:e12169.

75. Miller, N. A. and Najavits, L. M. Creating trauma-informed correctional care: A balance of goals and environment. *European Journal of Psychotraumatology* 2012 Dec 1;3(1):17246.

76. Kinner, S. A., Young, J. T., Snow, K. et al. Prisons and custodial settings are part of a comprehensive response to COVID-19. *Lancet Public Health* 2020 Apr 1;5(4): e188–9.

77. Burki, T. Prisons are 'in no way equipped' to deal with COVID-19. *The Lancet* 2020 May 2;395(10234):1411.

78. Hewson, T., Shepherd, A., Hard, J. and Shaw, J. Effects of the COVID-19 pandemic on the mental health of prisoners. *Lancet Psychiatry* 2020 Jul 1;7(7):568–70.

79. Kothari, R., Forrester, A., Greenberg, N., Sarkissian, N. and Tracy, D. COVID-19 and prisons: Providing mental health care for people in prison, minimising moral injury and psychological distress in mental health staff. *Medicine, Science and the Law* 2020 Jul; 60(3):165–8.

80. Kothari, R., Forrester, A., Greenberg, N., Sarkissian, N. and Tracy, D. K. Providing mental health services in prisons during the covid-19 pandemic – challenges and opportunities for growth. *Clinical Psychology Forum* 2020 Sep;2020 (333):18–23.

Introduction to Section 4

Section 4: Group Aspects

Many groups are more vulnerable to violence than others, with children, some ethnic minorities and the elderly more at risk than others. In this section, these aspects of vulnerability are examined closely. Children exposed to violence are perhaps the group who suffer most, as the effects of abuse and harm can scar them for the rest of their lives. Their inability to resist makes the need for safeguarding paramount, but intervention often takes place late when the damage has been done. Older people and those with intellectual disability are similarly vulnerable and the chapters in this section offer sound advice on management. Black, Asian and other minority groups (BAME) deserve a separate chapter. They are both more vulnerable to violence and perceived as more likely to express violence, a perception that is often wrong and can have racist overtones. There is controversy over the causes of violence in this group, but the authors present a balanced view containing sound advice.

13

Working With Violence in Children: A Developmental and Relational Perspective

Celia Sadie, Laura Steckley, Susan McGinnis
and Joanna Sales

Introduction

In this chapter, we set out to provide the reader with some direction about the management of violence when working with children, and how this feeds into the practices of assessment, formulation and treatment across the spectrum from preventative to reactive work. We look at current practice, signposting areas for practitioners to explore in depth elsewhere, often in other chapters of this book. While we focus on direct practice, it is vital to acknowledge that effective, meaningful work with children relies on good indirect practice (training, supervision, guidance, support, service development) being nurtured at an organisational level.

Children are in a constant state of change and growth; they learn and develop through interaction with others and with the systems of which they are a part. They are full of potential, yet limited by their lack of power to change the potentially damaging aspects of their world. When we encounter them as practitioners, we are meeting their distress in real time, not retrospectively, as we might with adults. Whatever is happening, or has happened, is immediate or in the very near past. Their responses may be raw and inarticulate but are no less an expression of their experience. For this reason, rather than speaking of 'violence' we will be referring to 'pain-based behaviour'.

The term 'pain-based behaviour' was coined by Anglin [1] to focus therapeutic attention on the psychosocial pain that underlies children's 'acting out' behaviour. In a grounded theory study of what makes for well-functioning residential childcare, he found that this pain was underacknowledged and often unaddressed. While violence is often assumed to be the product of anger, his findings revealed a much broader and more complex mix at its roots, including grief, loss, abandonment, anxiety, hopelessness, fear and terror. In his words, 'the ongoing challenge of dealing with such primary pain without unnecessarily inflicting secondary pain experiences on the residents through punitive or controlling reactions can be seen to be the central problematic for the care work staff' (p. 178). This, we believe, is equally true for the management of anyone coming into contact with violence, at any level of the system.

We argue that this is, in part, because witnessing and responding to the pain-based behaviour of children is very often difficult for those around them, including families, carers and professionals. We also argue that a cultural unconscious exists that cannot bear to acknowledge the fear, shame and despair that children experience and instead finds it more comfortable to gather those feelings under the umbrella of anger, which can then be 'managed'. This approach serves to locate the problem in the child and absolves us as a society, and those immediately around the child, from taking responsibility for the conditions from which these behaviours typically arise (i.e. from microsystem settings, such as families, to macrosystem forces, like poverty, inequalities and political ideologies such as 'austerity'). Dockar-Drysdale [2] refers to this as 'out there' thinking (p. 62), challenging us to 'tolerate' looking 'in here' at our own responsibility for violence: our defensiveness and our unconscious complicity in these systems. Strength is required not just for resisting one's own defences, but our collective ones as well.

Throughout the chapter, we acknowledge four main themes in our thinking:

- Work with children needs to be thought about differently from work with adults, because of their relative systemic powerlessness and undeveloped capacities.
- Pain-based behaviour is generated by experiences in relationships and can be understood, contained and resolved through them.
- Profound distress brings a request for relational containment, and this can be enabled by creating containing systems (support, reflective spaces, training, supervision) around staff that validate their experiences and provide spaces where they can make sense of children's communication.
- Pain-based behaviour can provoke feelings of fragmentation and splitting within the child, their family, carers, practitioners and teams, and our aim should be to find integrated, holistic ways of working together that can then support the process of nurturing the child's own sense of integration.

This chapter seeks to reinstate an understanding of, and attention to, the origins of pain-based behaviour that can easily be lost in the language and discourse around the management and prevention of violence in children, both in the research literature and in the practice of care, whether through child and adolescent mental health services (CAMHS), in children's homes or in secure settings. We seek to provide a counterpoint and a challenge to the prevailing tendency to focus responsibility within the individual and to initiate a dialogue wherein relational and reparative interventions can be considered, together with behavioural ones, as part of a process-informed response to pain-based behaviour.

Finally, we note that the missing voices here are those of the children themselves. Remarkably little research has been done asking children, parents and carers about what they have found helpful in being understood and supported in relation to pain-based behaviour. This will prove a vital source of future progress in this field.

Prevalence

Pain-based behaviour in children deserves a great deal of attention from practitioners and researchers because of the ripples of harm and disturbance it generates across multiple systems; because of what it tells us about the environments children are experiencing; and because intervening early prevents later harm. Rivara [3, p. 747] reminds us that 'decades of research by criminologists, sociologists and psychologists indicate that the basis for violence rests in childhood and that there is remarkable continuity of behaviour over time'. We know that children frequently experience and witness violence at home and in their communities: in the US-based NatSCEV survey [4], 60% of children surveyed had been exposed to violence in the previous year, 10.2% had experienced maltreatment and 9.7% had witnessed family violence. One in five had experienced maltreatment at some point in the past. The latest national UK survey [5] suggested that 18.7% of adults had experienced some form of childhood abuse, 7.6% had experienced physical abuse and 9.8% had witnessed family violence.

In turn, aggression and violence are common reasons for referral to CAMHS [6] and are frequently associated with diagnoses of attention-deficit/hyperactivity disorder (ADHD), conduct disorder, oppositional defiant disorder and autistic spectrum conditions. Childhood aggression is thought to be a risk factor for a wide range of difficulties in adolescence [7, 4]; whilst most aggression subsides in early childhood, around 15% [8] continue to show such difficulties into adulthood. This kind of pain-based behaviour can lead to school exclusions, peer difficulties, emotional distress and involvement in the criminal justice system. Early intervention is therefore of particular value. At the extreme end of the scale, we can see that there were 16,000 proven violent offences in the United Kingdom by under eighteens in the year ending March 2019; the 'dark figure of crime' including unreported or undetected offences is likely to be far higher [10].

Guidance

The National Institute for Health and Care Excellence (NICE) Guidelines regarding violence and aggression in children [11] offer a useful overview of practice in the area, making recommendations for preventative and anticipatory measures to reduce the risk of violence and aggression, to manage it by therapeutic means, and then ultimately to contain it via restraint, seclusion and tranquillisation. There is a natural degree of overlap with the guidance relating to the treatment of conduct disorder [6], which goes into greater depth regarding recommended psychosocial interventions. Key points are summarised as follows:

Prevention

- Staff should be trained to use restrictive interventions (e.g. restraint) suitable for children, but should avoid or minimise their use.
- Psychosocial strategies should be used wherever possible.
- Staff teams should be well-led, trained and supportive.
- Staff should provide meaningful therapeutic activities, should know their patients well and should work to balance safety with freedom and privacy.
- Safeguarding and collaboration are key principles.

Assessment

- Underlying mental health, cognitive, trauma-related, cultural or other relevant factors should be identified and relevant practice guidance followed

Management

- Age-appropriate interventions promoting self-soothing and self-control, and support and training for parents, should be offered.
- De-escalation should precede any more restrictive intervention.
- Punishment-based interventions are unacceptable.
- Mechanical restraint should not be used.
- Restraint, rapid tranquillisation and seclusion (never in a locked room) should only be used according to the guidance and with close medical monitoring.

The guidance is due to be updated following a surveillance proposal in 2019 that highlighted the need for a future review to consider the importance of trauma-informed care and support, and to offer a greater consideration of service users' human rights. In addition, the guidance will need to consider the introduction of the Bild Restraint Reduction Network (RRN) Standards (published in April 2019) [12], which are now mandatory for all training on restrictive interventions delivered to NHS-commissioned services.

Assessment

Understanding Pain-Based Behaviour in the Context of Development and Relationships

Assessing pain-based behaviour in children requires us to integrate numerous ideas and sources of information that the vast literature in this area has yielded, to inform the creation of contexts in which the child can feel able to tell us, in whatever ways they can, about what is going on. The starting point is to provide an environment in which the truth of what is going on can emerge, in terms of collaborative, exploratory and empathic relationships between professionals, the child and their network. Once that is in process, the mechanics of how the assessment takes place, and what components it may include, can be worked through. Good and meaningful assessment is multi-modal and takes into account the qualities of multiple levels and parts of the child's system, risk and protective factors and, crucially, the relational environment that surrounds the pain-based behaviour itself.

The principle that informs this chapter is that violence is never 'unprovoked' or 'random', but arises in the child as a response to a real or perceived threat to their psychological or physical integrity, in the context of a relationship or a network of relationships. Our role as practitioners is to understand this threat from the perspective of the child's experience and construction of it, and why the child has responded to it in the way he or she has.

In order to do this, we must hold in mind a sense of curiosity about where the child is, developmentally, at a given moment. This is as essential in our observations in spaces in which direct assessment takes place as it is in what we learn about the moments and conditions in which pain-based behaviour is being enacted. Depending on the qualities of those environments, neither will represent more than a snapshot of the child's capabilities, and information must be gathered from multiple sources and, most of all, from children themselves. This may include:

(i)   home and school observations
(ii) play- or discussion-based
(iii) assessment meetings with the child, with family members, siblings and sometimes peers if appropriate, in a clinic, at school, or in the home
(iv) interviews, including developmental histories, with parents (or other caregivers, including staff in residential care or custodial settings) and teachers
(v)   gathering and synthesis of past notes and reports
(vi) psychometric tests and symptom questionnaires, such as those listed here
(vii) specific observational assessments where indicated
(viii) consultations with other key professionals in the network.

Widely used measures of aggression and violence in children and adolescents

- Strengths and Difficulties Questionnaire [13]
- Child Behavioural Checklist [14]
- State Trait Anger Expression Inventory II [15]
- Beck Youth Inventories (BYI-II) [16]
- Brief Rating of Aggression By Children and Adolescents (BRACHA) [17]
- Structured Assessment of Violence Risk in Youth (SAVRY) [18] and the Structured Assessment of Protective Factors for Violence Risk in Juveniles (SAPROF-YV) [19]
- Disruptive Behaviour Rating Scale [20]

While in early childhood some forms of aggression may be seen as developmentally healthy expressions of emotions, such as excitement, frustration and loss, as children grow older we expect them to develop ways of expressing such emotions without doing harm to others.

Children who have experiences of developmental trauma, neglect, limited stimulation and educational opportunities, intellectual disability, illness and neurodevelopmental difficulties can be thrown off course from this normal and complex developmental process of growth, adaptation, refinement and integration. Growing up under challenging conditions can impede or distort development and leave children more vulnerable in their relationships and less able to express their feelings in safe and contained ways (e.g. through talking or seeking comfort); their feelings of distress remain unresolved.

Amongst the ways in which we might understand this, the concept of developmental integration is a useful one in understanding children's pain-based behaviour. Dockar-Drysdale [2] describes the process of developing as an integrated person through the experience of loving containment by the mother or primary caregiver, and states that 'the self is built from such experiences, so that where there are gaps in primary experience, there will be corresponding gaps in the self' (p. 65). Observing the characteristics of children in residential care, she noted two features: 'panic' and 'disruption'. The uniquely human drive to make sense of what is happening to us – what Stokoe [21] calls 'the Curiosity Drive' – means that children are constantly making meaning, in formative and powerful ways, of their experiences, and adapting accordingly, within the bounds of what is possible for them socially, cognitively, biologically and relationally. Where children are surrounded by difficult, frightening and unpredictable relationships, they may learn, consciously and unconsciously, that others cannot be trusted, that they must remain constantly on guard, that they must protect and defend themselves from shame or threat, that parts of themselves are intolerable or uncontrollable, and that their needs are only met when distress is amplified or suppressed. Some emotions may feel so overwhelming or unendurable that they can only be expressed as action: panic or disruption.

Risk and Protective Factors

The developing literature has much to offer in guiding the process of assessment, identifying key risk and protective factors that enrich our understanding of the child and prevent us from forgetting or turning a blind eye to things that matter, and creating frameworks (as shown later in the chapter) that enable us to consider multiple parts of each child's 'social ecology' in a holistic way.

Risk factors that repeatedly emerge from research into the lives and experiences of children who express their pain through violence include prior victimisation and experiences of violence, abuse and neglect at home, at school or in the community [22]. Socio-economic and family factors such as poverty, poor housing conditions, having parents who suffer with mental health difficulties, substance abuse, and/or involvement in offending, and who cannot easily foster the child's social competence, problem-solving or academic engagement, are commonly found [23]. Other studies identify the characteristics of the ways children think and feel, noting difficulties in understanding and managing social relationships, misperceiving others' behaviour as threatening and hostile [24] and a tendency towards 'moral disengagement' (i.e. dehumanising the victims of their violence, minimising the consequences of such behaviour and reconstructive violence as performed in the service of 'good' [25]). These might, of course, be understood as defensive adaptations to traumatic and disturbing experiences, and to feelings of shame and fear.

In contrast, protective factors appear to be the inverse, including internal qualities such as high empathy [26] and social and emotional competence [27]. Lösel and Farington [28] offer a comprehensive summary of direct and 'buffering' protective factors for youth violence, noting that social factors (such as living in a non-deprived and non-violent neighbourhood, medium socio-economic status, a positive school or class climate and 'strong school bonding'), family factors (such as a close relationship to at least one parent and intensive parental supervision) and individual factors (such as above-average intelligence, low impulsivity/easy temperament, enhanced anxiety, pro-social attitudes and academic achievement) acted in a dose–response relationship: the more protective factors in place, the lower the probability of violence.

Bringing these considerations together in a meaningful way, Bronfenbrenner's seminal ecological systems theory of human development [29] sparked a shift towards holistic approaches to child assessment that still exerts significant influence today. The seemingly simple model at the core of his theory (see Figure 13.1) offers an organising frame for

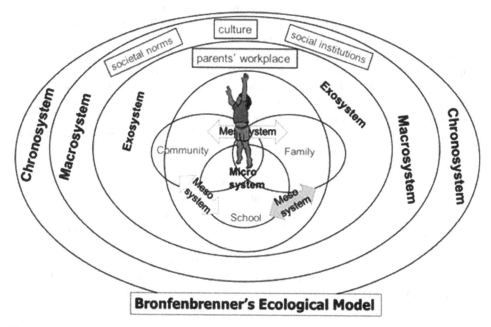

Figure 13.1 Bronfenbrenner's ecological model

assessing the multiple layers of influence on a child's development and the dynamic interplay between them. The ability to hold these complexities in an immediately comprehensible form not only makes this model elegant, but also strengthens its utility.

The *microsystem* holds immediate settings in which a child's life unfolds and tends to include family setting(s), school, community and, in the case of many of the children addressed in this chapter, alternative care settings. With the advent of social media and computer gaming, virtual settings (where children 'do' friendship and identity work) should also be considered [30]. Absences of one or more setting(s) should also be considered particularly relevant to understanding the developmental needs of children who display serious pain-based behaviour. The *mesosystem* comprises the interrelations between two or more settings in the child's microsystem: for example, the degree of mutual respect and good communication between parents and school personnel will influence a child's development in myriad ways. The *exosystem* refers to those settings in which the child is not an active participant, but where events occur which nevertheless exert influence. Settings in which parents experience a strong sense of well-being or significant assaults on their dignity, for example, or staff meetings in which a child is spoken about in a demeaning manner, would all be located in that child's exosystem. The *macrosystem* comprises the patterns manifest in the wider social institutions and ideologies common to a particular subculture or culture. Thus, seemingly intangible concepts such as gender norms or stigmatisation, as well as analyses of social policies (e.g. austerity), gain traction in the service of illuminating the particular experiences and needs of particular children while at the same time avoiding the tendency to locate their difficulties at the level of individual families. Bronfenbrenner later introduced the *chronosystem* to his model to explicitly address the dimension of time and the importance of identifying the impact of experiences and events on subsequent development [31]. Finally, children's active agency in their own development, and particularly their influence on the settings of their microsystem, is also explicitly recognised by Bronfenbrenner.

Thus, we encounter a tangled, complex network of relationships, settings, systems and events in the assessment of children's developmental needs, both generally and specifically related to their pain-based behaviour. Understanding this complexity is required to avoid the unnecessary infliction of secondary pain. This model supports the identification of those elements one might otherwise miss in assessments, and consideration of the dynamic ways in which they all interact and influence particular children's development over time.

A recent contribution specific to this area is the framework for assessment and intervention around violence (FAIV)[32] that unites Bronfenbrenner's model with specific considerations of client and practitioner factors. The model can encompass developments in practice, as it sets out core principles rather than specifics. A diagrammatic version of the model can be found in Figure 13.2:

Within a wider model such as the FAIV, structured professional judgement (as opposed to relying on clinical judgement, or actuarial risk assessment only) is widely understood to be the most reliable and meaningful method underlying an assessment. It combines attention to empirical risk factors (static, dynamic and protective, measured using a variety of inventories) with professional, clinical judgement and expertise gained from a comprehensive assessment of the child in question in the light of psychological theory [10]. It involves a step-by-step process whereby detailed background and current information is considered against structured evidence-based protocols, relevant future scenarios are explored, and potential interventions that help to manage the identified risks are suggested.

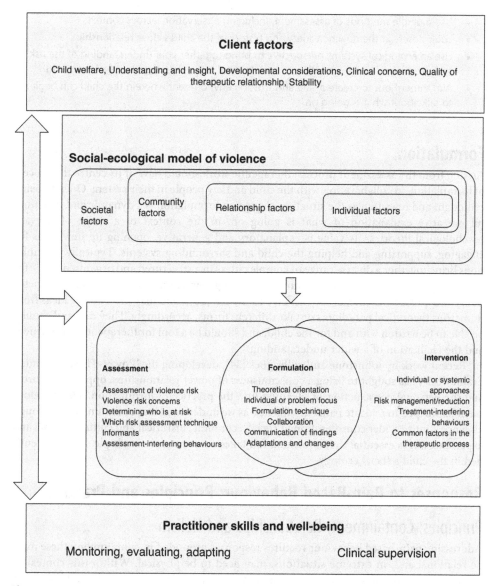

Figure 13.2 Framework for Assessment and Intervention with Violence (Morgan, 2015)

Practice points: Assessment

- Pay attention to the child's development (cognitive, emotional, physical, social) and the integration of their developmental capacities
- Analyse specific violent incidents, their contexts, antecedents, process and consequences, with close attention to the possible meanings of these from the child's perspective

- Use multiple methods of assessment, including observation, across contexts
- Look closely at the quality, variety and history of the child's close relationships
- Use an ecological systems perspective to bring together your understanding of the risk and protective factors operating at each layer of the child's experience of the world
- Aim throughout to create a safe and trusting environment wherein the child can begin to talk about what is going on

Formulation

Arising from the assessment process, therapeutic work should have at its centre the process of formulation, in collaboration with the child and key people in their system. Open to being rethought and rewritten as the situation changes, a formulation is a dynamic and meaningful narrative explanation of what is going on, in the context of a range of relevant psychological theories. Its value is explanatory and generative, opening up new ideas for engaging, supporting and helping the child and surrounding systems. Typically, formulations bring together a diverse range of complex ideas in a structured and organised way – for example, by dividing information into 'predisposing', 'precipitating', 'presenting', 'perpetuating' and 'protective' categories (the 'Five Ps model' [33]), and may incorporate ideas from numerous theoretical paradigms or take different forms, accordingly. They can, and should, be able to be written with and for the child, and should be a tool for therapeutic engagement and the facilitation of a wider understanding.

Recent work by Johnstone and colleagues [34], developing the 'Power-Threat-Meaning Framework', has sought to bring a consciousness of power relationships, oppression, threat and the personal construction of meaning into the practice of formulation. This development has helped to relocate pain – in this case as we understand it as communicated through violence – into a wider consideration of social, economic, historical and cultural factors and experiences. It is essential that a formulation takes account of the multiple systems identified in the child's social ecology.

Responses to Pain-Based Behaviour: Principles and Practice

Principles: Containment, Relationships and Holism

Addressing pain-based behaviour requires responses grounded in containment; these must be relational and, in extreme situations, may need to be physical. Within this context of containment practitioners can identify and meet unmet needs in the child and his or her system, and create the potential, ultimately, for healing and change.

Containment serves as a central theory through which we can make sense of children's pain-based behaviour and understand what practitioners need in order to respond helpfully and consistently. The term 'containment' is often used pejoratively to mean holding children within a status quo and lacking any real progress (or even intention of progress). The meaning of containment we are referring to here was developed by Wilfred Bion [35] and subsequently incorporated across a wide array of fields and disciplines. Bion identified the caring processes between primary caregiver(s) (in his day, the mother) and infant during the first few years of life as the basis for the development of thinking in order to manage raw experience and emotion. This ability develops further in toddlerhood through the introduction, or more extensive use, of oral interpretation by caregivers of toddlers' emotional states and experiences. Children who act out their pain through their behaviour are often unable, temporarily or throughout much of their day-to-day, to contain it.

Bion drew parallels between what happens between the primary caregivers and infant, and between the therapist and patient, to illuminate the processes involved in bringing about and/or restoring the capacity to think in the client. These processes include projective identification of unbearable (or uncontainable) feelings onto the caregiver, therapist or, for the sake of this discussion, practitioner. The practitioner who maintains calm receptiveness is able to absorb these feelings, to process them actively and cognitively, and to respond with empathic acknowledgement. In early years development, when this informs and infuses feeding, soothing and changing nappies, infants repeatedly experience the uncontainable being made containable. Similarly, when a practitioner absorbs and makes sense of the emotional communication of a child or young person and responds in a manner that begins to meet the expressed need, that child or young person's emotions and experiences become more thinkable and manageable – more containable. Put simply, the practitioner becomes a container for the child who, through repeated experiences of containment, becomes more able, more often, to contain (i.e. to use thinking to manage) his or her experiences and emotions.

Containment theory is a close kindred to attachment theory [36, 37] and Winnicott's theorising about the holding environment [38]. These are all beneficial perspectives for understanding pain-based behaviour. We argue that containment theory has greater elasticity in its explanatory power, in that it is just as usefully applied to indirect practice (i.e. processes that support practice at individual and organisational level) as it is to direct practice between practitioners and children. In direct practice, beyond significant dyadic relationships, processes of containment can be identified or cultivated in the network of relationships to which a child belongs, as well as in the rhythms, rituals, routines and even organisation of the physical environments within which the child's life unfolds. Moreover, containment is neither static nor a developmental milestone that one achieves; we all experience times where our ability to think clearly (or at all) becomes compromised. The capacity to use thinking to manage experiences and emotions fluctuates throughout life, not only due to the relative strength or fragility of one's developmental foundations, but to the ongoing, dynamic interplay of strengths, vulnerabilities, protections and adversities encountered throughout the life course.

Good therapeutic practice, whatever the modality, must involve the cultivation of a state of mind and style of interaction that is directly responsive to the cues of the child, and is based on a set of ideas and values about the child and the work that include empathy, genuineness, curiosity, acceptance, playfulness and flexibility [39]. This echoes Vygotsky's concept of the 'zone of proximal development' [40, p. 86]: in essence, the creation of a relational environment in which the child can flourish and reach their potential. A key principle is to cultivate a mode of working wherein the therapist attempts to meet the child and their family in their 'comfort zone' rather than requiring them to adjust themselves to expectations that may seem foreign or uncomfortable [41].

Current thinking adjures us to value the child, but not their challenging or aggressive behaviour. Whilst this way of using language may aid various therapeutic practices [42], it is problematic if it reflects a similar lack of integration in the practitioners' conceptualisation of what is going on. Seeing children as separate from their behaviour invites practitioners to separate their responses to behaviour from the personhood of the child. We take the view that pain-based behaviour is relational; it originates in relational experiences and is expressed in relation to others. It has meaning, history and context and is co-created and dynamic. Any useful and humane approach to a child in this kind of pain will address this meaning, history and context through the process of creating and sustaining a healing relationship, within a larger systemic context in which this way of working is supported. Within such a safe, contained and containing relationship there is scope for both empathy and challenge on the part of the practitioner and for children to explore the edges of their feelings and experiences. This process asks practitioners to hold simultaneously the ambivalence and complexity in the task of supporting a child's integration. Dockar-Drysdale [2] suggests that we as professionals must '*hold the violence and the child* together' (p. 67 [original emphasis]). The authors are reminded of a recent recruitment campaign for custodial officer roles in the youth estate that asked, 'Can you see the child and not the crime?' In fact, the essence of providing meaningful and containing holistic care to children who are being sanctioned for causing pain to others is to be able to see both the child *and* their experiences in their entirety. The most innovative approaches to practice embody exactly this commitment.

Practice

Preventative Work

Much has been written in recent years about the 'public health' approach to violence, wherein the emphasis is on prevention, as it might be with, for example, an infectious disease. Violence Reduction Units and similar initiatives in Glasgow, New York, Chicago and London have supported projects to strengthen local communities where violence has been prevalent through a variety of means, including reducing school exclusions, offering parenting programmes, enhancing after-school provision and developing initiatives that respond to specific local needs. Developing closer links between CAMHS services and schools, locating counselling services within school settings, offering training for teachers and providing spaces and opportunities to develop young people's social and emotional skills are all examples of promising preventative practice that addresses some of the systemic difficulties in the roots of much pain-based behaviour and attempts to offer support in accessible, inclusive ways.

Promising practice: The Well Centre

Recognising the need for a preventative, holistic and accessible health service for young people at risk of offending in Lambeth, south London, GP Stephanie Lamb set up a joint service with youth work and violence prevention organisation, RedThread, to offer a walk-in 'one-stop shop' for adolescents [43]. At the clinic, which opened in 2011 in a well-established local youth club, young people can see a GP, a CAMHS practitioner or engage with specialist youth workers trained in social prescribing who can address a range of unmet physical and mental health needs. A further clinic in Streatham extended their reach, as did a partnership with Lambeth Youth Offending Service. All young people are offered a biopsychosocial assessment, with a case-finding approach to tapping into mental health needs, with on-site counselling, sexual health, medical care and outreach services available, and in liaison with other services, such as housing, to enable coordinated care across the multiple systems around each young person. The service is valued by young people in the borough for its responsive, non-judgemental, holistic ethos and for the ease with which they can get the help they need without negotiating multiple referrals to disparate teams. The Well Centre has inspired the design of services in other boroughs, such as Spotlight, in Tower Hamlets.

An alternative trend – and, in the opinion of the authors, a counterproductive and potentially harmful one – is the use of 'zero-tolerance' and punitive systems, particularly evident in some secondary schools in the United Kingdom and America, where strict rules and behavioural sanctions including detention, isolation and exclusion are applied. Borgwald et al. [44] argue that zero-tolerance approaches are ineffective, counterproductive, unjust, overused, often racially disproportionate and likely to promote covert bullying and unhelpful stigmatising. In addition, they note that 'treating bullying as a crime and removing a child from the school is, in practice, transforming children from being children with behavioural problems into quasi-adults whose rights to an education are forfeited, a form of criminal punishment' (pp. 6–7). Such practices potentially preclude opportunities for forgiveness and repair, instead generating bitterness and reinforcing a sense of rejection. Exclusion from education deprives children of broader social contact and wide educational opportunities, leaving them more vulnerable to antisocial influences in alternative provisions such as pupil referral units (PRUs), and more exposed to difficulties at home and in their communities, propelling children along the 'PRU to prison pipeline' [45, 46].

Specific psychologically informed programmes aimed at the prevention of violence are not well-researched, possibly reflecting the early stages of the development of such interventions. The last Cochrane review in this area [47] attempted to evaluate programmes preventing gang involvement but was not able to proceed due to a lack of available studies meeting their criteria. The Gang Resistance Education and Training (GREAT) programme, a school-based American intervention in which children are taught a nine-week programme by law enforcement officers, yielded positive results in terms of pro-social attitudes and a decline in some forms of delinquency in a large-scale evaluation [48] but has not been used in the United Kingdom.

In treatment, educational and other social settings, initiatives such as the Enabling Environments programme [49], and the development of trauma-informed ways of working where principles of safety, trustworthiness, choice, collaboration and empowerment are genuinely integrated into working practices, promote conditions that are intended to prevent violence and encourage positive and therapeutic relationships. Some key principles specific to creating an environment that precludes violence in residential care for children are offered by Dockar-Drysdale, all of which require staff to be committed to taking up a caring, reflective, adult position:

Four principles for preventing violence in residential child care

1. to accept responsibility for keeping lines of communication always open, so that violent acting out can be converted into the communication of anger;
2. to contain and know our violent feelings so that we do not need to use children to act these out for us;
3. to respect the 'territorial imperative' and to provide insulation for children; and
4. to be responsible for containing children who are not themselves able to accept responsibility. [2, p. 68]

By the 'territorial imperative' and 'insulation', she refers to the need for privacy and ownership over physical space.

Treatment

Therapies, intervention and treatment (terms which are used fairly interchangeably in the literature depending on the dominant traditions within the given setting) to address aggression and violence may be delivered through a variety of services, including CAMHS, via social care and local authorities in residential child care, and through specialist services in community, educational and secure settings. Any intervention must be based upon the relevant practitioners being able to assess and formulate, keeping in mind the concept that any difficult and challenging behaviour may be based upon pain and trauma, whatever setting they may be working in.

Children and Young People's Mental Health Services

Access to mental health services in England and Wales is delivered through a tiered system.

- Tier 1 is about ensuring that all those working with children across a range of settings have a good understanding of the variety of ways in which emotional difficulties present, and the capacity to recognise these, respond appropriately and provide direction to sources of further help; thus, professionals working within education settings, social care and all health services seeing children must be trained in the presentation of emotional disorders, and be aware of how to refer on the children who require more specialised assessment.

- Tier 2 services are delivered across the community, with mental health practitioners being based in schools and other community services, to ensure greater, easier and more embedded access to help for children, in familiar settings; prevention and de-escalation of emotional difficulties is an underlying focus of these services, based upon the precept that more significant and enduring problems can be prevented and diverted.

- Specialist CAMHS represents Tier 3, with skilled mental health practitioners across a range of disciplines available in all areas, although the waiting times can be prohibitive, with children and their families experiencing considerable delays in accessing treatments and interventions. Professionals working within Tier 3 CAMHS will come from a range of disciplines: specialist mental health nurses, clinical psychologists, family therapists, specialist mental health social workers, child and adolescent psychiatrists. Assessments and treatments may be unidisciplinary or multidisciplinary.

- Tier 4 services are in place across larger geographical areas to provide specialist assessment and treatment, and inpatient care as necessary, including specialist eating disorder services.

- The advent of F-CAMHS (forensic CAMHS), since 2016, has led to the creation of a nationally commissioned network of specialist teams offering consultation, training, liaison and expert assessment to CAMHS teams around particularly complex children with forensic needs.

- In addition to mainstream mental health services, the Voluntary Sector also provides mental health services, often for circumscribed problems. For example, the NSPCC and Barnardo's provide services for survivors of sexual abuse and for young people showing harmful sexual behaviour.

Services across the tiers are commissioned through local clinical commissioning groups, but also through social services and models of joint funding. More recently schools, especially large academy groups, have become commissioners in their own right. Although the original thinking was for there to be a seamless, tiered service addressing the needs of children and young people, with fluidity and easy transition between the services, the commissioning models and fragmentation of funding has meant that it can be very difficult for families, and indeed professionals, to know where a young person's needs may best be met; unfortunately, young people can experience being 'bounced' between services and experience considerable delay before reaching the right professional to meet their specific needs. Additionally, families can experience internal waiting lists within services, which causes further delays to treatment.

It is important to understand that children displaying pain-based behaviour may present in a myriad of settings, and linking them in to the most appropriate intervention will depend upon how and when they present and a robust assessment and formulation.

Unfortunately, these children may find it difficult to access a service that will meet their needs. Specialist CAMHS will often reject referrals where challenging behaviour is the principal symptom, stating that they are not commissioned to meet the needs of this population. Children may be referred to alternative services or third-sector organisations, or simply knocked back. This process misses the core understanding that the visible behaviour often relates to underlying relational trauma and may reflect the operation of numerous biological, psychological and social factors that could have been addressed and de-escalated. By failing to link them with practitioners who understand about the difficult experiences that might have led to the development of pain-based behaviour, services deny children timely and helpful interventions. In order to ensure that these vulnerable children are picked up early, it is important to teach and train around pain-based behaviour, across all children and young people's mental health and specialist services, so that there can be broader discussions about the origin of the behaviours and better practice to change the course for the children involved.

In the following sections, we describe parent-, child- and system-focused interventions, including medication, that may be used to address pain-based behaviour.

Parent-Focused Interventions

Programmes offering training and support to parents are a well-researched mode of treatment, and some have shown considerable effectiveness in promoting parental resilience and reducing harsh practices [50, 51]. Several versions are used in CAMHS services, including the Incredible Years Programme [52] and the 'Triple-P' Positive Parenting Programme [53]. Often they involve multiple or alternative formats (group, individual and self-directed, with guidance by phone), and generally cover limit-setting, consistency, problem-solving, play, praise and the prioritisation of 'golden' or 1:1 'quality' time with carers. The most effective programmes are collaborative, leave room for parents to relate the teaching to their own experiences, are delivered in tandem with separate family therapy and are supported by the provision of creches, transport and other practical interventions that enable struggling families to attend. It often proves difficult, however, to engage families in these kinds of interventions, particularly where there are histories of mistrust in services or other circumstances that may act as a barrier. Fairly high rates of attrition and non-attendance in such groups [54] mean that these interventions cannot always reach those who are in the greatest need or at the highest risk. The Lighthouse programme [55], a therapeutic initiative for parents using mentalisation-based treatment (MBT), art and group-based discussion and currently running across various services in the west of England, is a new and promising development in this area.

Child-Focused Interventions

Structured, often manualised, cognitive behavioural therapeutic (CBT) interventions for children, delivered in both group and individual formats, have been widely studied and evaluated. With children, CBT for anger-related issues usually involves psychoeducation, relaxation strategies, problem-solving, social skills and conflict resolution training [56], and may involve complementary work with parents. The 'third wave' of cognitive therapies, incorporating (amongst others) mindfulness and compassion-focused approaches, may enhance the effectiveness of these interventions [57, 58]. Meta-analyses of the effects of group-based CBT for children [59, 60, 61] have generally found that multi-modal, skills-based treatments are the most effective, especially where they include problem-solving components. Dominant CBT programmes include the Anger Coping Program for younger children [62] and Aggression Replacement Training (ART) for adolescents [63].

Many of the more manualised interventions for children and parents assume that skills deficits are the problem, and that the solution can be found in learning more skills and the control to apply them. As Cochran et al. [41, p. 292] point out, however, 'the skills tend to be known, but not used, by such youth'. All practitioners in this field are familiar with the experience of working with young people who appear more than able to grasp ideas and describe how they can be manifested in positive behaviours but who struggle profoundly to feel any emotional charge in these conversations, or to feel there is any place for such skills in real life. Cochran et al. suggest that 'the self-defeating belief systems and environmental influences have largely solidified by teen years: thus a corrective therapeutic relational experience may be more effective than directives and skill teaching' (p. 292). Indeed, years of research have repeatedly told us that the therapeutic alliance is a greater predictor of positive change than the manifest content or technique of any therapy [63, 64], and that attention to multiple levels of the child's social ecology is more likely to effect change than focused attention to a specific set of skills.

While there is some evidence that CBT interventions for anger and aggression can be effective, the interventions evaluated in such studies are usually American, group-based and manualised, with male-only samples, and do not necessarily reflect the nature and form of CAMHS work in the United Kingdom. Nor are non-cognitive behavioural approaches such as psychodynamic or family therapy often included in the major studies, despite clinicians' experience of their value, which creates the obvious danger of their being disregarded in the allocation of funding, commissioning of services or further research.

Small-scale studies highlight the value of other approaches such as mentalisation-based therapy and mindfulness-based therapy [58, 65] and mind–body approaches such as yoga and biofeedback training, and we would recommend that practitioners in the area remain open and curious about such therapeutic approaches that intuitively, theoretically and anecdotally appear to benefit children showing pain-based behaviour but are yet to be evaluated on a large scale. Approaches designed for other groups of children, for example those affected by bereavement or loss, such as the Seasons for Growth programme and Tree of Life work [66, 67], may have great applicability to children whose distress is expressed through aggression and violence and who have often experienced significant losses.

Medication

Pharmacological interventions are not recommended in the research literature or in the NICE guidelines [6, 11] for the routine treatment of children presenting with violence or aggression; psychosocial interventions are the first-line treatment. However, as Squire et al. [68, p. 124] suggest, 'due to the lack of psychologically oriented practitioners within services and a predominance of a medical model of understanding behaviour' – and, we would add, because often the fear engendered by violent behaviour feels as if it requires a rapid and reactive response which medication easily supplies – 'this guidance is not necessarily followed widely'. It is important, nevertheless, to accept that there are occasions when the use of medication may be appropriate. For some children, there may be a comorbid difficulty that can be addressed by the use of medication; an improvement in this area may then enable them to engage with psychological treatment or to respond to changes in how they are treated by teachers or parents following systemic interventions. When there is thought to be comorbidity alongside underlying pain-based behaviour, medication may be considered. Treatment of comorbid ADHD, significant depression and crippling anxiety may be addressed through stimulant medication and SSRIs respectively, in keeping with NICE guidance. Prescribing should only be done by an experienced CAMHS psychiatrist, preferably as part of a multidisciplinary response to a good assessment and formulation; it is important that clinicians understand that this is a part of the treatment, and not the sole answer. Within specialist inpatient settings, medication may be used to manage particularly distressed and challenging behaviour; this needs to be done in keeping with local protocols and national guidance around the use of rapid tranquillisation in young people.

Systemic and Multi-modal Treatments

Functional family therapy [70] is a widely used and researched form of family therapy designed to support families to address and resolve aggressive and antisocial behaviour in children. It uses a three-stage programme focusing first on beliefs about change and patterns of relationships within the family, then on behavioural interventions, and finally on generalising change across systems. Early studies of its effectiveness showed promising results, but subsequent trials have not shown significant advantages over other forms of intervention [71].

Non-violent resistance (NVR) [72] is a family-based psychological intervention derived from the principles espoused by activists such as Mahatma Gandhi and Martin Luther King. It has been developed by Haim Omer, Peter Jakob and colleagues as a systemic intervention to support families and carers of people whose behaviour is violent or controlling. Delivered in regular sessions, in the form of guidance and coaching and often supported by telephone contact, it aims to redefine and strengthen family relationships and reduce conflict and violence. NVR rests on the idea of parental presence and non-engagement in escalating verbal or physical exchanges. The assumption is that without a violent counter-response, the aggressive child will find that their usual strategies become ineffective and wear out. It is explicitly relational: violence is not regarded as the inevitable expression of trauma, depriv-ation, uncontrollable impulsivity or illness, but as a relational phenomenon in which the parents/carers have acquiesced (usually without realising they are doing so) and continued to provide the means for it to perpetuate. NVR is widely used in Israel, Germany and, increasingly, the United Kingdom. In a German study in 2009 [73], NVR was compared with TEEN-Triple-P. Improvements were evident amongst both groups, with some advantages found in the NVR group. A more recent UK study [74] found that group NVR improved family relationships and reduced episodes of violence and aggression in the home.

Interventions such as multisystemic therapy (MST) [75] and multidimensional family therapy (MDFT) attempt to address more severe difficulties intensively, at multiple levels of the system (i.e. individual, parents, wider family, school, peer, community). MST is based on ecological systems theory [29] and the understanding that the child is an active participant enmeshed in a series of larger, connected systems that affect their experience. It is aimed at preventing children going into custody or other forms of care outside the family home, and at improving the quality of family relationships. MST typically involves considerable therapeutic resources, with teams of specially trained therapists who develop close, collaborative and flexible working relationships with families, staying in daily or even 24-hour, contact, visiting them at home, facilitating engagement with other helpful resources and offering therapeutic intervention at all levels (i.e. in school, with peers) according to the needs and wishes of the family. Interventions typically last several months and can be extended as needed. Where families remain engaged, these multi-modal, 'ecological', flexible, expertly delivered and responsive approaches produce some of the best outcomes [76].

Practice points: Treatment

- Treatment should be based on a thorough and meaningful assessment and a collaborative formulation that considers multiple contributory risk and protective factors across the systems around the child.
- Though Tier 3 CAMHS services are staffed with clinicians with appropriate skills and training to address pain-based behaviour, resource shortages and commissioning priorities mean that children may not be able to access them.
- Parent-focused interventions, including supportive skill-building groups, can be highly effective.
- Child-focused interventions should meet the child at their developmental level, and should be engaging, individualised and based on a meaningful and shared formulation of their difficulties. Medication can be helpful in specific circumstances, as part of a wider response.
- Systemic interventions such as MST, FFT and NVR may offer more ecologically valid and meaningful responses that work at multiple levels.
- Therapeutic responses should operate on the principle of developing safe, containing and communicative relationships around the child that foster the child's developmental integration and positive sense of self and other.

Restrictive Interventions

Criminalisation and Incarceration

The use of 'secure care' to manage and prevent violence in children represents an extreme form of physical containment. The United Kingdom's readiness to criminalise children is somewhat mitigated by sentencing guidelines that discourage custodial sentences and promote community orders and welfare interventions. There is a decreasing reliance on incarceration for children, though less so for crimes that involve violence. Since 2008, the number of children in custody in England and Wales has fallen from approximately 2,900 to 8,609. The 2017 Lammy Review [77] found that a disproportionate and rising number of these children are from Black and other minority racial and ethnic groups, reflecting the operation of structural racism in UK society and within the criminal justice system (51.9% of those in the YOIs were from minority groups, according to 2021 statistics, relative to 27% in youth custody in 2009, and 18% across the general population [78]). These children are housed in Young Offenders' Institutions (YOIs) (for 15–18 year-old boys), secure training centres (STCs) and secure children's homes (for 12–18 year-old boys and girls), on remand and while serving sentences of varying lengths. Of children in custody, 51% are detained for violent offences [9]. Over the last ten years the average sentence length has increased from approximately 11 months to 18 months, but this statistic disguises the rapidly growing proportion of young people in custody who are serving 'life' sentences (given a minimum tariff by the judge at their sentencing, after which release depends on the approval of the parole board, and a lifetime on licence). Minimum tariffs have increased dramatically over the past ten years, a trend Crewe et al. [79, p. 6] describe as reflecting 'the increased use of forms of expressive punishment designed to communicate moral outrage and a political culture that is less resistant to punitive demands, cultivated by the popular press'.

In England, Wales and Northern Ireland, the age of criminal responsibility (ACR; the age at which a child can be prosecuted and punished by law for an offence) is currently ten. This is the lowest ACR in Europe and one of the lowest in the world; it has been criticised by the UN as incompatible with their Convention on the Rights of the Child and 'not internationally acceptable' [80]. Scotland has recently moved to implement legislation raising the ACR to 12 (The Age of Criminal Responsibility [Scotland] Act, 2019). Mounting neurobiological and psychological evidence has shown that children do not reach emotional, moral or intellectual maturity until far later than ten, particularly where development is disturbed by trauma and adversity. Adolescence is a period in which risk-taking, impulsivity and boundary-breaking behaviour is developmentally and culturally normative [81], after which these behaviours naturally decline [82]. As Dockar-Drysdale [2, p. 65] notes, 'Roughly, one can equate degree of responsibility with degree of integration as an individual reached by the person who has committed the violent act. Unintegrated people of any age are unable to contain conflict, to make a choice, to feel personal guilt or compassion for others or to accept responsibility'. This understanding fundamentally questions the legitimacy of criminalising young people, let alone administering sentences that are sometimes longer than the lives they have already lived and coloured by systemic prejudices.

The fact of coming into custody suggests that containment in the systems of relationships, home, school, community and the community youth justice system has not been adequate. The level of violence or dangerousness that the child is thought to present is now to be met by what we might understand as 'the brick mother' [83]. While nominally preventing violence to the public, secure settings are notoriously violent places for both young people and custodial staff; in YOIs, between April 2018 and March 2019, there were 2,400 assaults, roughly equally split between peer-on-peer and staff assaults [9]. The vengeful paradigm that suggests that incarceration is an appropriate and curative response to violence is not validated by any known research. Reoffending rates for children who have been in custody were last measured at 69.3% in the United Kingdom (for the year ending in

March 2019) [9], and there is evidence that children who are treated most harshly in custody are the least likely to desist from crime [84].

Balancing popular pressure, the apparent protection of the public, long-established working practices in the prison service, adherence to human rights and standards supporting the humane and rehabilitative care of children, and advancing psychological theory and practice, is clearly a complex task. The upshot is a system that struggles to manage and address violence, much like an uncontained parent reacting chaotically to competing pressures; sometimes punitive, sometimes thoughtful, rarely consistent. In response to repeatedly critical reports from the prison inspectorate (HMIP) a damning review by Lord Taylor in 2016 [85] and campaigns by the Howard League and other organisations, the Youth Custody Service has introduced a set of reforms aimed at developing a more therapeutic, trauma-responsive system and training a skilled, professional and dedicated workforce, with the planned creation of 'Secure Schools' to replace the YOIs and the STCs in England and Wales. The standard service options for children in custody had already expanded over the last ten years, as specialist CAMHS services were increasingly commissioned to operate in secure settings. These brought a clinical perspective to the care children were offered, beyond formerly minimal mental health provision and the (largely cognitive behavioural) manualised offending behaviour programmes offered by established forensic psychology services. There have been numerous attempts to reduce violence in the youth estate – including staff training in restorative justice and de-escalation techniques, embedding conflict resolution teams, and limiting and supervising contact between the boys – with, unfortunately, limited success.

Promising innovations: SECURE STAIRS

A key element of the new Reform programme across the secure youth estate in England, SECURE STAIRS, is a framework for integrated care, devised, funded and shared jointly between HMPPS, NHS England and the Department for Education. It embodies a set of principles for developmentally sensitive, psychologically informed work with children and staff in secure settings [86, 87].

SECURE STAIRS (an acronym for the key principles of the framework) significantly expanded the funding for NHS therapeutic provision and trauma-informed training and support for custodial officers in youth secure settings, from its inception in 2016. The operationalisation of the framework differs across these settings but involves core components of formulation-based care for young people, and intensive training, reflective practice and clinical-style supervision for custodial staff. Its ambitious aim is the transformation of 'warehouses' to 'greenhouses', re-training custodial staff as 'therapeutic parents' and embedding cultures of benign enquiry, care and reflection in these establishments, drawing on a broadly systemic and psychodynamic understanding of organisational functioning and trauma [88, 89].

The programme draws on ideas from the literature on therapeutic communities to promote stable patterns of communal living and relating, establishing community meetings and valuing the voices of the boys alongside those of custodial staff. The idea of reparation is privileged, where the community offers the potential for forgiveness and reconciliation after damage or violence [90].

The expanded on-site CAMHS teams created by the SECURE STAIRS programme, working with custodial staff, can, when enabled to function within the complexity and rigidity of prison regimes, offer highly specialist, individualised, multisystemic therapeutic work, and enable 'through-the-gate' transitions with families and community services to address and resolve the systemic anxiety around release or transfer. A multi-site longitudinal outcome evaluation by the Anna Freud Centre is currently in progress.

Physical Restraint, Co-Regulation and De-Escalation

Children and adolescents in extreme states of distress or arousal, particularly when attacking another person, naturally need to be made safe and those around them protected. As a last resort, this may require physical restraint or holding [91]. Restraint must be undertaken by trained staff and must be 'appropriate to the situation, reasonable, proportionate and necessary, used for the shortest period possible'. During the restraint, 'vital observations are taken and recorded', and ideally carried out by a member of staff who is the same sex as the child [11, p. 183].

While restraint is rarely necessary in community CAMHS settings, it is more common in inpatient psychiatric and forensic adolescent units, and in secure settings. In the youth secure estate in England between 2018 and 2019, there were 6,300 restrictive physical interventions (a rise of 16% from the previous year) – an average of 46.6 incidents per 100 children in custody [9]. Restraint training, guidance and protocols, which include debriefing and multi-agency monitoring of video footage of restraints and the presence of medical staff to monitor the child's condition during and after restraint, are normal practice in these settings.

There is an increasingly strong emphasis on the use of de-escalation techniques as a way of averting violence, and for good reason. Physical restraint poses serious risks of physical and psychological harm to all involved, including death [92, 93]. Its misuse is associated with children's rights abuses [94] and the Committee on the Rights of the Child (2016) has criticised the United Kingdom for its lack of related monitoring [95]. Accordingly, young people should always have access to independent advocates and means of raising concerns via complaints or other processes.

In the United Kingdom, seclusion and isolation are no longer considered humane ways to deal with children in distress, although recent media reports have suggested that some schools here continue to use such practices. It is increasingly understood that co-regulation – the use of a relational space in which an adult in a caregiving role can help the child to regulate his or her emotions using proximity, vocal comfort and other strategies – is a more therapeutic and naturalistic response. The capacity to co-regulate, however, depends on an environment and a set of relationships that support staff to be able to work in this manner, as well as a knowledge of the child that includes an understanding of any sensory issues. It is also important to acknowledge that building and maintaining the kind of relationships that children can access when they become distressed is sometimes profoundly difficult, particularly when previous experiences have given them good reason to resist and/or test their relationships with adults. Staff should be closely familiar with the individual formulation for each child, which should encompass co-produced care plans that anticipate how that child is understood to respond to stressful events, and suggest what may help.

When feelings have built to a level at which they have erupted into pain-based behaviour that poses a serious risk of imminent harm it is essential, first, to remain *in relationship*, maintaining calm receptiveness and making yourself and the relationship as accessible as possible to the child through actively cognitively processing the communicated pain and empathically acknowledging it, even (and especially) as you assess it necessary to physically restrain the child. This can be one of the most complex and demanding requirements of professionals working with children who have chronic and severe psychosocial pain. The second essential component of good related practice (individually and organisationally) is *the provision of meaningful opportunities for understanding, resolution and reparation* afterwards. This has the power to contain and transform feelings of shame, confusion and hurt, and is a crucial part of enabling children to learn to express their pain in less harmful ways.

Physical restraint is one of the most extreme forms of containment that will occur in the settings to which this chapter is addressed. This is the case whether the restraint is carried out as a form of what we might call 'crude containment,' or whether it is part of the therapeutic processes theorised by Bion (and, subsequently, others), as discussed earlier. In a large-scale, in-depth, qualitative study of staff and young people's experiences of physical restraint in residential child care [96, 97], almost half of the 30 young people who shared their experiences of being physically restrained described *some* as having positive effects, either on how they felt afterwards or on their relationships with those who restrained them. Young people appeared to experience and make sense of restraints based on the degree of trust they had in the staff who restrained them – trust that staff were trying to avert recourse to restraint, that staff were trying to understand and help them, and that when they were restrained, it was done for the right reasons and in a way that did not deliberately hurt them. For trust to withstand the intense potential for restraint to rupture relationships, the two essentials outlined earlier come into sharper relief. To be clear, we are not suggesting that physical restraint itself is beneficial. Indeed, in the aforementioned study, *all* young people who shared experiences of being physically restrained spoke of negative experiences and/or impacts on their relationships with staff. Thus, it warrants repetition: physical restraint should only be used when less restrictive ways of resuming safety are proving ineffective or the immediacy and severity of risk is so great that there is not time to use them. When it is carried out relationally within wider systems and practices that are robustly containing, it can be a part of a wider experience of therapeutic containment.

The RRN has set out to reduce the reliance on coercive practices (including physical restraint) across education, health and social care settings, including both children's and adult services. Towards this end, they have developed training standards and a certification scheme, as well as an active network of committed practitioners and a repository of related resources [12].

Developing Protective Factors Through Legal and Ethical Practice

Throughout this chapter we have touched on the elements in children's lives that can lead to pain-based behaviour. Most of these – victimisation, abuse, neglect, poverty – are beyond childrens' power to change. Compounding these external influences are internalised beliefs about themselves and others as a result of inadequate attachment relationships and unmet needs which telegraph to children the message that they do not matter: 'These children are sensitive to humiliation; they have been exposed to a catastrophic loss of power' [98, p. 5]. The picture can look bleak. However, in Bronfenbrenner's macrosystem there exists a positive, protective and potentially developmental factor in the form of laws and guidance relating to children. These, in tandem with our professional ethical codes and frameworks, offer opportunities for practice that can plant the seeds of self-respect and agency in children.

Child law in all four nations of the United Kingdom takes a strong children's rights perspective, with many of its principles grounded in the UN Convention on the Rights of the Child (UNCRC), adopted by the United Kingdom in 1991. Statutes such as the Children Acts set out who has rights and responsibilities with regard to children. Case law such as

Gillick v. *West Norfolk and Wisbech Area Health Authority* draws on the principles of capacity, consent and privacy in the Convention to allow children the right to make choices about their own lives.

According to Psychological Interventions in Child and Adolescent Mental Health Services [99], the competence framework for CAMHS, one of the core competences for work with children and young people is 'knowledge of legal frameworks related to working with children/young people'. The competence required includes knowledge of capacity and informed consent, parental rights and responsibilities, participation, child protection, mental health, education, data protection and equality. These topics sound dry but they represent a vital and living resource for practitioners seeking to establish growth-enhancing relationships with children.

Capacity, Informed Consent and Confidentiality

In the United Kingdom, a child under 16 can consent to medical treatment if they understand the risks and benefits of what is being proposed. This right is found in the Age of Legal Capacity (Scotland) Act 1991 in Scotland and in *Gillick* v. *West Norfolk and Wisbech Area Health Authority* in the rest of the United Kingdom. There is no lower age limit for consent, although in Scotland there is a presumption of capacity at age 12. A relational (and therefore developmental) approach to assessing children's capacity makes it a collaborative process of informing children about their treatment in child-friendly language, checking their understanding, answering their questions and upholding their decisions. A parent cannot overturn the wishes of a child who has capacity in Scotland. In the rest of the United Kingdom, parents must make a request through the courts.

A child who has capacity and has given his or her consent to treatment is entitled to confidentiality within certain limits based in the child's right to protection. This right to confidentiality is found in case law (*Axon* v. *Secretary of State for Health* (The Family Planning Association: intervening) [2006]) and in Article 16 of the UNCRC, which says that children are entitled to privacy. Maintaining confidentiality and, when sharing information, requesting consent and discussing with the child what is being shared demonstrate respect for the child and can help to build trust.

Participation

Legal frameworks endorse a child's right to have a view when adults are making decisions that concern them, and for that view to be taken into account. This principle of participation is also articulated in Article 12 of the UNCRC: 'States Parties shall assure to the child who is capable of forming his or her own views the right to express those views freely in all matters affecting the child, the views of the child being given due weight in accordance with the age and maturity of the child' (www.unicef.org.uk/what-we-do/un-convention-child-rights). In practice, this means routinely consulting with children throughout your relationship with them, and making sure that their wishes are understood and implemented in accordance with their capacity.

Child Protection

Children have a right to be protected. This is a universal, ethical, moral and legal right. In legal terms, the responsibilities that pertain to safeguarding and child protection can be found in the Children (Scotland) Act 1995 and the Children and Young People (Scotland)

Act 2014 in Scotland, and in the Children Act 1989 and Children Act 2004 in the rest of the United Kingdom. The principle of protection is found in Article 19 in the UNCRC and addressed in detail in child protection guidance at national and local levels.

When practitioners take action to protect children it should be done with care and compassion: informing them, consulting them, respecting their choices as far as possible, supporting them throughout the process and acknowledging the impact of any loss or change that results.

Data Protection

The General Data Protection Regulation (GDPR) entitles children to the same data protection rights as adults, with additional specific rights:

- Children of any age may share their personal data in order to access free online preventative or counselling services.
- Children must be provided with clear child-friendly information presented in plain, age-appropriate language about how you will process their data.
- You must explain to children why you require the personal data you have asked for, and what you will do with it – including when and how you will share it – in a way which they can understand.
- You must tell children what rights they have over their personal data in language they can understand.

In relational terms this might take the form of writing case notes together with a child or young person at the end of sessions, using session rating outcomes measures with them or keeping a shared treatment diary.

Equality

Discrimination and unfair treatment of children can go unnoticed simply because they do not know their rights or because having a protected characteristic means that they become used to habitual bullying and day-to-day discriminations, like lack of wheelchair access, for example. Under the Equality Act 2010, children have the same protections as adults in all categories except age discrimination. Children are only protected from age discrimination in employment or, if under age 18, when using, or trying to use, services.

Living with a protected characteristic – and the resulting sense of difference – can be especially difficult for children and young people, for whom fitting in with their peers is important. A relational approach to equality means not making assumptions about the impact of a protected characteristic and instead taking time to understand the meaning of it for the individual child, valuing the child as a whole person and asking the child how they would like you to work with them.

Codes of Practice and Ethical Guidelines

The Royal College of Psychiatrists' *Good Psychiatric Practice: Code of Ethics* (2014) [100] sets out 12 principles for good professional practice. These principles do not distinguish between adults and children and are not limited by age, except Principle 5 which addresses issues of capacity and consent. According to the Code, all patients shall have their essential humanity and dignity respected. They shall have their consent sought, their confidentiality maintained and be enabled to make the best available choices about their treatment. The Code describes collaborative practice with patients, referring to ethical principles of benefi- cence, non-maleficence, justice and autonomy common to professional codes of practice across most of the helping professions. While recognising that children's autonomy and ability to self-determine can be limited by their age and circumstances, developmental practice endeavours to see the opportunities for growth in every encounter with them.

The law respects children's ability to make choices within the limits of their capacity, takes their views into account, protects them from harm, safeguards the information they share with us and ensures that they are treated equally and fairly. Ethical frameworks for good practice articulate the values that we hold as practitioners and that we bring to our work with children and young people: amongst these are a commitment to treating them with care, respect and fairness, and supporting them to discover what they are capable of. Together, the law and ethics represent a powerful resource for developing protective factors in children, such as self-worth, empathy and social competence.

It is perhaps too much to expect a child who has experienced little or nothing of these values and principles to suddenly, and miraculously, embrace them or to trust the person who offers them. It takes consistency, patience, trustworthiness, hope and even a degree of stubbornness to stick with the personhood of a child who has lived with pain and expresses it through behaviour: 'A good enough therapist [for children] has a dash of a caring grandmother combined with the forensic discipline of a scientist and the compassion of a spiritual leader, humbled to the healing powers of love and time' [98, p. 4].

The Impact of COVID-19

At the time of writing (early 2021), COVID-19 and the associated restrictions continue to affect the lives of young people in the United Kingdom and the provision of healthcare for them and their families. The pandemic seems to have provoked creative approaches to providing care and unexpected opportunities but has also highlighted, exacerbated and, in some cases, been used to justify the reinforcement of existing inequalities.

CAMHS teams have largely moved to providing assessment and therapy online, which seems to have had both advantageous (widening access to some, enabling greater flexibility) and disadvantageous effects (narrowing access to others, limiting the provision of specialist assessments, providing a different and potentially less 'real' experience of relating, raising confidentiality and privacy issues), and Social Care and Youth Offending Services were able to monitor children less closely. School closures affected children differently, with some children increasingly exposed to harm at home, others retreating with anxiety, and many of those with social, communication and other neurodevelopmental needs no longer able to access specialist provisions.

Anecdotal evidence from clinicians and youth offending teams suggested concerns about some of the most vulnerable young people disengaging, others waiting so long for treatment that they turned 18 before provision or transition to adult services could be arranged, and young people 'going missing' more than usual during the pandemic, poten- tially involved in county lines drug dealing and exploitation by criminal gangs. A joint report by organisations working with children affected by youth violence (RedThread, Street Doctors and MAC-UK [101]) on the impact of COVID-19 highlighted the loss of statutory support and rising feelings of depression, anxiety and isolation amongst the young people they interviewed.

For young people in custody, remand time lengthened as the courts shut, leaving some young people detained for extended periods. Attempts to promote early release in order to ease crowded conditions in custody resulted in few expedited releases. New entrants into custody – those known to be at the greatest risk of suicide – were segregated for 10–14 days in order to limit transmission. There was an immediate reduction in violence, mainly because boys were only unlocked in small 'household' groups, and were confined in their cells for much longer periods than usual. Family visits were stopped, then reinstated on a restricted basis (with no physical contact allowed), and video calls were made available. HMIP 'scrutiny' inspections determined that the boys felt safer, but also raised concerns about their access to fresh air, education and services. For some, confinement paradoxically provided an opportunity for them to establish more trusting and consistent relationships with officers stationed on their units but, for others, boredom and loneliness were acute. With low staffing, restrictions on face-to-face work and the withdrawal of the Independent Monitoring Board and most agencies working within the YOIs (apart from NHS physical and mental health care), services available to the boys were comparatively limited, and the usual levels of safeguarding scrutiny reduced.

The Impact of Pain-Based Behaviour on Practitioners and Systems

Working with children expressing pain through their behaviour demands a great deal from practitioners, not least because the experience of facing pain-based behaviour can itself be traumatising and arouses individual and organisational defences that can then get in the way of doing the work of care and containment. This is well documented in the psychoanalytic literature on violence and systems [102, 103] and, frequently, tragically enacted in the scandals of abuse and neglect in care homes, psychiatric hospitals and secure settings that regularly surface in the media. In order to do this work safely and therapeutically, staff must be well-trained, closely supervised, given reflective spaces in which to process the impact of the work and supported by systems of management – and, beyond this, political ideologies and cultural narratives – that understand, enable and value good work.

The central theme in this chapter is the value of understanding and working with children through a developmental, relational lens: paying attention to their social ecology and planning therapeutic work accordingly. Safeguarding – protecting and promoting the child's safety and that of those around them at all times – is central. Working at multiple levels means that multidisciplinary teamwork, good information-sharing and liaison and joined-up work with other services and agencies is crucial. Staffing must be at a level to meet these needs, both in terms of the size and the diversity of therapeutic teams, and in the care and containment provided to practitioners in order for them to do this very challenging work with humanity and integrity. As Dockar-Drysdale [2, p. 62] reminds us, 'We have to be careful that children find us when they reach out, and that they do not again find defences instead of people'.

In settings where we are dealing with pain-based behaviour, good systems of containment are particularly important, as painful and violent dynamics will otherwise be played out between staff or parts of the wider system, or in relation to the children. The greater the frequency, severity and duration of uncontained states experienced by children, the more likely the disruption to practitioners' and organisations' capacity to think clearly and respond helpfully. In offering a containing space for staff working with young children with severe disabilities, Mawson [103, p. 67] noticed that 'workers would frequently feel depressed, despairing of being able to make a worthwhile difference in these children's lives ... they would sometimes feel intensely persecuted by these feelings, even to the extent of experiencing at some level a measure of hostility towards the children themselves'.

The Healthy Organisation Model [21, 89] offers a framework for thinking about how processes of containment can operate in teams. Stokoe suggests that healthy functioning depends on several factors: first, clarity about the primary task and the shared principles that underlie the task. These may be represented through a mission statement, an operational policy and a team ethos that is mutually understood and agreed. Then, the organisation requires a decision-making system that delegates authority down through the hierarchy and welcomes and accepts the resultant anxieties up through the system as a source of valuable information. The provision of opportunities to discuss and work through these anxieties – in this case, through supervision, learning, reflective practice and other team meetings – and the organisational commitment to a position of curiosity and benign inquiry are essential to continuing healthy functioning as well as adaptation and the containment and transformation of the anxieties that naturally arise in the course of the work. In organisations in which these factors are not in place, or are endangered by the operation of external and internal pressures (e.g. painful experiences with children in their care, changes in institutional priorities, losses of funding, increases in workload), anxiety can become located in individuals and relationships, causing a toxic, blame-focused culture, rather than understood as an inevitable and meaningful signifier of a systemic problem and worked through together.

Conclusion

Our intention in this chapter has been to set out key principles and good practice in assessment, formulation and treatment, inviting practitioners to consider violence in children from a relational perspective wherein behaviour is understood to be a pain-based response to situations, settings and systems. We want to encourage those who encounter pain-based behaviour to see these children in context and to respond to them from a position of humanity and empathy, while bringing all of the professional knowledge, experience and skills we have to contain them, to provide the right care for them (and for ourselves as we support them) and to walk alongside them as they take steps towards fulfilling their potential.

References

1. Anglin, J. P. Creating 'well-functioning' residential care and defining its place in a system of care. *Child & Youth Care Forum* 2004; 33:175–92. https://doi.org/10.1023/B: CCAR.0000029689.70611.0f.

2. Dockar-Drysdale, B. The management of violence. *Residential Treatment For Children & Youth* 1998; 16(3):61–74.

3. Rivara, F. P. Understanding and preventing violence in children: Editorial. *Archives of Pediatric Adolescent Medicine* August 2002:156.

4. Finkelhor, D., Turner, H., Ormerod, R., Hamby, S. and Kracke, K. Children's exposure to violence: A comprehensive national survey. *Juvenile Justice Bulletin* October 2009. www.ncjrs.gov/pdffiles1/ojjd p/227744.pdf [Accessed 27.4.2022].

5. Office for National Statistics. Child abuse extent and nature, year ending March 2019,

Crime Survey for England and Wales. 2020. www.ons.gov.uk/peoplepopulationandcommunity/crimeandjustice/articles/childabuseextentandnatureenglandandwales/yearendingmarch2019 [Accessed 27.4.2022].

6. National Institute of Clinical Excellence. Antisocial behaviour and conduct disorders in children and young people: recognition and management. Clinical guideline [CG158] Published: 27 March 2013 Last updated: 19 April 2017. Available at www.nice.org.uk/Guidance/CG158 [Accessed 27.4.2022].

7. Lochman, J. E. Cognitive-behavioral intervention with aggressive boys: Three-year follow-up and preventive effects. *Journal of Consulting & Clinical Psychology* 1992; 60:426–32.

8. Piquero, A. R., Carriaga, M. L., Diamond, B., Kazemian, L. and Farrington, D. P. Stability in aggression revisited. *Aggression and Violent Behavior* 1992; 17(4):365–72.

9. Youth Justice Board/Ministry of Justice. Youth justice statistics 2018/19: England and Wales. London: Ministry of Justice, 2020. https://assets.publishing.service.gov.uk/government/uploads/system/uploads/attachment_data/file/862078/youth-justice-statistics-bulletin-march-2019.pdf [Accessed 27.4.2022].

10. Johnstone, L. and Gregory, L. Youth violence risk assessment: A framework. In A. Rogers, J. Harvey, and H. Law (eds.) *Young People in Forensic Mental Health Settings: Psychological Thinking and Practice.* Basingstoke: Palgrave Macmillan; 2015, pp. 96–122.

11. NICE. Violence and Aggression: Short-term management in mental health, health and community settings, updated edition, NICE Guideline NG10. 2015. www.nice.org.uk/guidance/ng10 [Accessed 27.4.2022].

12. Restraint Reduction Network. [website]. https://restraintreductionnetwork.org/ [Accessed 27.4.21].

13. Goodman, R. Psychometric properties of the strengths and difficulties questionnaire. *Journal of the American Academy of Child and Adolescent Psychiatry* 2001 Nov; 40 (11):1337–45.

14. Achenbach, T. *Manual for the Child Behavioral Checklist/4–18 and 1991 profile.* Burlington, VT: University of Vermont Press; 1991.

15. Spielberger, C. D. *State-Trait Anger Expression Inventory.* Orlando, FL: Psychological Assessment Resources; 1988.

16. Beck, A. T., Beck, J. S., Jolly, J. and Steer, R. *Beck Youth Inventories – Second Edition For Children and Adolescents (BYI-II).* Bloomington: Pearson; 2005.

17. Barzman, D. H., Brackenbury, L., Sonnier, L. et al. Brief Rating of Aggression by Children and Adolescents (BRACHA): Development of a tool for assessing risk of inpatients' aggressive behavior. *Journal of the American Academy of Psychiatry and the Law Online* 2011; 39:170–9.

18. Bartel, P., Bourm, R. and Fourth, A. *Structured Assessment for Violence Risk in Youth (SAVRY).* Consultation ed. Tampa: University of South Florida; 2000.

19. De Vries-Robbe, M., Geers, M., Stapel, M., Hilterman, E. and de Vogel, V. *SAPROF – Youth Version Manual.* 2014. www.saprof.com.

20. Sukhodolsky, D. G., Cardona, L. and Martin, A. Characterizing aggressive and noncompliant behaviors in a children's psychiatric inpatient setting. *Child Psychiatry and Human Development* 2005; 36:177–93.

21. Stokoe, P. *The Curiosity Drive.* Phoenix: London; 2020.

22. Duke, N. N., Pettingell, S. L., McMorris, B. J. andBorowsky, I. W. Adolescent violence perpetration: Associations with multiple types of adverse childhood experiences. *Pediatrics* 2010; 125 (4): e778–e786.

23. Blake, C. S. and Hamrin, V. Current approaches to the assessment and management of anger and aggression in youth: a review. *Journal of Child and Adolescent Psychiatric Nursing* 2007; Nov; 20(4):209–21.

24. Crick, N. R. and Dodge, K. A. A review and reformulation of social information processing mechanisms in children's social adjustment. *Psychological Bulletin* 1994; 115:74–101.

25. Espejo-Siles, R., Zych, I., Farrington, D. P. and Llorent, V. J. Moral disengagement, victimization, empathy, social and emotional competencies as predictors of violence in children and adolescents. *Children and Youth Services Review* 2020; 118, 105337.

26. Broidy, L., Cauffman, E., Espelage, D. L., Mazerolle, P. and Piquero, A. Sex differences in empathy and its relation to juvenile offending. *Violence and Victims* 2003; 18(5):503–16.

27. Contreras, L. and Cano, M. C. Social competence and child-to-parent violence: Analyzing the role of emotional intelligence, social attitudes, and personal values. *Deviant Behavior* 2016; 37 (2):115–25.

28. Lösel, F. and Farington, D. Direct protective and buffering protective factors in the development of youth violence. *American Journal of Preventive Medicine* 2012; 43:S8–S23.

29. Bronfenbrenner, U. *The Ecology of Human Development.* Cambridge, MA: Harvard University Press; 1979.

30. Gharabaghi, K. and Stuart, C. Life-space intervention: Implications for caregiving. *Scottish Journal of Residential Child Care* 2013; 12(3):11–19.

31. Bronfenbrenner, U. *Making Human Beings Human: Bioecological Perspectives on Human Development.* Thousand Oaks, CA: Sage; 2005.

32. Morgan, W. Violence among young people: A framework for assessment and intervention. In A. Rogers, J. Harvey and H. Law (eds) *Young People in Forensic Mental Health Settings.* London: Palgrave Macmillan; 2015, pp. 143–66.

33. Dudley, R. and Kuyken, W. Case formulation in cognitive behavioural therapy: A principle-driven approach. In L. Johnstone and R. Dallos (eds.) *Formulation in Psychology and*

Psychotherapy: Making sense of people's problems, 2nd ed. Hove: Routledge; 2014:18–44.

34. Johnstone, L., Boyle, M. with Cromby, J. et al. *The Power Threat Meaning Framework: Overview.* Leicester: British Psychological Society; 2018.

35. Bion, W. R. *Learning from Experience.* London: Karnac; 1962.

36. Ainsworth, M. D. S. and Bowlby, J. An ethological approach to personality development. *American Psychologist* 1991; 46:331–41.

37. Bowlby, J. *Attachment and Loss, Volume 1: Attachment.* New York: Basic Books; 1969.

38. Winnicott, DW. *The Maturation Process and the Facilitating Environment.* London: Hogarth Press; 1965.

39. Hanna, F. J, Hanna, C. A. and Keys, S. G. Fifty strategies for counseling defiant, aggressive adolescents: Reaching, accepting, and relating. *Journal of Counseling & Development* 1999; 7:395–404.

40. Vygotsky, L. S. *Mind in Society: The Development of Higher Psychological Processes.* Cambridge, MA: Harvard University Press; 1978.

41. Cochran, J. L., Fauth, D. J., Cochran, N. H., Spurgeon, S. L. and Marinn Pierce, L. Growing play therapy up: Extending child-centered play therapy to highly aggressive teenage boys. *Person-Centered and Experiential Psychotherapies* 2010; 9 (4):290–301.

42. White, M. The externalizing of the problem and the re-authoring of lives and relationships. In M. White (ed.), *Selected Papers.* Adelaide: Dulwich Centre Publications; 1988/9,. pp. 5–28.

43. Hagell, A. and Lamb, S. Developing an integrated primary health care and youth work service for young people in Lambeth: Learning from the Well Centre. *Journal of Children's Services* 2016; 11(3):233–43.

44. Borgwald, K. and Theixos, H. Bullying the bully: Why zero-tolerance policies get a failing grade. *Social Influence* 2013; 8(2–3):149–60.

45. Perera, J. How Black working-class youth are criminalised and excluded from the english school system: A London case study. *Institute of Race Relations* 2020. https://irr.org.uk/wp-content/uploads/2020/09/How-Black-Working-Class-Youth-are-Criminalised-and-Excluded-in-the-English-School-System.pdf [Accessed 7.11.2022].

46. Sundius, J. and Farneth, M. Putting kids out of school: What's causing high suspension rates and why they are detrimental to students, schools and communities. Open Society Institute – Baltimore. 2008. Retrieved 10 October 2020. www.opensocietyfoundations.org/publications/putting-kids-out-school-whats-causing-high-suspension-rates-and-why-they-are-detrimental [Accessed 27.4.2022].

47. Fisher, H., Gardner, F. and Montgomery, P. Cognitive-behavioural interventions for preventing youth gang involvement for children and young people (7–16). *Cochrane Database of Systematic Reviews* 2 CD007008:16 Apr. 2008.

48. Esbensen, F.-A. and Osgood, D. W. Gang resistance education and training (great): Results from the National Evaluation. *Journal of Research in Crime and Delinquency*, 1999; 36(2):194–225.

49. Cook, A. and Williams, S. Enabling Environments Quality Improvement Process. 2019. www.rcpsych.ac.uk/docs/default-source/improving-care/ccqi/quality-networks/enabling-environments-ee/the-enabling-environments-process-document-2019.pdf?sfvrsn=10b4616c_2 [Accessed 27.4.2022].

50. Scott, S. National dissemination of effective parenting programmes to improve child outcomes. *British Journal of Psychiatry* 2010; 51(12):1331–41.

51. Furlong, M., McGilloway, S., Bywater, T. et al. Behavioural and cognitive-behavioural group-based parenting programmes for early-onset conduct problems in children aged 3 to 12 years. *Cochrane Database of Systematic Reviews* 2012. www.cochranelibrary.com/cdsr/doi/10.1002/14651858.CD008225.pub2/full [Accessed 27.4.2022].

52. Drugli, M. B., Fossum, S., Larsson, B. and Morch, W.-T. Characteristics of young children with persistent conduct problems 1 year after treatment with the Incredible Years program. *European Child and Adolescent Psychiatry* 2010; 19(7):559–65.

53. Sanders, M. R. The triple P-positive parenting program as a public health approach to strengthening parenting. *Journal of Family Psychology* 2008; 22(4):506–17.

54. Scott, S., Spender, Q., Doolan, M., Jacobs, B. and Aspland, H. Multicentre controlled trial of parenting groups for childhood antisocial behaviour in clinical practice. *British Medical Journal* 2001; 323:194–7.

55. Byrne, G., Sleed, M., Midgley, N. et al. Lighthouse Parenting Programme: Description and pilot evaluation of mentalization-based treatment to address child maltreatment. *Clinical Child Psychology and Psychiatry* 2019; 24(4):680–93.

56. Sukholdolsky, D. G. and Scahill, L. *Cognitive Behavioural Therapy for Anger and Aggression in Children.* Guildford: New York; 2012.

57. Thompson, M. and Gauntlett-Gilbert, J. Mindfulness with children and adolescents: Effective clinical application. *Clinical Child Psychology and Psychiatry* 2008; 13(3):395–407.

58. Lee, J., Semple, R. J., Rosa, D. and Miller, L. Mindfulness-based cognitive therapy for children: A pilot study. *Journal of Cognitive Psychotherapy* 2008; 22(1):15–28.

59. Sukhodolsky, D. G, Kassinove, H. and Gorman, B. S. Cognitive-behavioural therapy for anger in children and adolescents: a meta-analysis. *Aggressive and Violent Behaviour* 2004; 9:247–69.

60. Candelaria, A. M., Fedewa, A. L. and Ahn, S. The effects of anger management on children's social and emotional outcomes: A meta-analysis. *School Psychology International* 2012; 33(6):596–614.

61. Ho, B. P. V., Carter, M. and Stephenson, J. Anger management using a cognitive-behavioural approach for children with special education needs: A literature review and meta-analysis. *International Journal of Disability, Development and Education* 2010; 57(3):245–265.

62. Lochman, J. E. and Wells, K. C. The Coping Power Program for preadolescent aggressive boys and their parents: Outcome effects at the 1-year follow-up. *Journal of Consulting and Clinical Psychology* 2004; 72 (4)P: 571–578.

63. Goldstein, A.P. and Glick, B. Aggression replacement training: Curriculum and Evaluation. *Simulation & Gaming* 2004; 25 (1):9–26.

64. Martin, D. G. *Clinical Practice with Adolescents*. Pacific Grove, CA: Brooks/ Cole; 2003.

65. Horvath, A. O., Del Re, A. C., Flückiger, C. and Symonds, D. Alliance in individual psychotherapy. *Psychotherapy* 2011; 48 (1):9–16.

66. Ingley-Cook, G. and Dobel-Ober, D. Innovations in practice: Group work with children who are in care or who are adopted: Lessons learnt. *Child and Adolescent Mental Health* 2013; 18 (4):251–4.

67. Ncube, N. *Tree of Life Practitioners Guide.* Johannesburg: Phola. 2017.

68. Riley, A. Exploring the effects of the 'Seasons for Growth' intervention for pupils experiencing change and loss. *Education and Child Psychology* 2012; 29 (3):33–53.

69. Squire, B., Jefford, T. and Swenson, C. C. Whole systems approaches. In A. Rogers, J. Harvey and H. Law (eds.), *Young People in Forensic Mental Health Settings: Psychological Thinking and Practice.* Basingstoke: Palgrave Macmillan, 2015, pp. 123–42.

70. Alexander, J. F. and Parsons, B. V. *Functional Family Therapy: Principles and Procedures.* Carmel, CA: Brooks/Cole, 1982.

71. Sexton, T. and Turner, C. W. The effectiveness of functional family therapy for youth with behavioral problems in a community practice setting. *Journal of Family Psychology* 2010; 24(3):339–48.

72. Omer, H. (2004) *Non-violent Resistance.* Cambridge: Cambridge University Press.

73. Ollefs, B., Von Schlippe, A., Omer, H. and Kriz, J. Adolescents showing externalising problem behaviour. *Effects of Parent Coaching (German).* Familiendynamik 2009; 3:256–65.

74. Newman, M., Fagan, C. and Webb, R. (2014) Innovations in practice: The efficacy of nonviolent resistance groups in treating aggressive and controlling children and young people: A preliminary analysis of pilot NVR groups in Kent. *Child and Adolescent Mental Health* 19(2), 138–41.

75. Henggeler, S. W., Schoenwald, S. K., Borduin, C. M., Rowland, M. D. and Cunningham, P. B. *Multisystemic Therapy for Antisocial Behaviour in Children and Adolescents.* London: Guilford Press; 2009.

76. Schaeffer, C. M. and Borduin C. M. Long-term follow up to a randomized clinical trial of multisystemic therapy with serious and violent juvenile offenders. *Journal of Consulting and Clinical Psychology* 2005; 73 (3):445–53.

77. Lammy, D. The Lammy Review: An independent review into the treatment of, and outcomes for, Black, Asian and Minority Ethnic individuals in the Criminal Justice System. HMG, Government of the United Kingdom. 2017.

78. Ministry of Justice. (2020). Youth Justice Statistics 2019–2020. www.gov.uk/govern ment/statistics/youth-justice-statistics-201 9-to-2020 [Accessed 27.4.2022].

79. Crewe, B., Hulley, S. and Wright, S. *Life Imprisonment from Young Adulthood: Adaptation, Identity and Time.* London: Palgrave Macmillan. 2020.

80. Houses of Parliament: Parliamentary Office of Science and Technology (2018). Age of Criminal Responsibility. Postnote, 577, June 2018.

81. Steinberg, L., Icenogle, G., Shulman, E. P. et al. Around the world, adolescence is a time of heightened sensation seeking and

immature self-regulation. *Developmental Science* 2018, Mar; 21(2).

82. Farrington, D. P. Age and crime. In M. Tonry and N. Morris (eds.) *Crime and Justice: An Annual Review of Research*, vol. 7. Chicago: University of Chicago Press, 1986, pp. 189–250.

83. Rey, H. *Universals of Psychoanalysis in the Treatment of Psychotic and Borderline States*. London: Free Association Books. 1994.

84. Howard League for Penal Reform. The Carlile Inquiry 10 years on: The use of restraint, solitary confinement and strip-searching on children. 2016. https://howardleague.org/wp-content/uploads/2016/06/Carlile-Inquiry-10-years-on.pdf [Accessed 27.4.2022].

85. Ministry of Justice. Review of the Youth Justice System in England and Wales. 2016. Available at https://assets.publishing.service.gov.uk/government/uploads/system/uploads/attachment_data/file/577105/youth-justice-review-final-report-print.pdf [Accessed 27.4.2022].

86. Sadie, C. and Stokoe, P. Creating therapeutic environments in youth custody: The SECURE STAIRS programme. *Monitor* 2020 (March): 20–3.

87. Taylor, J., Shostak, L., Rogers, A. and Mitchell, P. Rethinking mental health provision in the secure estate for children and young people: A framework for integrated care (SECURE STAIRS). *Safer Communities* 2018; 17(4):193–201.

88. Bloom, S. L. The sanctuary model of organizational change for children's residential treatment. *Therapeutic Community: The International Journal for Therapeutic and Supportive Organizations* 2005; 26(1):65–81.

89. Stokoe, P. The healthy and the unhealthy organization: How can we help teams to remain effective? In A. Rubitel and D. Reiss (eds.) *Containment in the Community: Supportive Frameworks for Thinking about Antisocial Behaviour and Mental Health*. The Portman Papers, Karnac: London, 2011, pp. 237–259.

90. Shnabel, N. and Nadler, A. A needs-based model of reconciliation: Satisfying the differential emotional needs of victim and perpetrator as a key to promoting reconciliation. *Journal of Personality and Social Psychology* 2008; 94(1):116–32.

91. NICE. 2019 surveillance of violence and aggression: Short-term management in mental health, health and community settings (NICE guideline NG10) Surveillance report. www.nice.org.uk/guidance/ng10/resources/2019-surveillance-of-violence-and-aggression-shortterm-management-in-mental-health-health-and-community-settings-nice-guideline-ng10-pdf-9097015205365 [Accessed 27.4.2022].

92. Nunno, M. A., Day, D. and Bullard, L. For our own safety: Examining the safety of high-risk interventions for children and young people. Child Welfare League of America. 2007.

93. Nunno, M. A., Holden, M. J. and Tollar, A. Learning from tragedy: A survey of child and adolescent restraint fatalities. *Child Abuse and Neglect*. 2006 (Dec); 30 (12):1333–42.

94. National Childrens Bureau: Making a Difference. Report on the Use of Physical Intervention across Children's Services. London: NCB. 2004. Available at www.ncb.org.uk/sites/default/files/uploads/files/physical_intervention_across_childrens_services.pdf [Accessed 27.4.2022].

95. UN Committee on the Rights of the Child (CRC), General comment No. 20 (2016) on the implementation of the rights of the child during adolescence, 6 December 2016, CRC/C/GC/20. www.refworld.org/docid/589dad3d4.html [Accessed 27.4.2022].

96. Steckley, L. Containment and holding environments: Understanding and reducing physical restraint in residential child care. *Children and Youth Services Review* 2010; 32(1):20–128.

97. Steckley, L. Catharsis, containment and physical restraint in residential child care. *British Journal of Social Work* 2018; 48 (6):1645–63.

98. Batmanghelidjh, C. (2004). Therapy: A pretension too far? *Counselling in Education Journal*, Summer 2004.

99. University College London. Psychological Interventions in Child and Adolescent Mental Health Services. Welcome to the competence framework for child and adolescent mental health services. Available at www.ucl.ac.uk/pals/research/clinical-educational-and-health-psychology/research-groups/core/competence-frameworks-11 [Accessed 27.4.2022].

100. Royal College of Psychiatrists. Good Psychiatric Practice: Code of Ethics. 2014. www.rcpsych.ac.uk/docs/default-source/improving-care/better-mh-policy/college-reports/college-report-cr186.pdf?sfvrsn=15f49e84_2 [Accessed 27.4.2022].

101. Russell, L., Poyton, J., Lake, J. and Rennalls, S. Living Through a Lockdown. 2020. www.redthread.org.uk/living-through-a-lockdown/ [Accessed 27.4.2022].

102. Adshead, G. Mirror mirror: Parallel processes in forensic institutions. In J. Adlam, A. Aiyegbusi, P. Kleinot, A. Motz and C. Scanlon (eds.) *The Therapeutic Milieu Under Fire: Security and Insecurity in Forensic Mental Health*. Jessica Kingsley: London; 2012, pp. 97–115.

103. Mawson, C. Containing anxiety in work with damaged children. In V. Roberts and A. Obholzer (eds.) *The Unconscious at Work*. Oxon: Routledge; 1994, pp. 67–74.

Management of Violence in Older Adults

Jonathan Waite and Juliette Brown

Introduction

Violence from older adults is a challenge for healthcare services and a risk to older adults in services. Risk factors include those common to working-age adults, including substance misuse, active psychotic symptoms and inadequate care, and others more typical in older age, including cognitive impairment, acute confusion and pain. Aggression is a barrier to good care and a challenge to manage in older adults as they are more vulnerable to adverse medication effects. Medication must be used with caution. Prevention of violence, as mentioned many times in this book, is better achieved through sensitive person-centred care and good management of risk, with non-pharmacological management preferred. Rather than separating organic from functional illness in this chapter, we emphasise that the principles of a person-centred and preventive approach and management through non-pharmacological measures (except in cases of risk) apply regardless of the underlying cause of aggression. It is very important with older adults to make a thorough assessment of the triggers to aggression, including underlying pain or physical illness.

How Big Is the Problem?

Hospitals

A detailed analysis of five-year data on physical assaults against NHS staff in England [1] found that acute hospitals assaults are overwhelmingly committed by patients who are over 75 years of age. In mental hospital facilities, the prevalence of aggressive behaviour is less skewed to older patients, but around one-third of assaults are by people over 65 years. One study on inpatient wards totalling 50 beds for people with dementia and older adults with serious mental illness found an act of physical violence met the threshold for reporting on average every six days and resulted in a staff injury every eight days [2].

The Healthcare Commission's National Audit of Violence 2006–2007 [3, 4] included for the first time incidents of violence in hospital services for older people, in addition to those occurring in units for adults of working age. The findings were disturbing but not widely publicised. While the quality of nursing care was reported to be extremely high, physical violence remained a frequent event. Nurses working in older people's services were more likely to have experienced physical assault (64% had been assaulted) than those employed in services for adults of working age.

Around two-thirds of patients in general hospitals are over 70, many with mental as well as physical disorders. Staff starting to work with these patients identified learning how to manage agitation and aggression as their highest priority in training [5]. More than 50% of people with dementia are reported to be aggressive at some point during a hospital admission [6].

Delirium, a major risk factor for aggressive behaviours in older adults, has a prevalence in the community of 1–2%, rising to 14% in people over the age of 85. In the acute hospital setting, conservative estimates suggest that at least 20% have delirium. If confusion has an acute onset, or represents a significant change from baseline in dementia, it should be treated as possible delirium.

Relatively few of the recent international studies of violence directed against healthcare workers have included the age of the perpetrator in their analyses [7–10]. Research conducted in Macau [11] found that direct care of elderly patients was the strongest predictor of workplace violence.

Violence from older adults in healthcare settings affects the physical and psychological health of staff, fellow patients and the perpetrators of aggression themselves, as these are more likely to be treated with restraint and rapid tranquillisation. Restrictive interventions are likely to increase the risk of falls, injury and prolonged length of stay and increase the risk of death, and are also extremely traumatising for the patient, highlighting the importance of preventive practice.

Care Homes

About 430,000 people live in care homes in the United Kingdom, and one-third of people with dementia are thought to live in care homes. Data on care home populations are not routinely collected in the United Kingdom, but in Scotland about 90% of care home places are for older people [12]. Even in homes not specifically registered to provide care for people with mental disorders, the majority of residents have dementia. Behaviours that challenge family and other informal carers are an important factor in people with dementia being 'placed' in care homes [14]. There are no reliable recent data on the prevalence of violent episodes in UK care homes. One staff survey found that 85% of staff reported being psychologically abused in the past month, and 60% had been physically assaulted [15]. Similar rates have been reported from surveys in Switzerland and Japan [16, 17].

Care home staff report finding aggression the most challenging behaviour to deal with. They also report finding person-centred approaches more helpful than medication or other guideline-specific interventions. These approaches included a thorough assessment and knowledge of the person as an individual, the application of this knowledge, identification of triggers to violence, having time to spend with residents and using an appropriate style of communication [18].

Care home residents may exhibit violence towards their peers as well as care home staff [19]. Attacks are often precipitated by communication issues or invasion of personal space.

Older People in the Community

More than 850,000 people in the United Kingdom are thought to have dementia, making this by far the most prevalent serious mental disorder [20]. The majority are living at home. Nearly all will develop behavioural or psychological symptoms as a result of their dementia [21]; about 20% are reported to exhibit physical aggression [22, 23]. More than a third of family carers experience abuse from the person they are looking after, and at least 6% are subject to physical violence [24]. Violence and aggression that follow from the cognitive challenges of dementia are a major source of stress for carers. Psychoeducation and support for carers can delay care home placement for the person with dementia [25, 26].

Carers, both formal and informal, should be supported to understand the effects of dementia, including changes in the ability to recognise and regulate emotion, and to exercise judgement and behavioural inhibition. Agitation can reflect both an impaired ability to tolerate frustration and a communication of underlying distress. Emotional and psychological experiences of cognitive impairment are still often overlooked. Dementia affects self-esteem and self-mastery. Pre-existing traumatic experiences, psychiatric illness, coping strategies and interpersonal styles interact both with the disease process and with environmental factors and super-imposed physical illness and pain to contribute to behaviours that challenge [27]. Dementia and other severe mental illness in older adults with diminished cognitive reserve can be associated with a reduced ability to regulate anxieties and operate effective defences, giving rise to persecutory delusions.

A central tenet of dementia care is the application of a social model of disability, recognising that while the disease process is not yet treatable, social and environmental adjustments improve the experience and quality of life of people with dementia and their carers. Principles of dementia care include provision of reliable, attentive, attuned, facilitating environments in which people can flourish regardless of cognitive impairment. In this context, aggression and violence can be seen as a failure to meet basic needs, whether physical or psychological.

Recent NHS initiatives, including the Community Mental Health Framework for Adults and Older Adults following from the NHS Long-Term Plan (2019), aim to deliver community-based healthcare recognising the role of carers in supporting people with dementia as well as those with serious mental illness. Support for carers in managing aggression at home remains an important factor in reducing both care home placements and acute admissions.

What Is the Current Guidance?

It is curious that the National Institute for Health and Care Excellence (NICE) 2015 guideline on violence and aggression [28] does not offer any specific advice on managing aggression in older people. Mental health trusts commonly adapt local policies to the older adult population, in line with the recommendations detailed in this chapter. There is no specific guidance from NICE on a holistic approach to violence in older adults that reflects evidence on prevention.

For individuals with dementia, the Royal College of Nursing (RCN) and Scottish Intercollegiate Guidelines Network (SIGN) have produced guidance [29, 30]. Excellent advice for lay carers (which is also relevant for health and social care professionals) has been published by the Alzheimer's Society [31].

The NICE dementia guideline [32] emphasises the need for a structured assessment of triggers to distress, including clinical or environmental causes (e.g. pain, delirium or inappropriate care), prior to considering antipsychotics in those people living with dementia who are at risk of harming themselves or others or are experiencing agitation, hallucinations or delusions that are causing them severe distress. A decision aid on antipsychotic medicines is available from NICE to support discussion on the use of antipsychotics [33].

In an inpatient setting, medication will on occasion be required to manage acute distress and risk to self or others. NICE guidance and local policies on rapid tranquillisation in older adults should be followed. Typically, these would suggest the use of haloperidol and lorazepam, preferably in oral form and at lower doses than for younger adults. The guidance is otherwise in agreement with the recommendations detailed in Chapter 4. Particular considerations apply to those with Parkinson's disease or a suspected or confirmed Lewy Body Dementia, in whom antipsychotics may worsen motor symptoms or cause a sensitivity reaction.

Vignette: George is a 78-year-old writer with a diagnosis of bipolar affective disorder. His childhood was characterised by physical violence between his parents. When he is well he feels he does not need medication and declines depot medication. He increases his use of cannabis and alcohol. When he is noted to have deteriorated, with increasing disinhibition, verbal abuse and threats toward his neighbours, his community team and inpatient team liaise to manage an admission under the Mental Health Act, where he requires the minimum effective doses of rapid tranquillisation while he is re-established on his regular treatment. Ward staff are fully aware of his experience of violence in childhood and his heightened perception of threat, and are able to use de-escalation techniques and oral medications to avoid the need for more restrictive practices.

A key driver in recent guidance has been the concern that medication has been indiscriminately prescribed for older people in care homes and hospitals [34]. In 2009, the UK Department of Health commissioned a policy review on antipsychotic use in dementia. The report concluded that usage was unacceptably high. In response to this report, the Alzheimer's Society [35] and the RCN [36] produced good practice guidance on reducing the use of antipsychotics. In the years following the guidance, an audit on prescribing practices showed a reduction in prescribing of antipsychotics for people with dementia. There is evidence that during the COVID-19 pandemic antipsychotic prescribing in care homes increased in the absence of family visits and structured activities and an increase in isolation of patients. Specialist community teams reported a decrease in care home liaison referrals during the period. Some of the increase in use may have been in the management of delirium or palliative care [37].

NICE guidance on delirium [38] recommends use of the Confusion Assessment Method for diagnosis. Delirium can be diagnosed in the presence of (a) acute confusion and fluctuating course and (b) inattention, plus one or other of (c) disorganised thinking or (d) altered level of consciousness (i.e. if the patient is hyper-alert, drowsy or difficult to rouse). The Single Question in Delirium is 80% sensitive to a delirium: Do you think this person has been more confused lately? (asked of a carer). This guidance has been summarised usefully in the context of COVID-19 in joint British Geriatrics Society and Royal College of Psychiatrists Old Age Faculty guidance [39]. A set of recommendations on the management of older people in the emergency department from the British Geriatrics Society and the Royal College of Emergency Medicine – The Silver Book – has also been endorsed by the Royal College of Psychiatrists [40]. Prevention of delirium and identification of delirium are the most effective strategies for managing violence in older adults in the acute hospital setting.

Overuse of alcohol and other substance misuse is an under-recognised phenomenon in older adults. [41] Withdrawal rather than intoxication is most likely to precipitate violence and agitation in older adults. It is recommended to use tools such as the CIWA (Clinical Institute Withdrawal Assessment – Alcohol, revised) (widely available) to identify and treat withdrawal. Those at risk of complications of alcohol withdrawal include people with frailty, cognitive impairment or multiple comorbidities, and those who lack social support. Many may require admission for treatment, including treatment of thiamine deficiency, and prevention of Wernicke's encephalopathy and Korsakoff's syndrome. A regimen determined by the severity of withdrawal signs and symptoms is advised to reduce the risk of agitation [42].

Reducing the Risk of Violence

Violence in older adults can be reduced by an understanding of risk factors leading to agitation and aggression. Drivers of violence and aggression relating to the environment, to the individual (including risk factors for delirium) and to carers are outlined in Table 14.1. An interaction of different factors is commonly found.

Table 14.1 Risk factors for violence and aggression in older adults

Environmental	Individual	Carer
Overcrowding	Neurodegenerative disorders	Caregiver stress
Loss of personal space	Unmet emotional or psychological needs	Poor communication between staff and patient
Unfamiliar environment	Feeling threatened	Out-pacing
Lack of attention to basic needs – hunger, thirst, toileting, fatigue	New functional losses – aphasia, agnosia	Lack of understanding of trauma
Noise	Active psychosis / paranoia	Poor knowledge of the patient
Heat / cold / climate (heatwaves)	Intoxication	Lack of emotional awareness
Lack of access to natural environment	Drug or alcohol withdrawal	Conflicts between staff and carer
Over-stimulation	Sensory impairment	Task-based care
Staffing levels	History of personal trauma (sexual, physical or emotional abuse)	Poor staff engagement
Lack of privacy	History of violence	Inconsistency
Changes in environment (new care setting)	Medication side effects	Values and attitudes
Lack of activity	Physical illness	
Changes in carers	New onset of confusion [see risk factors for development of delirium, later in this chapter]	
	Reduced frustration tolerance – particularly associated with mania, frontotemporal dementia, vascular dementia, post-stroke or in those with Parkinson's disease	

Environmental factors may provoke or exacerbate violence, for example:

- noise
- heat
- cold
- interference by other residents

These factors may interact with poor hearing and eyesight to increase levels of suspicion and fear.

Violence and aggression has been shown to increase in relation to extremes of temperature, including during heatwaves. Environmental determinants due to global warming (including prolonged heatwaves) are likely to become increasingly relevant in the care of older adults.

Physical discomfort is often a trigger, including:

- pain
- constipation
- breathlessness
- urinary retention

Pain is under-recognised and under-treated in people with dementia in all settings. In a longitudinal study of self-reported and observed pain in people with dementia in the acute setting, pain was found to be common, poorly treated and associated with behavioural and psychiatric symptoms of dementia (BPSD) [43]. In an important study in nursing care, Husebo et al. [44] found a significant reduction in agitation as measured by the Cohen-Mansfield Agitation Inventory in people with dementia in nursing care when pain was proactively treated over eight weeks in a stepwise approach. The effect size in reducing agitation with the use of analgesia is significantly greater than with the use of antipsychotics.

Violence may be the first sign of physical illness; urinary tract infection is the most commonly observed condition but the presentation of disease in confused older people is notoriously non-specific. Sometimes the diagnosis becomes apparent on physical examination, but negative findings do not exclude the possibility of serious illness. There is a real dilemma in the community in deciding on investigation for an underlying cause, and determining what the best environment will be, especially with regard to the most appropriate care. New onset of confusion should prompt assessment for causes of delirium, including pain, acute brain injury (infection, stroke, head injury), acute deterioration of a physical condition, constipation, urinary retention, dehydration, acute infection, hypoxia, metabolic abnormalities, recent surgery, hip fracture, poor nutritional status, medication contributing to a confusional state, sensory impairments and end of life procedures.

Assessment of potential triggers should include analysis of the circumstances in which agitation and aggression occur. Agitation around moving and handling may relate to untreated pain. Unprovoked aggression can indicate unmet needs or goals. The loss of ability to express needs or goals (including meaningful activity) verbally can lead to agitation and aggression.

Practising Trauma-informed Mental Healthcare

Increasingly, the relevance of trauma and trauma-informed care is being recognised in mental healthcare and acute healthcare settings [45, 46]. In particular, experiences of childhood trauma dispose individuals to a chronically elevated cortisol response and a heightened perception of threat. These responses are likely to be triggered by the experience of receiving healthcare, and can lead to further trauma. Trauma makes it harder for people to feel safe, and triggers a stress response that may in the past have been adaptive but now can dispose to serious mental illness and re-traumatisation:

> Aspects of a situation that may seem benign to someone with no history of trauma can trigger overwhelming feelings of distress in a trauma survivor, leading the individual to behave in ways that might be labelled as, for example, 'oppositional', 'non-compliant', 'delinquent' or 'hostile'. If an organisation reacts to these behaviours with seclusion, exclusion, restraint or force, further trauma may result. [47, p. 4].

Vignette: Sophia is a 73-year-old former doctor with a mixed Alzheimer's and vascular dementia. She lives at home with her partner. She is referred by her GP to the local community mental health team due to concerns about carer stress. She is agitated and physically aggressive around personal care tasks, including toileting. There is a risk to her skin integrity. During sensitive collateral history taking, Sophia's history of prolonged sexual abuse by a family member at a young age is shared by her partner. In collaboration with him, a support worker is allocated to help carers develop a more trauma-informed and person-centred approach to her personal care that includes provision of consistent same-sex carers who position themselves in her sightline at all times, moderate their vocal cues and slowly and calmly communicate their actions to her during personal care. This approach helps her to remain calm during personal care and allows her to remain in her own home without the use of sedative medications.

Trauma-informed approaches have been seen to reduce violence and aggression in psychiatric settings. Practically, this involves the realisation of the extent of trauma experiences, the recognition of signs and symptoms and the introduction of trauma-informed practice and measures to reduce re-traumatisation.

We should also recognise that working with older adults, and with people who can be unpredictably aggressive, is difficult for carers, and they should be supported through high-quality supervision.

Practical Management of Violence in Older Adults

The application of basic principles of person-centred care and behavioural management minimises the risk of violence. These principles, along with preventive measures and management of risk factors, apply in all settings and to older adults with severe mental illness with or without cognitive deficits, those with cognitive impairment and dementia and those with delirium.

An assessment should be made of the triggers to aggression and agitation. A particularly useful tool in dementia is the PIECES framework developed in Canada, which takes the assessor through domains including physical, intellectual, emotional, capacity-based, environmental and social [48]. An example of how this might be applied is given in the Hearing Aid MDTea podcast episode on Management of BPSD [49]. The Hearing Aid MDTea podcasts are a series of open-access podcasts aimed at healthcare professionals working with older adults. The podcasts present the evidence base, recent advances and established best practice in healthcare for older adults. Each episode reviews an aspect of caring for older adults from the perspective of the group's multidisciplinary team 'faculty.'

Observational tools and person-centred care help staff and family think about what the experience of the person might be and focus on difficult feelings associated with the experiences of dementia, severe mental illness and functional decline – including helplessness, fear and shame. An ABC timelines approach can be effectively used in care homes, in particular looking at events pre- and post-aggression and the details of the agitation itself to identify triggers, and develop alternative approaches. Tools that encourage observation and reflection from caregivers are likely to foster a containing function of the kind referenced by writers such as Margot Waddell in relation to older adults [50].

Non-Pharmacological Measures

Non-pharmacologic strategies are recommended first-line treatments except where there is imminent risk. According to the Lancet Commission on Dementia Prevention, Intervention, and Care (2020), the best evidence for management of neuropsychiatric symptoms is in specific multi-component interventions, noting that 'psychotropic drugs are often ineffective and might have severe adverse effects' [51, p. 414]. Psychosocial interventions are likely to include a combination of person-centred care, medication management, activities, and carer support and education. These interventions have been shown in nursing care in particular to deliver major reductions in agitation without the side effects associated with medications.

Livingston at al. [52] found that person-centred care and adapted dementia care mapping reduce symptomatic and severe agitation in care homes. The effects could be seen immediately and persisted for up to six months [53]. Communication skills training [54] has been shown to be effective for up to six months. Activity programmes may alleviate agitation in the short term. There is also some evidence of short-term benefit from sensory interventions involving touch. Music therapy has also been shown to produce short-term benefits [55, 56, 57]. Staff education can help. A systematic review found that non-pharmacologic approaches with the strongest evidence are those involving family caregiver interventions, which have greater effect than antipsychotics [58].

Programmes such as WHELD (Well-being and Health for People Living with Dementia) – based on the most practical and effective therapies and including person-centred care, management of agitation and non-drug approaches – have been shown to be effective. A large-scale, multicentre randomised controlled trial of the programme in 69 care homes showed significant benefit to quality of life, agitation and overall neuropsychiatric symptoms, at a reduced cost compared with treatment as usual [59]. Psychological therapies should be offered to people with mild to moderate dementia where suitable to treat depression and support adjustment to the diagnosis.

Sensitive assessment of the circumstances surrounding agitation is most likely to yield effective non-pharmacological treatment strategies. If agitation is new, a physical cause should always be considered. If delirium is suspected, management of the underlying cause is essential, by treating infection, hydration, nutrition, constipation, pain, retention and immobility, and identifying medications that can cause confusion. These include tricyclic antidepressants, antimuscarinics, antihistamines, opioids, benzodiazepines, gabapentin, theophylline and hyoscine. In the acute setting, a dementia and delirium team may be available to provide further expertise and support. In acute psychiatric settings, geriatricians are increasingly part of multidisciplinary teams.

Pharmacological Treatments

Acetylcholinesterase inhibitors (donepezil, galantamine and rivastigmine) have a role in mild–moderate Alzheimer's disease, to improve cognitive function and activities of daily living, and also in Parkinson's dementia, Lewy Body Dementia and mixed dementias. They are not thought to reduce agitation. In practice, memantine is often added at a more severe stage in order to reduce the severity of behavioural symptoms despite limited evidence. According to the British Association for Psychopharmacology, selective serotonin reuptake inhibitors may help behavioural (but not cognitive) features of frontotemporal dementia [60].

Antipsychotic medication has a short-term effect in reducing levels of aggression in dementia [61, 62]. The best evidence is for risperidone in doses of 1 mg daily to treat psychosis and aggression. There is also data to support the use of aripiprazole [63]. Risperidone is the only licensed medication for aggression in dementia. There are likely to be adverse effects if treatment is continued and no major benefits [64]. Adverse outcomes of the use of antipsychotics include increased risks of Parkinsonism, sedation, respiratory infection, DVT, PE, a 1.5–1.7 relative risk of death, and 3 times increased risk of stroke in addition to 2–4 times increased risk of cognitive decline. Olanzapine and quetiapine are ineffective in the treatment of agitation in dementia [65]. Pimavanserin, a 5-HT2A inverse agonist not yet licensed in the United Kingdom, has shown promising results [66]. In the HARMONY trial, including people with Alzheimer's disease, dementia with Lewy bodies, Parkinson's disease dementia, vascular dementia and frontotemporal dementia, psychotic symptoms were reduced without sedation or worsening cognition.

If delirium is present and cannot be effectively managed without medication, NICE guidance recommends uses of haloperidol at a dose of 0.5 mg 2-hourly, up to a maximum of 5mg/24 hours. A baseline ECG is recommended due to risk of prolongation of the QTc interval. In Parkinson's disease, in cases of central nervous system depression or clinically significant cardiac disorders haloperidol is to be avoided. Lorazepam is recommended if there is a contraindication to haloperidol. Lorazepam can be used at a dose of 0.5 mg 2-hourly up to a maximum of 3 mg/24 hours.

In all cases, low dosing and slow titration is recommended. In addition, in the acute inpatient setting, the support of a registered mental health nurse in close observations and regular review by liaison psychiatrist or dementia and delirium team will be helpful.

> **Vignette:** Martin is a 68-year-old former labourer with no psychiatric history who is referred to a community mental health team following an admission to the acute hospital which involved a prolonged ITU admission with delirium. He is referred to manage the reduction in antipsychotic treatment. Back in his familiar environment, he is able to describe the experience of delirium. He recalls thinking staff had been sent to murder him. He vividly describes thinking he must try to escape from the window of the hospital ward, and try to carry the man in the adjacent bed out of the window with him. Back at home he is oriented and shocked at his behaviour on the ward. Medication is reduced without any recurrence of symptoms.

Anticonvulsants have only been subjected to small-scale trials in older adults with challenging behaviour. A study of carbamazepine showed some benefit but also adverse effects; valproate was used for some time to treat agitation but studies did not confirm benefit [67, 68]. Trazodone has been widely used to treat agitation, although the largest study did not demonstrate significant benefit [69]. There is evidence of harm. Citalopram led to a reduction in agitation in patients with Alzheimer's in the CitAD trial [70], with worsening cognitive function and QT interval prolongation at higher doses. Banerjee et al. [71] were unable to show benefit in depressive symptoms in patients with dementia treated with sertraline or mirtazapine. There is some limited evidence for short-term use of melatonin in behavioural symptoms of dementia.

There is little evidence on rapid tranquillisation in older people or people with dementia. Intramuscular lorazepam (1 mg) has been shown to be effective in reducing agitation and excitation, without producing sedation, cardiac conduction abnormalities or extrapyramidal system side effects [72].

Responding to Violent Behaviour

The following bullet points are offered as a general outline. Fuller accounts are given in other chapters in this volume; guidance issued by the Alzheimer's Society on the management of aggressive behaviour in dementia is clear and informative.

- Do not make things worse.
- Always remain calm and professional.
- Often doing nothing is the best strategy – say nothing and walk away.
- If it is necessary to remain, sit down and adopt a relaxed posture, maintain eye contact. Explain what you are doing.
- Minimise physical contact – this may be misinterpreted as a threat.
- Do what you can to calm things down.
- Ensure that other people are not at risk, give the person as much space and quiet as possible.
- If the person is amenable, do what you can to reassure them; try to reduce their fears.
- If physical restraint is needed, follow the principles detailed in Chapter 8.
- Afterwards, discuss what happened with a trusted colleague or mentor as part of the post-incident management.

Conclusion

Given the risks associated with management of violence in older adults, and the potential for traumatisation and re-traumatisation, prevention is paramount. The first-line management should be a detailed assessment to identify any treatable cause of the aggression (e.g. delirium, pain, etc.); this should include taking the history of the problem, observing the behaviour and discussing current and past behaviour with the carer or team. Pain should be proactively treated.

Person-centred care is likely to be an effective approach for giving confidence to mental health professionals in their interactions with older patients, reducing agitation and minimising violence.

Antipsychotic medication should not be a first-line treatment except in circumstances of extreme risk and harm. It is important to remember that older people with disturbed behaviour often have physical disorders. To make a physical assessment and diagnosis, it is justified to resort to the use of medication to allow an adequate physical assessment, if experienced medical and nursing staff are unable to de-escalate the situation causing violence. The prescription of tranquillising medication should be reviewed once the assessment has been completed and effective treatment has been initiated. Sometimes it will be necessary to continue medication for longer periods of time, to ensure the safety of carers and those who live with the patient, but this should always be subject to regular review.

References

1. Dixon, D. A five year analysis of physical assaults against NHS staff in England. SIRS / RPA Violence Report 2010 – 2015. NHS Protect. 2015. http://webarchive .nationalarchives.gov.uk/20170726163554/ https://www.nhsbsa.nhs.uk/crime-prevention/nhs-protect-statistics [Accessed April 25, 2021].

2. Brown, J., Fawzi, W. and McCarthy, C. et al. Safer Wards: Reducing violence on older people's mental health wards. *BMJ Quality Improvement Reports* 2015 4(1). u207447.w2977.

3. Healthcare Commission. National Audit of Violence 2006–7: Final Report – Working Age Adult Services. Royal College of Psychiatrists' Centre for Quality Improvement. 2008.

4. Healthcare Commission. National Audit of Violence 2006–7: Final Report – Older People's Services. Royal College of Psychiatrists' Centre for Quality Improvement. 2008.

5. Griffiths, A., Knight, A., Harwood, R. et al. Preparation to care for confused older patients in general hospitals: A study of UK health professionals. *Age and Ageing* 2014; 43:521–7.

6. Sampson, E. L., White, N., Leurent, N. B. et al. Behavioural and psychiatric symptoms in people with dementia admitted to the acute hospital: prospective cohort study. *British Journal of Psychiatry* 2014; 205:189–96.

7. Cheung, T. and Yip, P. S. F. Workplace violence towards nurses in Hong Kong: Prevalence and correlates. *BMC Public Health* 2017; 17:196.

8. Johansen, I. H., Baste, V., Rosta, J. et al. Changes in the prevalence of workplace violence against doctors in all medical specialties in Norway between 1993 and 2014: A repeated cross sectional survey. *BMJ Open* 2017; 7:e107757.

9. Shafran-Tikva, S., Zelker, R., Stern, Z. and Chinitz, D. Workplace violence in a tertiary Israeli hospital: A systematic analysis of types of violence, the perpetrators and hospital departments. *Israel Journal of Health Policy Research* 2017; 6:43.

10. Claudius, I. A., Desai, S., Davis, E. and Henderson, S. Case-controlled analysis of patient-based risk factors for assault in the health care workplace. *Western Journal of Emergency Medicine* 2017; 18:1153–58.

11. Cheung, T., Lee, P. H. and Yip, P. S. F. Workplace violence towards physicians and nurses: Prevalence and correlates in Macau. *International Journal of Environmental Research and Public Health* 2017; 14:879.

12. Information Services Division. Care Home Census 2011: Interim Analysis. NHS National Services Scotland. 2011.

13. Alzheimer Society. Dementia UK: Updated Second Edition. Alzheimer's Society. 2014.

14. Donaldson, C., Tarrier, N. and Burns, A. The impact of the symptoms of dementia on caregivers. *British Journal of Psychiatry* 1997; 170:62–68.

15. Zeller, A., Dassen, T., Kok,G. et al. Factors associated with resident aggression toward caregivers in nursing homes. *Journal of Nursing Scholarship* 2012; 44:249–57.

16. Zeller, A., Hahn, S., Needham, I. et al. Aggressive behavior of nursing home residents towards caregivers: A systematic literature review. *Geriatric Nursing* 2009; 30:174–87.

17. Ko, A., Fukahori, H., Igarashi, A. et al. Aggression exhibited by older dementia clients toward staff in Japanese long-term care. *Journal of Elder Abuse and Neglect* 2012; 24; 1–16.

18. Mallon, C., Krska, J. and Gammie, S. Views and experiences of care home staff on managing behaviours that challenge in

dementia: A national survey in England. *Aging and Mental Health* 2018; 25:1–8.

19. Ferrah, N., Murphy, B. J, Ibrahim, J. E. et al. Resident-to-resident physical aggression leading to injury in nursing homes: A systematic review. *Age and Ageing* 2015; 44:356–64.

20. Prince, M., Knapp, M., Guerchet, M. et al. Dementia UK: Update Second Edition report produced by King's College London and the London School of Economics for the Alzheimer's Society, 2014.

21. Savva, G. M, Zaccai, J., Matthews, F. E. et al. Prevalence correlates and course of behavioural and psychological symptoms of dementia in the population. *British Journal of Psychiatry* 2009; 194:212–19.

22. Burns, A., Jacoby, R. and Levy, R. Psychiatric phenomena in Alzheimer's Disease. IV: Disorders of behaviour. *British Journal of Psychiatry* 1990; 157:86–94.

23. Lyketsos, C. G., Steinberg, M., Tschanz, J. T. et al. Mental and behavioral disturbances in dementia: Findings from the Cache County Study on Memory in Aging. *American Journal of Psychiatry* 2000 57:708–14.

24. Cooper, C., Selwood, A., Blanchard, M. and Livingston, G. Abusive behaviour experienced by family carers from people with dementia: The CARD (caring for relatives with dementia) study. *Journal of Neurology, Neurosurgery, and Psychiatry* 2010; 81:592–6.

25. Andrén, S. and Elmståhl, S. Effective psychosocial intervention for family caregivers lengthens time elapsed before nursing home placement of individuals with dementia: A five-year follow-up study. *International Psychogeriatrics* 2008 Dec;20 (6):1177–92.

26. Banerjee, S., Murray, J., Foley, B. et al. Predictors of institutionalisation in people with dementia. *Journal of Neurology, Neurosurgery, and Psychiatry* 2003; 74 (9):1315–16.

27. Brown, J. Prognosis and Planning. In S. Evans, J. Garner and R. Darnley-Smith (eds.) *Psychodynamic Approaches to the Experience of Dementia*. London, Routledge, 2020, pp. 41–55.

28. National Institute for Health and Care Excellence. Violence and Aggression: short-term management in mental health, health and community settings (NG10). NICE. 2015.

29. Royal College of Nursing. Restraint Revisited: Rights, Risk, Responsibility: Guidance for Nursing Staff. RCN. 2004.

30. Scottish Intercollegiate Guidelines Network. Risk reduction and Management of delirium. 2019. www.sign.ac.uk/media/1423/sign157.pdf [Accessed 25.04.2022].

31. Alzheimer's Society. Aggressive behaviour (Factsheet 509LP). 2017. http://alzheimer webstg.prod.acquia-sites.com/sites/defaul t/files/pdf/factsheet_dementia_and_aggres sive_behaviour.pdf [Accessed 25.04.2022].

32. National Institute for Health and Care Excellence. Dementia: assessment, management and support for people living with dementia and their carers. NICE guideline [NG97] 2018. www.nice.org.uk/guidance/ng97 [Accessed 25.04.2022].

33. National Institute for Health and Care Excellence. Antipsychotic medicines for treating agitation, aggression and distress in people living with dementia. www .nice.org.uk/guidance/ng97/resources/ant ipsychotic-medicines-for-treating-agitation-aggression-and-distress-in-people-living-with-dementia-patient-decision-aid-pdf-4852697005 [Accessed 25.04.2022].

34. Banerjee, S. The use of antipsychotic medication for people with dementia: Time for action. Department of Health. 2009.

35. Alzheimer Society. Reducing the Use of Antipsychotic Drugs: A Guide to the Treatment and Care of Behavioural and Psychological Symptoms of Dementia. Alzheimer Society. 2011.

36. Sturdy, D. Antipsychotic drugs in dementia: A best practice guide. Royal College of Nursing and Nursing Standards. 2012.

37. Howard, R., Burns, A. and Schneider, L. Antipsychotic prescribing to people with

dementia during COVID-19. *The Lancet Neurology* 2020; 19(11):892.

38. NICE. Delirium: prevention, diagnosis and management. Clinical guideline [CG103] 2010 (2019). www.nice.org.uk/guidance/CG103 [Accessed 25.04.2022].

39. British Geriatrics Society and Royal College of Psychiatrists Good Practice Guide. Coronavirus: Managing delirium in confirmed and suspected cases. 2020. www .bgs.org.uk/sites/default/files/content/attac hment/2020-03-26/BGS%20Coronavirus% 20-%20Managing%20delirium%20in%20c onfirmed%20and%20suspected%20case s_0.pdf [Accessed 25.04.2022].

40. British Geriatrics Society & Royal College of Emergency Medicine. *The Silver Book: Quality Care for Older People with Urgent and Emergency Care Needs*. British Geriatrics Society. 2012.

41. Royal College of Psychiatrists College Report CR211. Our Invisible Addicts. 2018. www.rcpsych.ac.uk/improving-care/cam paigning-for-better-mental-health-policy/ college-reports/2018-college-reports/our-invisible-addicts-2nd-edition-cr211-mar-2 018 [Accessed 25.04.2022].

42. NICE. Alcohol-use disorders: diagnosis and management of physical complications. Clinical guideline [CG100] 2010 (updated: 12 April 2017). www .nice.org.uk/guidance/cg100 [Accessed 25.04.2022].

43. Sampson, E. L., White, N., Lord, K. et al. Pain, agitation, and behavioural problems in people with dementia admitted to general hospital wards: A longitudinal cohort study. *Pain* 2015 Apr;156 (4):675–83.

44. Husebo, B. S., Ballard, C., Sandvik, R., Nilsen, O. B. and Dag, A. Efficacy of treating pain to reduce behavioural disturbances in residents of nursing homes with dementia: cluster randomised clinical trial. *BMJ* 2011; 343 :d4065.

45. Sweeney, A., Clement, S., Filson, B. and Kennedy, A. Trauma-informed mental healthcare in the UK: What is it and how can we further its development? *Mental Health Review Journal* 2016:21: (3) 174–92.

46. Sweeney, A., Filson, B., Kennedy, A., Collinson, L. and Gillard, S. A paradigm shift: Relationships in trauma-informed mental health services. *BJPsych Advances* 2018; 24: (5) 319–33.

47. Wilton, J. and Williams, A. Centre for Mental Health: Engaging with complexity. 2019. www.centreformentalhealth.org.uk/s ites/default/files/2019-05/CentreforMH_E ngagingWithComplexity.pdf [Accessed 25.04.2022].

48. PIECES Tool. www.interiorhealth.ca/sites/ Partners/SeniorsCare/DementiaPathway/ MiddleDementiaPhase/Documents/PIECE S-ABCtool.pdf [Accessed 25.04.2022]

49. MDT podcast Episode 5.05 BPSD Management 2018 http://thehearingaid podcasts.org.uk/5-05-bpsd-management-5 / [Accessed 25.04.2022].

50. Waddell, M. Discussion of Sandra Evans' chapter 'Where is the unconscious in dementia?'. In *The Organic and the Inner World. Psychoanalytic Ideas series*. 2009. Karnac, London, pp. 103–8.

51. Livingston, G., Huntley, J., Sommerlad, A. et al. Dementia prevention, intervention, and care: 2020 report of the Lancet Commission. *The Lancet Commissions* 2020; 396:10248:413–46.

52. Livingston, G., Kelly, L., Lewis-Holmes, E. et al. Non-pharmacological interventions for agitation in dementia: systematic review of controlled trials. *British Journal of Psychiatry* 2014; 205:436–42.

53. Chenoweth, L., King, M. T., Jeon, Y. H. et al. Caring for aged dementia care resident study (CADRES) of person-centred care, dementia care mapping and usual care in dementia: A cluster randomised trial. *Lancet Neurology* 2009; 8:317–25.

54. McCallion, P., Toseland, R. W, Lacey, D., and Banks, S. Educating nursing assistants to communicate more effectively with nursing home residents with dementia. *Gerontologist* 1999; 39:546–58.

55. Cooke, M. L., Moyle, W., Shum, D. H. et al. A randomized, controlled trial exploring the effect of music on agitated behaviours

and anxiety in older people with dementia. *Aging and Mental Health* 2010; 14:905–16.

56. Lin, Y., Chu, H., Yang, C. Y. et al. Effectiveness of group music intervention against agitated behavior in elderly persons with dementia. *International Journal of Geriatric Psychiatry* 2012; 26:670–8.

57. Sung, H. C., Lee, W. L., and Li, T. L. A group music intervention using percussion instruments with familiar music to reduce anxiety and agitation of institutionalized older adults with dementia. *International Journal of Geriatric Psychiatry* 2012; 27:621–7.

58. Kales, H., Gitlin, L., and Lyketsos, C. G. Assessment and management of behavioral and psychological symptoms of dementia. *BMJ* 2015; 350:h369.

59. Ballard, C., Orrell, M., Moniz-Cook, E. et al. Improving mental health and reducing antipsychotic use in people with dementia in care homes: The WHELD research programme including two RCTs. *Programme Grants for Applied Research* 2020; 8(6).

60. O'Brien, J. T., Holmes, C., Jones, M. et al. Clinical practice with anti-dementia drugs: A revised (third) consensus statement from the British Association for Psychopharmacology. *Journal of Psychopharmacology* 2017;31(2):147–68.

61. Lonergan, E., Luxenberg, J., Colford, J. M. et al. Haloperidol for agitation in dementia. *Cochrane Database of Systematic Reviews* 2002; 2: CD002852.

62. Ballard, C. G., Birks, J. and Waite, J. Atypical antipsychotics for aggression and psychosis in Alzheimer disease. *Cochrane Database of Systematic Reviews* 2006; 1: CD003476.

63. Schneider, L. S., Dagerman, K. and Insel, P. S. Efficacy and adverse effects of atypical antipsychotics for dementia: meta-analysis of randomized, placebo-controlled trials. *American Journal of Geriatric Psychiatry* 2006; 14:191–210.

64. Ballard, C. G. and Howard,R. Neuroleptic drugs in dementia: Benefits and harm. *Nature Reviews Neuroscience* 2006; 7:492–500.

65. Ballard, C. G., Hanney, M. L., Theodoulou, M. et al. The dementia antipsychotic withdrawal trial (DART-AD): Long-term follow-up of a randomised placebo-controlled trial. *Lancet Neurology* 2009; 8:151–7.

66. Cummings, J., Ballard, C. G., Tariot, P. et al. Pimavanserin: Potential treatment for dementia-related psychosis. *Journal of Prevention of Alzheimers Disease* 2018; 5 (4):253–8.

67. Tariot, P. N, Erb, R., Podgorski, C. A. et al. Efficacy and tolerability of carbamazepine for agitation and aggression in dementia. *American Journal of Psychiatry* 1998:155:54–61.

68. Lonergan, E., Luxenberg, J., Colford, J. M. et al. Valproate preparations for agitation in dementia. *Cochrane Database of Systematic Reviews* 2009; 3:CD003945.

69. Teri, L., Logsdon, R. G., Peskind, E. et al. Treatment of agitation in dementia: A randomized placebo controlled trial. *Neurology* 2000; 55:1271–8.

70. Porsteinsson, A. P, Drye, L. T, Pollock, B. G. et al. Effect of citalopram on agitation in Alzheimer disease: the CitAD randomized clinical trial. *JAMA* 2014; 311 (7):682–91.

71. Banerjee, S., Hellier, J., Dewey, M. et al. Sertraline or mirtazapine for depression in dementia (HTA-SADD): A randomised, multicentre, double-blind, placebo-controlled trial. *The Lancet* 2011; 378:403–11.

72. Meehan, K. M., Wang, H., David, S. R. et al. Comparison of rapidly acting intramuscular olanzapine, lorazepam and placebo: A double-blind randomized study in acutely agitated patients with dementia. *Neuropsychopharmacology* 2002; 26 (4):494–504.

Management of Violence in People With Intellectual Disability

Mervyn Yong, Laura Humphries, Ingrid Bohnen, Alina Bakala and Anusha Wijeratne

Introduction

Violent behaviour displayed by individuals with intellectual disability (ID) is one of the biggest challenges to services. It is one of many manifestations of the more widely researched subject of challenging behaviour. Violent behaviours observed in people with an ID may include punching, slapping, pushing, pulling, kicking, pinching, scratching, pulling hair, biting, head butting, using weapons, throttling and sexual violence. Violence occurs in a variety of settings. It can happen in inpatient wards but also in community settings, including family homes and community-based settings run by organisations in statutory, independent and voluntary sectors. Children with an ID and severe challenging aggressive behaviours may be placed in residential schools.

Violent behaviour has many serious consequences for both individuals with ID and their formal and informal carers. This is a major obstacle to social integration. Violent behaviour is also one of the main reasons for referral to mental health professionals and services. Often violent behaviour leads to multiple admissions to institutions and psychiatric facilities. Staff working with individuals ID who display challenging behaviour, including violent behaviour, may experience high levels of stress and burnout [1, 2].

Epidemiology

Rates of violent and aggressive behaviour vary considerably across studies, ranging from 2% to 51% of the ID population [3–5]. The differences in prevalence of violence in various studies are due to methodological variations that include factors such as study settings (e.g. institutional vs. community), level of ID (profound ID to mild ID as well as borderline ID), time-span surveyed (e.g. past month, past year or more) and age group (children, adolescents or adults) [6].

Aetiology

Biological Factors

Violent behaviour in people with ID can be driven by factors which apply to those without an intellectual disability (e.g. coexistent mental illness, substance abuse and certain personality disorders). Additional factors arising from the presence of ID, such as impaired communication, poor regulation of frustration and anxiety, can compound or act independently to trigger violent behaviour [7]. Differences in interpretation of emotional cues, interpersonal attributions and beliefs about the likely outcome of aggression can be contributory factors [8]. There is also evidence to show that those with more mental and physical health problems are more likely to display aggressive behaviour than those with fewer and less severe problems [9].

Some specific biological factors which have been investigated for their role in precipitating aggression in people with ID include epilepsy, pain and menstruation [10–12]. There is also some evidence that certain syndrome groups (e.g. Cri du Chat, Smith-Magenis, Prader-Willi, Angelman, Cornelia de Lange and Fragile X syndromes) are more associated with aggression than others [13].

Developmental Disorders

The prevalence of autism spectrum disorders (ASD) in the ID population is thought to be between 20–30% [14]. In those with severe ID, the presence of some of the core features of ASD and attention-deficit/hyperactivity disorder were shown to be associated with aggression [15, 16]. A study in young people with ASD showed that those with sensory problems, sleep problems and self-injury displayed higher levels of aggression [17]. Another study suggested there may be more difficulties with cognitive shifting in those with ASD who present with aggressive behaviour [18].

Psychosocial Factors

People with ID are also more likely than the wider population to be ascribed low social status and to encounter stigmatisation by their peers [19, 20]. Environmental factors such as overcrowding, high staff turnover and inadequate staff training may also contribute to violent behaviour. Moreover, people with ID are more likely to be exposed to more severe forms of maltreatment. People with ID with a history of victimisation or abuse are at high risk of exhibiting violent behaviour [21]. Gardener and Moffatt [22] offered a multi-modal explanation of aggression in people with ID that stressed the importance of individual setting conditions, environmental setting conditions and maintaining factors.

A large national audit conducted from 2003 to 2005 on the management of violence in inpatient services for people with learning disabilities showed that aspects of the unit environment, such as noise, temperature and access to quiet spaces, had a significant impact on the risk of violence occurring [23]. Support being available for staff following a violent incident, good staff morale and good quality of communication to service users (especially regarding their stay and treatment) were found to be significantly positive factors [24].

Assessment

The National Institute for Health and Care Excellence (NICE) guidelines on Challenging Behaviour in people with Learning Disabilities (2015) recommend that all relevant biopsychosocial factors are explored in a multidisciplinary way. This includes a functional assessment of behaviour, with the aim to establish the relationship between behaviour and the function it serves for an individual. This is achieved through a process of data collection through observation of the trigger of the behaviour, identifying the behaviour itself and identifying the consequence of the behaviour which continues to maintain it [25].

A past history of aggression or aggression trigger factors should be sought, including a history of abuse or trauma and previous response to management of violence or aggression. Cognitive, language, communication and cultural factors that may increase the risk of violence or aggression should also be identified [25].

Any underlying mental health problems should be identified and treated in line with relevant NICE guidelines, including any coexisting physical health and sleep problems.

Risk Assessment

Evaluation of the key domains of risk assessment and management that apply to the general population is important, but additional consideration should also be given to biological psychological and social factors that can raise distress and anxiety in people with ID.

Objective instruments of violent risk assessment have been mostly validated in the offender population with learning disability. The Violence Risk Appraisal Guide (VRAG), Historical Clinical Risk-20 (HCR20), Short Dynamic Risk Scale (SDRS) and Emotional Problem Scale (EPS) would appear to have some value in the evaluation of risk for future violent incidents when applied in a wide variety of settings, including high/medium/low secure and community [26–30]. Readers should however note the limited predictive value of these instruments as described in Chapter 4.

Prevention

Central to prevention is establishing a robust formulation of the biopsychosocial needs of an individual with ID and a comprehensive assessment of risk. ID teams should focus on planned, proactive and responsive risk management with ongoing positive-behaviour support.

Therapeutic consideration should be afforded to inherent factors of ID that lower the threshold for violence. These include poor problem-solving skills, impaired regulation of negative emotional experiences, reduced understanding of socially acceptable behaviour and empathic difficulties. A prevention care plan should be holistic and address all biological, psychological, sensory and social factors that may contribute to violent aggression in each individual. One suggested way of minimising the impact of environment on behaviour is to train both staff and the patient to make the best use of the environment (also see Chapter 4).

Management

It is essential that good-quality services are commissioned and provided which ensure that people with additional and complex needs are appropriately cared for so that they can lead fulfilling lives in the community. Services should be local, provide individualised support, ensure innovative day opportunities and offer short breaks as respite for family carers. Additional specialist services are required locally which can support good mainstream practice as well as directly serve a small number of people with the most challenging needs. These services are usually found as part of a community ID team [31].

Rarely, specialist interventions in inpatient services will be most suitable to manage behaviours of high risk.

Interventions

The NICE guidelines 2015 (NG11) recommend personalised interventions tailored to a range of settings with clear targeted behaviours and agreed outcomes. Strategies that do not lead to change within a specified time frame should be modified. There should be assessment and modification of environmental factors that could trigger or maintain the behaviour, including assessing the responses of staff, family and carers to the challenging behaviour [25].

Psychological Interventions

Psychological treatments have the strongest empirical support. However, even where staff are well-organised to undertake psychological treatment of aggressive challenging behaviour, the results are often short lived [32]. One reason for this is the difficulty staff often have in maintaining appropriate levels of organisation and skill in their interaction with the service user over time.

Positive Behaviour Support

This is a person-centred approach to working with people with challenging behaviour, the aim of which is to replace difficult behaviour with functionally equivalent 'replacement' behaviours while at the same time looking at the environmental and social factors that influence or maintain the behaviour and increasing communication skills for the individual [33].

Cognitive Behavioural Therapy

There is growing evidence for individual and group-based cognitive behavioural therapy (CBT) for anger management in people with ID, including randomised controlled trial evidence for its use in both forensic secure and community settings [34, 35]. The use of CBT does rely on language, which may reduce its utility in people with significant communication difficulties, and there have been no standardised approaches developed for use in this population. There is also some literature emerging about the use of modified dialectical behaviour therapy.

De-Escalation

This is defined as the purposeful use of a complex range of communication and therapeutic intervention skills based on a knowledgeable understanding of the causes of violence and aggression which is aimed at the prevention, reduction or management of the probability of violent or aggressive behaviour.

Family Work

There can be a role for addressing relationship patterns in the system around the person, including family therapy [36].

Medical Management

Medical intervention (mainly drug treatment) for aggressive challenging behaviour can be effective where there is an underlying mental health or physical health problem which has been correctly diagnosed. Psychotropic medication can also be used to attenuate some problems associated with violent behaviour where no medical or psychiatric cause is identified, but the evidence base for this is limited and there remain concerns that psychotropic drugs of all kinds are overprescribed.

A Cochrane review of antipsychotic medication for challenging behaviour analysed nine randomised controlled trials and concluded that there was no evidence of whether antipsychotic medication helps or harms adults with learning disability and challenging behaviour [37]. The NACHBID RCT of neuroleptics in the treatment of aggressive challenging behaviour for people with intellectual disabilities study showed that there were no significant important benefits conferred by treatment with risperidone or haloperidol, and treatment with these drugs was not cost effective [38].

The Maudsley Prescribing Guidelines in Psychiatry (MPGP) comment that, despite the limited evidence base, there is 'a significant body of other evidence' to support the use of antipsychotics, including second-generation antipsychotics such as risperidone, aripiprazole and olanzapine, for behavioural disturbance [39]. It is likely that antipsychotics have some effect on the underlying anxiety and arousal states that are associated with an aggressive incident and therefore indirectly influence the manifestation of violence in a person.

Furthermore, Sheehan and Hassiotis's [40] systematic 2017 review of the available evidence on the reduction or discontinuation of antipsychotics used for challenging behaviour in adults with ID concluded that, although the relevant evidence was limited, withdrawal of medication led to behavioural deterioration for some people, with no evident personal characteristics distinguishing the group who experienced adverse side effects. However, there is not always a re-emergence of problem behaviours on reducing or stopping antipsychotic medication, and in some cases a reduction in medication may even be associated with an improvement in presentation.

Withdrawal of antipsychotic medication should be gradual, and patients should be closely monitored for any withdrawal symptoms or changes in behaviour.

So where does this leave clinicians?

Psychotropic medication continues to be used in clinical practice for challenging behaviour, and recent NICE guidelines 2015 (NG11) advise that antipsychotic medication can be considered for challenging behaviour if the risks are very severe, but this should be reviewed regularly to assess response and should be part of an overall multidisciplinary team approach to management [25].

The severity of the behaviour disturbance is the key to prescription. Clearly, angry and violent actions liable to harm self or others may require drug intervention, including rapid tranquillisation in some cases, but most challenging behaviour is much milder in severity, and ways of managing it without recourse to drug therapy are now recognised to be more appropriate.

If psychotropic medication for people with intellectual disability and challenging behaviour is used, then prescribers should adhere to four key prescribing standards as outlined by practice guidelines FR/ID/09 from the Royal College of Psychiatrists [41].

These are as follows:

1. Clear documentation of the indication and rationale for the prescription, including whether it is off-label, polypharmacy or high dose.
2. Consent-to-treatment procedures (or best-interest decision-making processes) should be followed and documented.
3. Regular monitoring of treatment response and any side effects (preferably every three months or less, at a minimum every six months).
4. Regular review and evaluation of the need for continuation or discontinuation of psychotropic medication (preferably every three months or less, at a minimum every six months) or whenever there is a request from patients, carers or other professionals.

Prescribers should also consider advice given in a useful guide on the use of psychotropic medication in ID produced by the MPGP [39].

Stopping over-medication of people with an ID, autism or both (STOMP) was a campaign launched in 2016 by NHS England in collaboration with several Royal College organisations, aimed at urging a change in culture around prescribing psychotropic medication for challenging behaviour in people with an ID, emphasising a more judicious approach to prescribing with an emphasis on building support for alternatives to medication [42]. A recent survey by the Royal College of Psychiatrists reported that antipsychotic medications were less likely to be initiated since the STOMP initiative was launched and alternative psychotropics, most commonly antidepressants, were prescribed for the management of challenging behaviour [43]. Certain key factors that could hamper attempts at antipsychotic withdrawal include deterioration in challenging behaviours, family and carer concern, inadequate multi-agency and multidisciplinary input and lack of psychosocial interventions.

Following the success of STOMP, which focused on the adult population, a similar initiative – *Supporting Treatment and Appropriate Medication in Paediatrics* (STAMP) – was launched to support children and young children with an ID, autism or both [44]. A recently released RCPsych position statement outlines the college's position on STOMP and STAMP: the aim is to support professionals to provide 'the best quality prescribing regime possible' for people with ID and or autism [44, pp. 7–10]. The position statement emphasises that the effective use of psychotropic medication needs to be for the right indication, for the right reason and with appropriate monitoring for side effects, in order to improve the quality of life of the individual concerned. Clinicians are asked to carefully weigh up the disadvantages versus advantages of prescribing psychotropic medication following a holistic approach to management, taking into consideration the significant metabolic and extrapyramidal side effects associated with psychotropic medication and the impact on the physical health of the individual concerned. The report references evidence that people with ID have poorer health than their non-disabled peers [45].

Rapid Tranquillisation

Most of the evidence for the use of rapid tranquillisation comes from studies amongst patients with psychiatric illnesses; therefore, the inference drawn for its use amongst people who have learning disabilities has to be interpreted with caution [46]. Judicial use of medication, including the intramuscular route, can be recommended in the management of acute violence where other methods have failed, there is a danger of imminent risk and to do so is in the patient's best interests. Prior medical examination and ongoing medical monitoring is important due to high levels of comorbidity with physical illness in this patient population. There is a significantly increased prevalence rate of epilepsy in people with ID, and possible changes to seizure threshold with neuroleptic administration need to be considered.

The NICE guidelines 2015 (NG10) recommend intramuscular lorazepam or combined intramuscular haloperidol with intramuscular promethazine for rapid tranquillisation. If the patient is antipsychotic-naïve, has evidence of cardiovascular disease including a prolonged QT interval or does not have a recent electrocardiogram, administration of intramuscular lorazepam is preferred instead. Monitoring of the patient's vital signs, consciousness level and any side effects are required at least hourly until there are no concerns about their physical health status [47].

Electroconvulsive Therapy

There is little to no research on the use of electroconvulsive therapy (ECT) in managing violence in people with ID. Even in common clinical practice it is only used in exceptional circumstances.

Restrictive Interventions

If all attempts to defuse the risks that arise from violent behaviour have failed and in the event of imminent violence, it may be necessary to use physical interventions, seclusion or segregation from other residents as a last resort. There is recent guidance from the Care Quality Commission on the proper assessment, implementation and review whenever there has been use of restrictive practice [48]. The rationale, conduct and review should be clearly documented in the individual's care plan. The Mental Health Act Code of Practice (2015) states that physical intervention should be used as a last resort and never as a matter of course [46]. It should be used proportionally in an emergency when there seems to be a real possibility that significant harm would occur if intervention is withheld [49]. Conditions such as heart or respiratory disease, which are prevalent amongst people who have ID, contribute to the potential hazards associated with the physical restraint. The NICE guidelines (NG10) recommend that whenever restrictive intervention is used the person should be monitored closely and continuously to ensure their physical and emotional comfort [47]. Its use should be documented as part of an incident record to be used in personal and organisational debrief procedures.

Autism Spectrum Disorder

Some studies have shown that individuals with ID and comorbid autism are more likely to display aggressive behaviour compared to those without autism [6, 50]. Management of individuals with comorbid autism adopts a similar approach to individuals with intellectual disabilities. Evidence-based studies for non-pharmacological treatment include functional behaviour assessments, functional communication training and reinforcement strategies. In those requiring pharmacological treatment, there is evidence to support the use of second-generation antipsychotics in reducing aggression [51].

According to a review done by the British Association for Psychopharmacology, risperidone and aripiprazole have both been shown to help reduce irritability and aggressive behaviour in children with ASD [52]. Treatment efficacy in adults with ASD, however, is less well studied and the evidence base is limited. Therefore, the decision for pharmacotherapy in adults with ASD should be made cautiously, on a case-by-case basis, with close monitoring of side effects and after consideration of alternatives.

Transforming Care

NHS England published a national plan, Building the Right Support [53], in October 2015; this originated following the Winterbourne View scandal in 2011, which highlighted abuse and neglect of people with intellectual disabilities in a private hospital in South Gloucestershire, England. The agenda of this plan was to improve community health and care services for people with intellectual disabilities and autism who display challenging behaviour by closing inappropriate and outmoded inpatient facilities. The Department of Health aimed to close a minimum of 45–65% of CCG-commissioned inpatient capacity and 25–40% of NHS England-commissioned inpatient capacity by 2018 [53].

There were concerns about the implementation of the policy without having the prior required investment and development of the appropriate community services. The pressure to discharge and keep hospital admissions as short as possible would affect patients' rehabilitation, and community services were not resourced properly to manage ongoing risks [54]. Another consequence noted from the rapid bed-closure policy for people with ID and forensic needs was that they were instead admitted to generic mental health services or sent to prison. In addition to the lack of specialist assessment and treatment available, they were at an increased vulnerability risk of exploitation from other, more able service users because of their disabilities [54].

Legislation

The principles of the Mental Capacity Act 2005, Mental Health Act 1983 as amended in 2007 and Human Rights Act 1998 need to guide all assessment care and treatment decisions in this vulnerable patient population. In those who lack capacity, best interests should be considered and safeguarding procedures applied in order to ensure the person's safety. Best-interest decision-making should be person-centred, involve families or the individual's support network, and the process should be recorded and regularly reviewed according to NICE guidance 2018 [55]. Independent advocacy services can support the decision-making task and must be offered as described in the Care Act 2014, Mental Capacity Act 2005 and Mental Health Act 2007.

COVID-19 Pandemic

A report published by Public Health England in November 2020 reviewed deaths of people with intellectual disabilities from COVID-19 and factors impacting on mortality risks. The mortality rates in people with intellectual disabilities were up to six times higher than for the general population [56].

People with ID are less likely to have capacity to understand and follow social restriction guidance, including use of personal protective equipment, which could cause distress and potentiate aggression. In addition to their increased physical, mental and social vulnerability, they would be more prone to anxiety, distress and deterioration of challenging behaviours. For people with autism, disturbance in routine caused by socio-environmental restrictions or increased obsessional thinking about COVID-19-related information can lead to depression, anxiety, agitation and aggression. Access to services which normally provide behaviour and psychological interventions would be significantly limited due to the impact of social restriction measures [57].

On the positive side, the changes forced on people with ID as a consequence of COVID-19 offer both carers and residents the opportunity to make environmental adjustments that may be of benefit. A randomised trial of collaborative environmental improvements (nidotherapy) carried out with 200 people with ID in care homes who showed challenging behaviour demonstrated benefits somewhat greater that those achieved by the enhanced care programme [58].

Conclusion

People with an ID require a tailored, person-centred approach alongside close collaborative working with multidisciplinary and multi-agency services. The challenging behaviours displayed impacts detrimentally not only on the patient, but also on services, family and social networks, and all interested parties need to work together to ensure that the appropriate care needs of the individual are met. Assessments and interventions need to be inclusive, evidence-based and take on a holistic approach. Any usage of pharmacological interventions should be carefully considered, regularly reviewed and closely monitored for any potential adverse effects and long-term health implications. Care services and support available to individuals, family and carers should be efficient, equitable and well resourced, with the aim of improving overall health and social outcomes, in addition to empowering patients and providing advocacy where indicated.

References

1. Jenkins, R., Rose, J. and Lovell, C. Psychological well-being of staff working with people who have challenging behaviour. *Journal of Intellectual Disability Research* 1997; 41:502–11.

2. Male, D. B. and May, D. S. Burnout and workload in teachers of children with severe learning difficulties. *British Journal of Learning Disabilities* 1997; 25:117–21.

3. Borthwick-Duffy, S. A. Prevalence of destructive behaviors: A study of aggression, self-injury, and property destruction. In T. Thompson and B. D. Gray (eds.) *Destructive Behavior in Developmental Disabilities: Diagnoses and Treatment*. California: SAGE Publishing; 1994, pp. 3–22.

4. Emerson, E., Kiernan, C., Alborz, A. et al. The prevalence of challenging behaviors: A total population study. *Research in Developmental Disabilities* 2001; 22:77–93.

5. Crocker, A. G., Mercier, C., Lachapelle, Y. et al. Prevalence and types of aggressive behaviour among adults with intellectual disabilities. *Journal of Intellectual Disability Research* 2006; 50:652–61.

6. McClintock, K., Hall, S. and Oliver, C. Risk markers associated with challenging behaviours in people with intellectual disabilities: A meta-analytic study. *Journal of Intellectual Disability Research* 2003; 47:405–16.

7. Bhaumik, S., Nadkarni, S. S., Biswas, A. B. and Watson, J. M. Service innovations: Risk assessment in learning disability. *Psychiatric Bulletin* 2005; 29:28–31.

8. Larkin, P., Jahoda, A. and MacMahon, K. The social information processing model as a framework for explaining frequent aggression in adults with mild to moderate intellectual disabilities: A systemic review of the evidence. *Journal of Applied Research in Intellectual Disabilities* 2013; 26 (5):447–65.

9. Crocker, A. G., Prokić, A., Morin, D. and Reyes, A. Intellectual disability and co-occurring mental health and physical disorders in aggressive behaviour. *Journal of Intellectual Disability Research* 2014; 58 (11):1032–44.

10. Creaby, M., Warner, M., Jamil, N. and Jawad, S. Ictal aggression in severely mentally handicapped people. *Irish Journal of Psychological Medicine* 1993; 10:12–15.

11. Tenneij, N. H. and Koot, H. M. Incidence, types and characteristics of aggressive behaviour in treatment facilities for adults with mild intellectual disability and severe challenging behaviour. *Journal of Intellectual Disability Research* 2008; 52:114–24.

12. Rodgers, J., Lipscombe, J. and Santer, M. Menstrual problems experienced by women with learning disabilities. *Journal of Applied Research in Intellectual Disabilities* 2006; 19:364–73.

13. Powis, L. and Oliver, C. The prevalence of aggression in genetic syndromes: A review.

Research in Developmental Disabilities 2014; 35(5):1051–71.

14. Emerson, E. and Baines, B. Health inequalities and people with learning disabilities in the UK. *Tizard Learning Disability Review* 2011; 16(1):42–8.

15. Matson, J. L. and Adams, H. L. Characteristics of aggression among persons with autism spectrum disorders. *Research in Autism Spectrum Disorders* 2014; 8(11):1578–84.

16. Davies, L. E. and Oliver, C. Self-injury, aggression and destruction in children with severe intellectual disability: Incidence, persistence and novel, predictive behavioural risk markers. *Research in Developmental Disabilities* 2016; 49–50:291–301.

17. Mazurek M O, Kanne S M & Wodka E L. Physical aggression in children and adolescents with autism spectrum disorders. *Research in Autism Spectrum Disorders* 2013; 7(3):455–65.

18. Visser E M, Berger H J C, Prins J B, et al. Shifting impairment and aggression in intellectual disability and autism spectrum disorder. *Research in Developmental Disabilities* 2014; 35(9):2137–47.

19. Crocker, J., Major, B. and Steele, C. Social stigma. In S. T. Fiske, D. T. Gilbert and G. Lindzey (eds.) *Handbook of Social Psychology*. Boston, MA: McGraw-Hill; 1998, pp. 504–533.

20. Dovidio, J. F., Major, B. and Crocker, J. Stigma: Introduction and overview. In T. F. Heatherton, R. E. Kleck, M. R. Hebl and J. G. Hull (eds.) *The Social Psychology of Stigma*. New York: Guilford Press; 2000, pp. 1–28.

21. Strand, M., Benzein, E. and Saveman, B. I. Violence in the care of adult persons with intellectual disabilities. *Journal of Clinical Nursing* 2004; 13:506–14.

22. Gardner, W. I. and Moffatt, C. Aggressive behaviour: Definition, assessment, treatment. *International Review of Psychiatry* 1990; 2:91–100.

23. Healthcare Commission. Final report: National Audit of Violence (2003–2005).

London: Healthcare Commission, 2005. [online]. www.wales.nhs.uk/documents/FinalReport-violence.pdf [Accessed 27.4.2022].

24. Deb, S. and Roberts, K. The evidence base for the management of imminent violence in Intellectual Disability services. *Occasional Paper OP57*. Royal College of Psychiatrists, 2005.

25. National Institute for Health and Care Excellence (NICE). Challenging behaviour and learning disabilities: Prevention and interventions for people with learning disabilities whose behaviour challenges: NICE Guideline (NG11). 2015.

26. Quinsey, V. L., Harris, G. T., Rice, M. E. and Cromier, C. A. *Violent Offenders: Appraising and Managing Risk*. Washington, DC: American Psychological Association; 1998.

27. Webster, C. D., Eaves, D., Douglas, K. S. and Wintrup, A. *The HCR-20: The Assessment of Dangerousness and Risk*. Vancouver: Simon Fraser University and British Colombia Forensic Psychiatric Services Commission; 1995.

28. Quinsey, V. L., Book, A. and Skilling, T. A. A. Follow-up of deinstitutionalized men with intellectual disabilities and histories of antisocial behaviour. *Journal of Applied Research in Intellectual Disabilities* 2004; 17:243–53.

29. Prout, T. H. and Strohmer, D. C. *Emotional Problem Scale*. Lutz, FL: Psychological Assessment Resources, Inc.; 1991.

30. Lindsay, W. R., Hogue, T. E., Taylor, J. L. et al. Risk assessment in offenders with intellectual disability: A comparison across three levels of security. *Int J Offender Ther Comp Criminol* 2008; 52:90–111.

31. Mansell Report 2007. Department of Health: Services for people with learning disabilities and challenging behaviour or mental health needs (project report). https://research.kent.ac.uk/tizard/wp-content/uploads/sites/2302/2019/01/dh2007mansellreport.pdf.

32. Totsika, V., Toogood, S., Hastings, R. P. and McCarthy, J. The effect of active support interactive training on the daily

lives of adults with an intellectual disability. *Journal of Applied Research in Intellectual Disabilities* 2010; 23(2):112–21.

33. Horner, R. H., Dunlap, G., Koegel, R. L. et al. Toward a technology of 'nonaversive' behavior support. *Journal of the Association for Persons with Severe Handicaps* 1990; 15:125–32.

34. Nicoll, M., Beail, N. and Saxon, D. Cognitive behavioural treatment for anger in adults with intellectual disabilities: A systematic review and meta-analysis. *Journal of Applied Research in Intellectual Disabilities* 2013; 26(1):47–62.

35. Willner, P., Rose, J., Jahoda, A. et al. A cluster randomised controlled trial of a manualised cognitive behavioural anger management interventions delivered by supervised lay therapises to people with intellectual disabilities. *Health Technology Assessment* 2013; 17(21):1–173.

36. Brown, J. F., Hamilton-Mason, J., Maramaldi, P. and Barnhill, L. J. Exploring perspectives of individuals with intellectual disabilities and histories of challenging behaviours about family relationships: An emergent topic in a grounded theory focus group study. *Journal of Mental Health Research in Intellectual Disabilities* 2016; 9 (3):1–24.

37. Brylewski, J. and Duggan, L. Antipsychotic medication for challenging behaviour in people with learning disability. *Cochrane Database of Systematic Reviews* 2004; (3): CD000377.

38. Tyrer, P., Oliver-Africano, P., Romeo, R. et al. Neuroleptics in the treatment of aggressive challenging behaviour for people with intellectual disabilities: A randomised controlled trial (NACHBID). *Health Technology Assessment* 2009; 13:1–54.

39. Taylor, D. M., Barnes, T. R. E. and Young, A. H. *The Maudsley Prescribing Guidelines in Psychiatry* 13th ed. Chichester: John Wiley & Sons; 2018.

40. Sheehan, R. and Hassiotis, A. Reduction or discontinuation of antipsychotics for challenging behaviour in adults with intellectual disability: A systematic review. *The Lancet Psychiatry* 2017; 4(3):238–56.

41. Royal College of Psychiatrists (2016). Psychotropic drug prescribing for people with intellectual disability, mental health problems and/or behaviours that challenge: practice guidelines. Faculty report FR/ID/09. 2016.

42. NHS England (2016). Stopping over medication of people with a learning disabilty, autism or both (STOMP). www .england.nhs.uk/learning-disabilities/impr oving-health/stomp/ [Accessed 27.4.2022].

43. Deb, S., Nancarrow, T., Limbu, B. and Sheehan, R. UK psychiatrists' experience of withdrawal of antipsychotics prescribed for challenging behaviours in adults with intellectual disabilities and/or autism. *BJPsych Open* 2020; 6(5): e112.

44. Royal College of Psychiatrists. Position statement. PS05/21. Stopping the overmedication of people with intellectual disability, autism or both (STOMP) and supporting treatment and appropriate medication in paediatrics (STAMP). [online] 2021. www.rcpsych.ac.uk/docs/de fault-source/improving-care/better-mh-policy/position-statements/position-statement-ps0521-stomp-stamp.pdf?sfvrs n=684d09b3_6 [Accessed 27.4.2022].

45. Emerson, E. and Bains, S. Health inequalities and people with intellectual disability in the UK 2010. Improving Health and Lives: Intellectual Disability Observatory. 2010.

46. Royal College of Psychiatrists. The evidence base for the management of imminent violence in Intellectual Disability settings. Occasional Paper OP57. London: Royal College of Psychiatrists. 2005.

47. National Institute for Health and Care Excellence (NICE), Violence and aggression: Short-term management in mental health, health and community settings: NICE Guideline (NG10). 2015.

48. Care Quality Commission (2020). Out of sight – who cares? A review of restraint, seclusion and segregation for autistic people, and people with a learning

disability and/or mental health condition. www.cqc.org.uk/sites/default/files/202012 18_rssreview_report.pdf.

49. Department of Health, UK. The Code of Practice: Mental Health Act 1983. London: The Stationery Office. 2015.

50. Tsakanikos, E., Costello, H., Holt, G., Sturmey, P. and Bouras, N. Behaviour management problems as predictors of psychotropic medication and use of psychiatric services in adults with autism. *Journal of Autism and Developmental Disorders* 2007; 37(6):1080–5.

51. Fitzpatrick, S. E., Srivorakiat, L., Wink, L. K., Pedapati, E. V. and Erickson, C. A. Aggression in autism spectrum disorder: Presentation and treatment options. *Neuropsychiatric Disease and Treatment* 2016; 12:1525–38.

52. Howes, O. D., Rogdaki, M., Findon, J. L. et al. Autism spectrum disorder: Consensus guidelines on assessment, treatment and research from the British Association for Psychopharmacology. *Journal of Psychopharmacology* 2018; 32 (1):3–29.

53. NHS England. *Building the Right Support: A National Plan to Develop Community Services and Close Inpatient Facilities for People with a Learning Disability and/or Autism who Display Behaviour that Challenges, including those with a Mental Health Condition.* NHS England, 2015.

54. Taylor, J. L., McKinnon, I., Thorpe, I. and Gillmer, B. T. The impact of transforming care on the care and safety of patients with intellectual disabilities and forensic needs. *BJPsych Bulletin* 2017; 41:205–8.

55. National Institute for Health and Care Excellence (NICE), Decision making and mental capacity: NICE Guideline (NG108). 2017.

56. Public Health England. Deaths of people identified as having learning disabilities with COVID-19 in England in the spring of 2020. November 2020.

57. Courtenay, K. and Perera, B. COVID-19 and people with intellectual disability: Impacts of a pandemic. *Irish Journal of Psychological Medicine* 2020; 14:1–6

58. Tyrer, P., Tarabi, S. A., Bassett, P. et al. Nidotherapy compared with enhanced care programme approach training for adults with aggressive challenging behaviour and intellectual disability (NIDABID): Cluster-randomised controlled trial. *Journal of Intellectual Disability Research* 2017, 61:521–31.

16 The Relationship Between Violence and Mental Health Inequality in the Black, Asian and Minority Ethnic Communities

Masum Khwaja and Eric Baskind

Introduction

Much has been written about the differences in managing violence in mental health practice in those from ethnic minority backgrounds. In this account we discuss the mental health inequalities in the Black, Asian and Minority Ethnic (BAME) communities and how these relate to the particular issue of restraint.

Race, culture and ethnicity are not the same and, without wanting to appear patronising, we would like readers to be reminded of the differences between the terms:

- Race is a classification of people based on physical or biological characteristics, such as skin colour, facial features, blood type and stature.
- Culture is defined as the values, beliefs, attitudes, art, languages, symbols, rituals, religion and behaviours unique to particular group of people and passed from one generation to the next. Culture has been called 'the way of life for an entire society'.
- Ethnicity is a classification of people based on national origin and/or culture; members of an ethnic group may share a common heritage, geographic location, language, social customs and beliefs.

The term BAME has been criticised for being an umbrella term that pools together individuals from diverse backgrounds. However, ethnic groupings are useful for monitoring, discussing and addressing discrimination and inequalities, and as there is as yet no universally accepted alternative terminology this is the term we have chosen for the book. At least it is widely understood. We hope readers will agree that in considering inequality we should not get distracted by trying to find a 'terminology that perfectly captures one's identity' but focus instead on identifying 'the ways in which people, by virtue of their race or citizenship or ethnicity, are put at systemic disadvantage in Britain – and fixing these injustices' [1].

In discussing mental health inequality in BAME groups, we need to acknowledge that some other groups in society, who may or may not identify as BAME (such as asylum seekers, travellers and the LGBTQ+ community), also face discrimination and have higher rates of mental health problems than the general population [2, 3, 4].

BAME Mental Health Inequality

There is clear evidence that the mental health of those from BAME backgrounds is often worse than for their white counterparts [5]. It is also known that more white people receive treatment for mental health issues than people from BAME backgrounds and that they have better outcomes [6]. The reasons for this are multifactorial and may include the impact of mental health stigma, racism and discrimination, and social and economic inequalities [7].

A disproportionate number of BAME patents have died as a result of excessive force, restraint or serious medical neglect. 'Big, Black and Dangerous' is the subtitle of a report published almost 30 years ago: the 1993 Report of the Committee of Inquiry into the deaths of three African-Caribbean patients, Michael Martin, Joseph Watts and Orville Blackwood, all of whom died in Broadmoor Hospital after being placed in seclusion cells [8]. The report showed that Black people were more likely to have police involvement in their admissions to hospital, more likely to be detained and more likely to receive secure care. The impression that these patients were 'big, black and dangerous' was given so frequently to the committee that they included it in the title of their report [8].

In October 1998, the death of David 'Rocky' Bennett at the Norvic Clinic in Norwich, a forensic unit providing medium secure services to the counties of Norfolk, Suffolk and Cambridgeshire, raised particular issues concerning the use of interpersonal restraint in BAME patients [9]. On the night of his death, Bennett was removed from his ward after fighting with another patient who had 'racially' abused him. While resisting the move, Bennett assaulted a nurse. Five nurses then used restraint measures, holding Bennett face down while immobilising his arms, ankles and upper chest for an estimated 25 minutes. After some time, the nurses realised that he was no longer struggling and was not breathing. They were not able to revive him and he was pronounced dead a short time later.

The report of the Inquiry into Bennett's death noted, amongst other things, that the nurses were not aware of Bennett's cultural needs and treated him as a 'lesser being' [10]. The report also noted that 'unless there are sufficient resources and sustained management, which is both dedicated and committed, these problems cannot be solved. At present people from the black and minority ethnic communities, who are involved in the mental health services, are not getting the service they are entitled to. Putting it bluntly, this is a disgrace' [10, p. 58].

The 2002 Sainsbury Centre for Mental Health review of the relationship between mental health services and African and Caribbean communities reported a 'circle of fear', with 'black people mistrusting services, and staff often wary of the black community, fearing criticism and not knowing how to respond, and fearful of young black men'. This circle of fear, 'is fuelled by prejudice, misunderstanding, misconceptions and sometimes racism' [11, p. 6]. The report acknowledged that young Black men in particular are heavily over-represented in the most restrictive parts of the mental health service and generally have a negative experience of services. Furthermore, these same communities were not 'accessing the primary care, mental health promotion and specialist community services which might prevent or lessen their mental health problems. They are getting the mental health services they do not want but not the ones they do or might want' (p. 6).

Twenty years on from the Sainsburys Report, disparities in the use of the Mental Health Act (MHA) persist, as highlighted in the 2018 Independent Review of the Mental Health Act which confirmed that Black people were four times more likely to be detained and eight times more likely to be subject to a community treatment order than white people [12]. Black people of Afro-Caribbean or African heritage were also disproportionately subjected to use of section 136, had longer average lengths of stay in hospital, higher rates of repeat admissions, higher rates of seclusion, were less likely to be offered psychological therapies and had higher drop-out rates from cognitive behavioural therapy for psychosis [12].

The review concludes that 'profound inequalities' exist for people from ethnic minority communities in 'accessing mental health treatment, their experience of care and their mental health outcomes'. The reasons behind this are multiple, involving 'longstanding experience of discrimination and deprivation' and 'structural factors that engender racism, stigma and stereotyping'. The authors consider that there is 'no single or simple remedy to resolve this situation' (p. 20).

Amongst the review's recommendations is the development and rollout of an organisational competence framework (OCF) and patient and carer (service user) experience tool across health and care organisations. In response to the recommendation, NHS England and NHS Improvement have developed the Patient and Carers Race Equalities Framework (PCREF) [13]. The framework is an important part of NHS England and NHS Improvement's Advancing Mental Health Equalities Strategy (discussed later in the chapter) and is being used to support NHS trusts to improve ethnic minority community experiences of care in mental health services. The framework has three components:

- *Statutory and regulatory obligations* – expectations on all mental health trusts in fulfilling their statutory duties under core pieces of legislation, such as the Health and Social Care Act and the Equalities Act;
- *Organisational competency* – a competency framework to support trusts to improve patient and carer experience for ethnic minorities;
- *Patient and carers feedback mechanism* – to embed patient and carer voice at the heart of the planning, implementation and learning cycle.

In *Community Care*, Steven Gilbert [14], who has a diagnosis of bipolar affective disorder and was one of the vice-chairs of the review, explains the thinking behind the framework and some of the other recommendations made.

The NHS Race and Health Observatory was established in 2020 [15] after an issue of *The British Medical Journal* (BMJ) highlighted the continuing problem of racism in medicine [16]. The Observatory 'works to identify and tackle ethnic inequalities in health and care by facilitating research, making health policy recommendations and enabling long-term transformational change'.

In February 2022, the Observatory published their rapid review of ethnic health disparities [17]. The review identified evidence of health inequalities faced by ethnic minority communities, including in:

- Seeking help for mental health issues
- Improving access to psychological therapies (IAPT);
- Receipt of cognitive behavioural therapy (CBT) for psychosis;
- Compulsory admission and 'harsher treatment' (e.g. prone restraint and seclusion) during admission (particularly for 'Black groups').

A striking finding of the review was that Black children were ten times more likely to be referred to Children and Adolescent Mental Health Services (CAMHS) via social services than via a general practitioner. Commenting on the review, Smith and Mohan [18] highlight this statistic, explaining that 'clearly there are barriers to accessing primary care that are not noticed, that are neglected, and thus remain unaddressed. This inaction in the face of need is the very essence of systemic discrimination.' Furthermore, marginalisation and exclusion from society start early in a person's life, and by the time patients get to mental health services they've often been 'failed many times over by institutions across education, health, social services, housing, and the justice system' [18].

The illegal killing of George Floyd in Minneapolis, Minnesota, USA by the hands of a policeman on 25 May 2020 'reopened a psychological wound for black people and revealed unique challenges within mental health services' [19]. George Floyd's tragic death gave rise to Black Lives Matter (BLM) protests across the globe. The protests energised the call for discrimination to be robustly addressed within mental health services and in society in general.

The BLM movement is often criticised by those who say in response to BLM higlighting discrimination and racial inequality experienced by Black people, that 'white lives matter also'. The inference being that that those supporting BLM are not valuing white lives, when in reality the movement is simply asking for Black lives to be valued equally to those of their white neighbours. Researchers use the term 'racial gaslighting' to describe a way of maintaining a pro-white/anti-Black balance in society by labelling those that challenge acts of racism as psychologically abnormal [20].

There remains a need to challenge false narratives and narrow review and interpretation of evidence to undermine the existence of racism [21]. For example, the recent report of the Commission on Race and Ethnic Disparities concluded that there was 'no evidence of systemic or institutional racism' in the United Kingdom [22]. The report was heavily criticised by, amongst others, the Royal College of Psychiatrists (RCPsych) who stated: 'The report implies that, in the claimed absence of structural or institutional factors, individuals or families are to blame for the negative experiences and discrimination they face and that the authors have relied on outdated information and selective review of the available evidence to make their recommendations, meaning the methodology, as well as the conclusions, are flawed' [23].

In evaluating the contribution of racism in this debate, one needs to consider underlying inequality, differences in help-seeking behaviour and educational attainment, as well as systemic and institutional racism. What is undeniably true is that research on inequality shows that socio-economic factors are the major determinants of both mental and physical health across all racial groups [24]. Furthermore, over the last decade austerity has had a detrimental effect on health equity in England, especially for the poorest in society. However, to quote Michael Marmot [25], 'outcomes, on the whole, are even worse for minority ethnic population groups and people with disabilities' (p. 5). This point is reinforced by a recent MIND survey of 14,000 adults over the age of 25 which showed that existing inequalities in housing, employment, finances and other issues have had a greater impact on the mental health of people from different BAME groups than on white people during the coronavirus pandemic [26]. A literature and evidence review of racial disparities in mental health commissioned by NHS England also concluded that black and minority ethnic communities are 'disproportionately impacted by social detriments associated with mental ill health. From accessing treatment to receiving mental health support, through to assessment and treatment, inequality and discrimination remains rife for black and minority ethnic communities' [27, p. 24].

Although the impact of racism must be fully acknowledged, it is equally important that we do not assume that the inequalities identified (e.g. the differences in detention rates) are entirely due to racism. There is no published study that can demonstrate unequivocally that race is the most important factor contributing to increased detention, and so blame directed solely on racism is premature. The complexity of researching health inequalities for causal factors is well-made in a recent systematic review and metanalysis considering ethnic variations in compulsory detention under the MHA [28]. The review found that BAME and migrant groups are at a greater risk of psychiatric detention than are majority groups, and that the 'most common explanations for the increased risk of detainment in BAME populations included increased prevalence of psychosis, increased perceived risk of violence, increased police contact, absence of or mistrust of general practitioners, and ethnic disadvantages' (p. 313). The authors advised that 'attempts to explain increased detention in ethnic groups should avoid amalgamation and instead carry out culturally specific, hypothesis-driven studies to examine the numerous contributors to varying rates of detention' (p. 305). There are no studies that have been published that are able to avoid such amalgamation of possible contributory factors and they are going to be difficult, if not impossible, to separate.

Those working in mental health also face discrimination. The RCPsych has explored evidence related to the disproportionate impact of coronavirus (COVID-19) on BAME healthcare staff and linked this to reporting from the Workforce Race Equality Standard and wider evidence which demonstrates that BAME healthcare staff are disadvantaged within the UK healthcare system [29].

COVID-19 was one of the drivers for the NHS to expedite action against ethnic health inequalities as it became clear that BAME groups were significantly more likely to die from COVID-19 and societal inequalities were likely to play a role [30].

In 2020, NHS England and NHS Improvement published the first Advancing Mental Health Equalities Strategy [31]. The strategy summarises the core actions that need to be taken to create more equitable access, experience and outcomes in mental health services in England. The importance of organisations improving their understanding of the communities they serve is emphasised.

The strategy document describes four workstreams aimed at:

- *supporting local health systems* by, for example, rollout of NHS-led provider collaboratives and by ensuring that patients do not fall through gaps in commissioning and service provision;
- gathering more *accurate, comprehensive and transparent data* at a national level to inform strategy;
- developing a *diverse and representative workforce* at all levels of the system, and one equipped with the skills and capabilities to advance mental health equalities;
- *tracking and assuring delivery of the Advancing Mental Health Equality Strategy* to be undertaken by the Advancing Mental Health Equalities Taskforce, which has as its membership an alliance of leaders and experts by experience from the mental health sector.

In January 2021, the RCPsych published an Equality Action Plan with 29 key actions, which will be rolled out between now and the end of 2023 [32]. The action plan acknowledges the findings of the independent review of the MHA. Professor Kimberlé Crenshaw's theory of intersectionality is referenced in the plan. This is the theory that those who possess more than one characteristic that can lead to under-representation or underprivilege (e.g. LGBTQ + and BAME) 'are hit harder' than those who do not because of a 'multiplier effect' as a result of the mix of their characteristics. The action plan commits to 'delivering equality for all college staff and equality of opportunity for members' and to 'promoting equality of access, experience and outcomes for mental health patients and carers' (p. 10).

The RCPsych's three-year Advancing Mental Health Equality (AMHE) collaborative, which launched in July 2021, is part of the action plan and is aimed at supporting mental healthcare providers to reduce mental health inequalities in their local areas [33]. The collaborative offers tailored support for organisations, including help to:

- *Identify* population groups and inequalities to focus on
- *Design* services that improve access, experience and outcomes for the target group(s)
- *Deliver* a new service
- *Evaluate* the impact of the changes that will be introduced, and how to sustain improvements that are made.

As inequality is continuing to widen in most Western countries, this needs to be addressed as a priority. Whilst the statistics are disheartening, the recent commitment shown by the NHS and RCPsych to tackling inequality is to be welcomed, and there are already some excellent projects around the country committed to addressing the long-term inequality of mental health care for the BAME community and other discriminated groups in society [34, 35]. We all deserve equitable access to high-quality mental health services and treatment regardless of our background.

BAME and Restraint

Much has been written about Black people being subjected to stereotypical assumptions and being perceived to be more threatening than white people [36–39]. The stereotyping of young Black males as 'dangerous, violent and volatile' is a long-standing trope that is ingrained in the minds of many in our society. People with mental-health needs also face the stereotype of the mentally ill as 'mad, bad and dangerous' [36].

Recent data on police Taser use is a cause for concern. Home Office data, albeit based on police officer perception, indicates that Black people are more likely to have a Taser used against them than white people. Black people are involved in around 20% of Taser incidents in three years' worth of data despite making up less than 4% of the population [40]. In 2019–20, Black people were subjected to Taser use at a rate between five and eight times higher than white people [41]. This can be contrasted with the data on Asian people, who were involved in 6% of Taser incidents in 2017/18, and in 7% of incidents in both 2018/19 and 2019/20. People of mixed ethnicity were involved in 3% of Taser incidents in all three years [41]. Although much of this data relates to the use (but not necessarily the discharge) of a Taser, there is no reason to suspect that other uses of force are different. Indeed, Home Office data indicates that Black people were involved in 16% of use-of-force incidents in 2018–19 and 2019–20 despite representing less than 4% of the population [42]. As well as the stereotypical assumptions described earlier, this disproportionality is often explained by police officers describing the Black men they have restrained as having 'superhuman strength' (see also Chapter 10) and, often incorrectly, as the 'biggest man I have ever encountered' [36]. It is hardly surprising, therefore, to see that these perceptions translate into disproportionate uses of force against Black men, even in cases where no force can objectively be justified [43]. The tragic death of Kevin Clarke, an acutely mentally unwell Black man who was restrained by up to nine officers from the Metropolitan Police in 2018, illustrates the dehumanising effect restraint can have, to the almost total exclusion of the well-being of the person restrained. Mr Clarke should have been treated as a medical emergency rather than being forcibly restrained [43]. The inquest jury concluded that Mr

Clarke was generally cooperative up until the point when police officers laid hands on him and restrained him.

Restraint training has improved considerably over the years, but much more is needed to educate staff and others about the needs of those whose presentation or behaviour all too often leads to restraint (see Chapter 1). Improvement is necessary in other areas as well. For example, the Care Quality Commission (CQC) has reported that there was a higher proportion of people from a Black or Black-British background in prolonged seclusion on CAMHS wards: 24%, compared with 6% of all people on CAMHS wards in England. Similarly, for learning disability wards, 11% of those in prolonged seclusion were from Black or Black-British backgrounds, compared with 5% of all people on these wards [44].

Organisations should implement mandatory training covering the nature of discrimination, including race issues, ensuring sufficient attention is paid to confronting discriminatory assumptions and stereotypes. This will help ensure that staff are able to challenge the stereotypes which often lead to restraint techniques or other coercive measures being more likely to be used. Consideration should also be given to how this training could take the form of a meaningful two-way dialogue allowing staff to hear first-hand the experiences of people from BAME backgrounds.

Organisations should also ensure that issues of race and discrimination are considered as an integral part of their work to help ensure the well-being of everyone who uses their services. This requires careful monitoring at a senior level, with a 'lessons learnt' approach in appropriate cases and managers being alert to whether any discriminatory attitudes may have caused or contributed to adverse outcomes. Discrimination issues should be addressed robustly in line with the organisation's policies. Managers should be alert to similar cases involving the same staff.

Conclusion

Socio-economic factors, such as housing, income, education, employment, and social isolation, remain the major determinants of both mental and physical health for all population groups, with the impact being disproportionately greater for the BAME community.

Recent reviews of evidence suggest that there remain profound inequalities for people from BAME communities in access to, experience of and outcomes in mental health care that are grounded in structural, institutional and interpersonal racism in society. Furthermore, other groups in society, who may or may not identify as BAME, such as asylum-seekers, travellers and the LGBTQ+ community, also face discrimination and have higher rates of mental health problems than the general population. Those who possess more than one characteristic that can lead to under-representation or underprivilege face a 'multiplier effect' and are likely to face greater hardship and discrimination.

Tackling the social determinants of mental health inequality ultimately requires coordinated action by government at the societal level. However, organisations and individuals working with people with mental illness have a responsibility to identify and address, wherever possible, inequality of mental health care for discriminated groups in the population they serve.

The RCPsych AMHE collaborative offers tailored support for organisations who wish to consider how they can improve access, experience and outcomes for those from minority backgrounds. Initiatives may range from relatively straightforward interventions, such as ensuring that robust interpreting services and appropriate staff training (e.g. to reduce restrictive practices in the BAME community) are in place, through to the commissioning of a service specifically designed to work with a particular minority ethnic group.

The PCREF is an organisational competency framework developed to support organisations to improve ethnic minority community experiences of care in mental health services. One of the core components of the framework is patient and carer feedback.

Mental health stigma, racism and prejudice exist in every society and in all ethnic groups, and all of us have a responsibility to challenge prejudices within our communities and organisations. Doing so will build a fairer, and healthier, society for us all.

References

1. Mistlin, A., So, the term BAME has had its day. But what should replace it? The Guardian. [online] 8.4.2021. www .theguardian.com/commentisfree/2021/ap r/08/bame-britain-ethnic-minorities-acronym [Accessed 8.5.2022].

2. Mental Health Foundation. Mental health statistics: Refugees and asylum seekers. [online] www.mentalhealth.org.uk/explor e-mental-health/statistics/refugees-asylum-seekers-statistics [Accessed 8.5.2022].

3. The Traveller Movement. The Traveller Movement – policy briefing addressing mental health and suicide among Gypsy, Roma and Traveller communities in England. England. [online] 2019. https:// wp-main.travellermovement.org.uk/wp-content/uploads/2021/08/Mental-Health -and-Suicide.pdf [Accessed 8.5.2022].

4. NHS. Mental health support if you're lesbian, gay, bisexual or trans (LGBTQ+). [online] July 2020. www.nhs.uk/mental-health/advice-for-life-situations-and-events/ mental-health-support-if-you-are-gay-lesbian-bisexual-lgbtq/ [Accessed 8.5.2022].

5. Institute of race relations. Health and mental health statistics. [online]. https://irr .org.uk/research/statistics/health/ [Accessed 8.5.2022].

6. Cabinet Office. Race Disparity Audit Summary Findings from the Ethnicity Facts and Figures. October 2017. [online] Revised March 2018. https://assets.publish ing.service.gov.uk/government/uploads/sy stem/uploads/attachment_data/file/68607 1/Revised_RDA_report_March_2018.pdf [Accessed 8.5.2022].

7. Mental Health Foundation. Black, Asian and minority ethnic (BAME) communities. [online] July 2021. www .mentalhealth.org.uk/a-to-z/b/black-asian-and-minority-ethnic-bame-communities [Accessed 8.5.2022].

8. Special Hospitals Service Authority. Report of the Committee of Inquiry into the death in Broadmoor Hospital of Orville Blackwood and a review of the deaths of two other Afro-Caribbean patients 'big, black and dangerous?', 1993.

9. Institute of Race Relations. Rocky Bennett – killed by institutional racism? [online] 2014. https://irr.org.uk/article/roc ky-bennett-killed-by-institutional-racism/ [Accessed 8.5.2022].

10. Blofeld, J., Sallah, D., Sashidharan, S. et al. Independent inquiry into the death of David Bennett. Cambridgeshire Strategic Health Authority. [online] 2003. http://im age.guardian.co.uk/sys-files/Society/docu ments/2004/02/12/Bennett.pdf [Accessed 8.5.2022].

11. Sainsbury Centre for Mental Health. Breaking the Circles of Fear: A review of the relationship between mental health services and African and Caribbean communities. [online] 2002. www .centreformentalhealth.org.uk/sites/defaul t/files/publication/download/breaking_th e_circles_of_fear.pdf [Accessed 8.5.2022].

12. Department of Health and Social Care. Modernising the Mental Health Act – final report from the independent review. Published December 2018. [online] Last updated 14 February 2019. www.gov.uk/g overnment/publications/modernising-the-

mental-health-act-final-report-from-the-independent-review [Accessed 8.5.2022].

13. National Collaborating Centre for Mental Health. Patient and Carer Race Equality Framework. [online 2018]. www .healthylondon.org/wp-content/uploads/2 021/05/nccmhpatientandcarerraceequality frameworknovember2018-1.pdf [Accessed 8.5.2022].

14. Haynes, L. Community care: How treatment of ethnic minority groups in mental health system can be improved following independent review. [online] 2019. www.communitycare.co.uk/2019/01/ 17/treatment-ethnic-minority-groups-mental-health-system-can-improved-review/ [Accessed 8.5.2022].

15. Kmietowicz, Z. NHS launches Race and Health Observatory after BMJ's call to end inequalities. *BMJ*, 2020;369:m2191. https:// doi.org/10.1136/bmj.m2191. PMID: 32482618.

16. British Medical Journal. Racism in medicine. [online 2020] www.bmj.com/ra cism-in-medicine [Accessed 7.5.2022].

17. NHS Race and Health Observatory. Ethnic Inequalities in Healthcare: A Rapid Evidence Review [online February 2022] www.nhsrho.org/publications/ethnic-inequalities-in-healthcare-a-rapid-evidence-review/ [Accessed 7.5.2022].

18. Smith, S. and Mohan, R. The NHS is not an island – tackling racial disparities in healthcare *BMJ* 2022; 377 :o944. https://doi .org/10.1136/bmj.o944.

19. Lola, J., The Black Lives Matter movement has reopened a psychological wound for black people and revealed unique challenges within mental health services. BBC. [online] August 2020. www.bbc.com /future/article/20200804-black-lives-matter-protests-race-mental-health-therapy [Accessed 8.5.2022].

20. Wolstenholme, R. The hidden victims of gaslighting. BBC. [online] November 2020. www.bbc.com/future/article/20201123-what-is-racial-gaslighting [Accessed 8.5.2022].

21. Dissanayaka, N. Centre for Mental Health. Racial disparity in mental health:

Challenging false narratives. [online] July 2020. www.centreformentalhealth.org.uk/r acial-disparity-mental-health-challenging-false-narratives [Accessed 8.5.2022].

22. Commission on Race and Ethnic Disparities. The report of the Commission on Race and Ethnic Disparities. The Commission's report into racial and ethnic disparities in the UK. March 2021. [Online] Updated April 2021. www.gov.uk/govern ment/publications/the-report-of-the-commission-on-race-and-ethnic-disparities [Accessed 8.5.2022].

23. Iacobucci, G. What did the Commission on Race and Ethnic Disparities say on health? *BMJ* 2021; 373: n943. https://doi.org/10 .1136/bmj.n943.

24. Marmot, M. and Wilkinson, R. G. *Social Determinants of Health*. 2nd ed. Oxford: Oxford University Press.

25. The Health Foundation. Health Equity in England: The Marmot Review 10 Years on. February 2020. www.health.org.uk/publica tions/reports/the-marmot-review-10-years-on [Accessed 8.5.2022].

26. MIND. Existing inequalities have made mental health of BAME groups worse during pandemic, says MIND. [online] July 2020. www.mind.org.uk/news-campaigns/news/ex isting-inequalities-have-made-mental-health -of-bame-groups-worse-during-pandemic-says-mind/ [Accessed 8.5.2022].

27. Bignall, T., Jeraj, S., Helsby, E. and Butt, J. Racial disparities in mental health: Literature and evidence review. [online 2019] https://raceequalityfoundation .org.uk/wp-content/uploads/2020/03/men tal-health-report-v5-2.pdf [Accessed 7.5.2022].

28. Barnett, P., Mackay, E., Matthews, H. et al. Ethnic variations in compulsory detention under the Mental Health Act: A systematic review and meta-analysis of international data. *Lancet Psychiatry* 2019 Apr;6(4):305– 17. https://doi.org/10.1016/S2215-0366 (19)30027-6. Epub 2019 Mar 4. PMID: 30846354; PMCID: PMC6494977.

29. RCPsych. Task and Finish group. Ending racial inequalities exposed by the COVID-19 pandemic for mental health staff.

[online] July 2020. www.rcpsych.ac.uk/do cs/default-source/about-us/covid-19/reco mmendations_-ending-racial-inequalities-exposed-by-covid-19-for-mh-staff_t-f-group_220720_final.pdf?sfvrsn=ecd0ef_2 [Accessed 8.5.2022].

30. RCPsych. Written evidence submitted by the Royal College of Psychiatrists (MRS0475). [online]. 2020. https://com mittees.parliament.uk/writtenevidence/48 94/pdf/ [Accessed 7.5.2022].

31. NHS England. Advancing mental health equalities strategy. [online]. 2020. www .england.nhs.uk/publication/advancing-mental-health-equalities-strategy/ [Accessed 8.5.2022].

32. RCPsych. Equality Action Plan 2021-23. [online]. 2021. www.rcpsych.ac.uk/docs/d efault-source/about-us/equality-diversity-and-inclusivity/equality-action-plan--january-2021.pdf [Accessed 17.10.2022].

33. RCPsych. Advancing Mental Health Equality Improvement Collaborative. [online]. 2020. www.rcpsych.ac.uk/about-us/equality-diversity-and-inclusion/advan cing-mental-health-equality-collaborative# [Accessed 7.5.2022].

34. NICE. Innovative ways of engaging with Black and Minority Ethnic (BME) communities to improve access to psychological therapies. [online]. December 2017. www.nice.org.uk/sharedlearning/inn ovative-ways-of-engaging-with-black-and-minority-ethnic-bme-communities-to-improve-access-to-psychological-therapies [Accessed 8.5.2022].

35. Taraki Wellbeing. Home page. www .taraki.co.uk/about [Accessed 8.5.2022].

36. Angiolini, E. Report of the Independent Review of Deaths and Serious Incidents in Police Custody [online]. 2017; https://ass ets.publishing.service.gov.uk/govern ment/uploads/system/uploads/attach ment_data/file/655401/Report_of_Angiol ini_Review_ISBN_Accessible.pdf [Accessed 8.5.2022].

37. Vox. Study: People see Black men as larger and more threatening than similarly sized white men [online] 2017. www.vox.com/i

dentities/2017/3/17/14945576/Black-white -bodies-size-threat-study [Accessed 8.5.2022].

38. Trawalter, S., Todd, A. R., Baird, A. A., Richeson, J. A. Attending to threat: Race-based patterns of selective attention. *Journal of Experimental Social Psychology* 2008 Sep;44(5):1322–7. https://doi.org/10 .1016/j.jesp.2008.03.006. PMID: 19727428; PMCID: PMC2633407.

39. Wilson, J. P., Hugenberg, K., Rule, N. O. Racial bias in judgments of physical size and formidability: From size to threat. *Journal of Personality and Social Psychology* 2017 Jul;113(1):59–80. https://doi.org/10 .1037/pspi0000092. Epub 2017 Mar 13. PMID: 28287752.

40. Gov.uk. Population of England and Wales. 2018. [online] Last updated August 2020. www.ethnicity-facts-figures.service.gov.uk /uk-population-by-ethnicity/national-and-regional-populations/population-of-england-and-wales/latest [Accessed 8.5.2022].

41. Home Office. Police use of force statistics, England and Wales: April 2019 to March 2020. https://assets .publishing.service.gov.uk/government/uplo ads/system/uploads/attachment_data/file/94 5435/police-use-of-force-apr2019-mar2020-hosb3720.pdf [Accessed 8.5.2022].

42. Home Office. Police Use of Force Statistics. 2018 [online] Last updated December 2020. www.gov.uk/government/collec tions/police-use-of-force-statistics [Accessed 8.5.2022].

43. Baskind, E. 'I Can't Breathe: Black and Dead in Custody', BBC Panorama, commenting on the death of Kevin Clarke, an acutely-unwell Black man who was restrained by up to nine Metropolitan Police Service officers. [online] 2021 www .bbc.co.uk/programmes/m000r6z2 [Accessed 8.5.2022].

44. Care Quality Commission. Out of sight – who cares?: Restraint, segregation and seclusion review. [online] 2020. Available from www.cqc.org.uk/publications/themed-work/rssreview [Accessed 19.09.2021].

Introduction to Section 5

Section 5: Violence and Society

This section is concerned with the highly important subject of the interaction of violence with society as a whole. If we can improve the outcomes of children involved in violence, have good ways of linking programmes of treatment with societal understanding and can overcome the pain and anger of victims who have been exposed to violence, we will have moved a long way.

The evidence that those with mental illness are much more likely to be victims of violence than its perpetrators is repeated several times in this book, and we make no apology for this; it needs to be repeated over and over again until society understands.

Professionals working in health, social care and the justice system require a robust understanding of when to share confidential information; the information-sharing chapter (Chapter 18) has been expanded from the first edition and provides information on legislation and guidance to be considered when sharing information about patients and information sharing by organisations supporting victims of crimes committed by mentally disordered offenders. The chapter includes discussion of the new Victims' Code and of liaison with victims.

The notion of home as a place of calm and quiet support is a chimera for so many people, and for too long we have ignored the impact of violence in all its forms in this setting. Domestic violence is mentioned in several chapters, most notably the safeguarding chapter (3) in Section 1 and the community chapter (9) in Section 3. The final chapter in this section, on the victims of violence, also gives special attention to the problem of domestic violence and provides a wealth of information on the support and interventions available.

Chapter 7

Criminal and Youth Justice Liaison and Diversion Systems

Bradley Hillier and Heidi Hales

Introduction

It has been shown many times in this book that the relationship between mental disorder and violence is complex, dynamic and many-layered. But in this context there is a clear over-representation of those with severe mental illness (SMI) interacting with the criminal justice system (CJS) [1]; it is estimated that up to 5% (1 in 20) violent offences are committed by those with SMI [2]. Consequently, those who work with people with SMI are likely at some stage to find themselves interacting with different authorities and receiving requests to share information to inform the justice process (before, during and after arrest). They will also be expected to facilitate multi-agency risk management structures in the community. In the last 15 years there has been significant policy and service development in the way the CJS and associated agencies work with mentally disordered offenders (MDOs). This has taken place against the background of an existing legal framework already designed to take mental health factors into account.

In this chapter we review the development of policy and practice in England and Wales (E&W) concerning MDOs and their needs, followed by consideration of the pathway of an individual with SMI as they encounter the various levels of the CJS: from the police to the courts through to sentencing and disposal. We will also consider the particular differences that pertain when the individual is a child or young person (CYP), and broader fora wherein information sharing occurs for the purpose of public protection in the community context.

The Policy Background

In 1992, the British government published *The Health of the Nation: A Strategy for Health in England* [3], setting out improvements in five strategic areas, including mental health. This report required health authorities to include MDOs in their plans, and an associated report focusing specifically on MDOs [4] espoused principles which were groundbreaking at the time; namely, that MDOs should receive care provided by health and social care services (as opposed to the CJS), according to individual need, as close to home as possible, in the community where possible, and in conditions of no greater security than necessary. In short, their access to health and care should not in any way be forfeited as a consequence of violence being part of their illness. This required an expansion of healthcare in the community and secure settings, across forensic and non-forensic services and organisational boundaries. It led to the provision of care in prisons (and Immigration Removal Centres [IRCs]) being commissioned by NHS England and assessed by national quality standards. Alongside this was an increase in the number of medium secure services, as recommended by the Butler Report [5], with specifications later formalised [6] and a concomitant expansion of lower-security, 'step-down' services. Community forensic services developed later to provide a complete forensic 'pathway'. At the time of writing, specialist community forensic teams (SCFTs) are being developed across England [7] in what is likely to be a national specification for community forensic services in due course.

One of the most important pieces of policy guiding the current landscape and framework of the interaction of MDOs within the CJS has been the Bradley Report [8], which emphasises Liaison and Diversion (L&D) services, aiming to identify MDOs at an early stage in the CJS process and considering alternatives to this where possible; as of March 2020 there was 100% coverage, with NHS-commissioned services in police stations and courts [9]. Furthermore, time frames were described for the transfer to hospital of sentenced and remand prisoners suffering from acute mental illness. The recommendations of this report remain the current gold standard.

The Crisis Care Concordat [10] is an important agreement focusing on the role of multiple services to prioritise the mental health needs of individuals interacting with statutory services and other agencies, which continues to guide service provision.

Liaison and Diversion Services

L&D services describe the process whereby people of all ages are screened and assessed for mental health problems, intellectual disability, substance misuse and other issues as early as possible in their contact with the CJS in England. Information gained from these assessments (which include liaison with other services) can be used to arrange for mental health treatment if needed or to offer advice to the police or court. This does not necessarily mean that an MDO will *not* experience any criminal sanctions for their behaviour, but rather that mental health factors can be taken into consideration to inform the pathway. This may lead to an alternative to the CJS (e.g. hospital admission and 'no further action' [NFA]), or may allow medico-legal aspects to be scrutinised (e.g. assessment of fitness to plead and any special measures needed). This ensures that the MDO receives a fair assessment of all aspects of their problem. It can also allow factors to be taken into consideration for sentencing.

We now consider the different interfaces in which an MDO interacts with the CJS and the ways in which mental health factors can be taken into consideration. It is important to note that L&D services themselves are often integrated within police custody and court settings.

Police Street and Custody Liaison and Diversion

In 2008, up to 15% of police incidents were thought to involve people with mental health problems [11]. In 2019, research carried out by the BBC [12] identified that, between 2014 and 2018, there had been an approximate 28% increase in 'mental health incidents', rising from 385,206 to 494,159.

Mental health services have developed more formal health-based places of safety (HBPoS), using A&E departments as places of safety in preference to police cells. The Mental Health Act 1983 (amended 2007) (MHA) [13] provides powers under Sections 135 and 136 to convey an individual with suspected mental disorder to a HBPoS for assessment as an alternative to arrest, with a view to considering admission to hospital. However, if the offence is serious, this may not be appropriate, or mental health factors may not be easily identifiable at arrest. The mental health alternatives to arrest may include signposting to these services and/or alerting the Multi-Agency Safeguarding Hub (MASH) who can inform mental health services of individuals who have had police contact and who they consider may have mental health problems.

In 2013, a Street Triage pilot initiated a trial of mental health practitioners going out with police; the evaluation [14] found that this did reduce the use of Section 136 detentions, and it led to a broader roll-out of this model. The Bradley Report noted that police stations can be a crucial place for early identification of MDOs. Since the Bradley Report, there has been significant development of police custody-based L&D services, often consisting of a psychiatric nurse or similar healthcare practitioner. Prior to this, the forensic medical examiner (FME) service, commissioned by the police service, was often the only form of custody-based health practitioner. The provision of on-site mental health specialism allows access to screening and assessment by mental health professionals at the early stages of the CJS process, and for these professionals to advise the police on mental health alternatives that may be available to them. These include detention under the MHA civil sections, with police being able to make a charging decision at a later stage when an individual has received treatment. Similarly, information obtained from health services at this early stage can inform the ongoing CJS process, such as whether an individual is fit to be interviewed.

If an individual reports or is identified as having mental health problems and/or being 'mentally vulnerable', and if the alleged offence is serious enough to warrant further investigation and interview, the Police and Criminal Evidence Act 1984 (PACE) [15] becomes relevant. If the individual is deemed fit to be interviewed, the formal requirement is for an appropriate adult (AA) to be present in addition to any legal representation. A particular area of concern identified in the Bradley Report was the availability of appropriate adults when this need was identified, and this was further emphasised by McKinnon and colleagues [16]. From a legal perspective, lack of this safeguard can lead to miscarriage of justice, unsound verdict and failed prosecution. Since that time, although L&D practitioners in police stations can raise awareness of this need, there remain ongoing concerns that the use of appropriate adults is still low [17].

These 'all age' L&D services based in police custody can be very busy. Efficient services rely on good working relationships with the police custody officers, local mental health services and the local approved mental health practitioner (AMHP) service. Priority is given to those who are acutely unwell. Arranging a private but safe place to assess a person, building up a therapeutic rapport in a police station and then liaising with local services to arrange a MHA assessment and possible admission can be a complex process. This is most difficult when the person is not local and so there are no easy routes to hospital admission. Every effort should also be made to review those of reduced mental capacity, for example those with intellectual difficulties, so that any additional support can be offered if needed.

Youth Justice Liaison and Diversion

Liaison and diversion services cover all ages. There is a requirement that all young people under 18 who are arrested have a mental health screen. This requirement is interpreted differently across the country. In some areas this is a paper screen, noting any current or past Child and Adolescent Mental Health Service (CAMHS) contact and details of current clinicians. This is helpful in assessment and can lead to additional sessions or offering appointment reviews to those previously known to CAMHS but now closed.

In London, L&D services are commissioned to complete a face-to-face screen for all children who are arrested or involved with youth offending services (YOS). Each London borough has a youth justice liaison and diversion (YJLD) worker, located in the youth offending team (YOT) but supervised by health, to complete these screens and follow up on referrals. The L&D clinicians in police custody can complete the screen if available and hand the information on to the YJLD worker, or the YJLD worker can be called in. However, many young people are 'street arrested' and not taken to police custody, and police are asked to 'process' those taken to custody as quickly as possible. There is often insufficient time to complete a screen. The screen can be completed later for those receiving YOT triage or a community resolution, as it is permissible for this to be done whilst the young person is engaging with the YOT team. It can also be completed for those remanded into custody. There is a more detailed assessment (comprehensive health assessment tool [CHAT]) on arriving in custody. However, some may be missed, including young people released under investigation (RUI), who may be at risk as they are often being investigated for serious offences which require time to collect evidence. Similarly, those who are released with no further action may be vulnerable to further risk behaviours if their needs are not identified and met. See Figure 17.1 for an overview of this process in London.

Consent for contact and information sharing is complex. Parents may not want contact with health services linked to a police arrest or for the GP to be informed of the arrest. Difficulties can also arise when a decision to refer to community services for further support

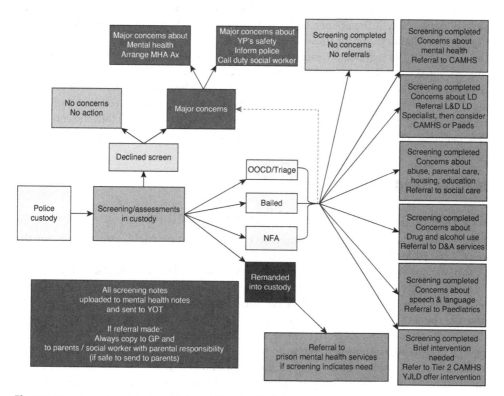

Figure 17.1 London Youth Justice Liaison and Diversion flow chart

is made. Because of long wait lists and high threshold criteria in many community services, there can be long delays before acceptance. The strength of screening programmes lies in the availability of early intervention services for those who qualify.

Court Liaison and Diversion

Court L&D services were the original L&D services, developed organically in various areas across the United Kingdom by innovative clinicians, managers and commissioners. Now more formalised within the 'all age L&D services' in England, these teams usually consist of a (forensic) psychiatrist and psychiatric nurse as a minimum, with more well-developed services including specialist practitioners in intellectual disability and neurodevelopmental disorders, using an agreed national template which has been produced in conjunction with the senior judiciary.

Originally it was thought that having L&D services in police custody suites would remove the need for court L&D services. However, there are still several roles, specific to L&D teams, in court. As police custody L&D services are not all available on a 24-hour basis, those arrested at night are not seen until the next morning. For those being taken to court, the assessment is better completed in court cells.

Court L&D teams are available to the judiciary and legal representatives to consider specific mental health issues that arise in court, such as fitness to participate, to plead and to stand trial. For those returning to court whilst on remand in prison, assessment and diversion to hospital from court may be quicker than referral pathways from prison and may be possible through a civil section of the MHA, avoiding criminalising the unwell person, particularly if the offence is not serious. Court L&D teams in courts that manage high-profile offenders and/or those attending for long trials are available. These can assess the mental state of defendants and support them at times of high stress during the legal process. Finally, L&D services in court may be best placed to assist in the identification of psychiatric experts required to inform the legal process. They can also liaise with appropriate services over the individual's mental health, and are particularly relevant to hospital teams when a mental health disposal is under consideration. Box 17.1 details the competencies expected of L&D practitioners in Crown Court as per the current L&D Service Specification [18].

Mental Health Powers of the Court

Assessment and Disposal to a Mental Health Setting

Both police and court L&D teams undertake and co-ordinate MHA assessments; for the court L&D teams this is mainly at magistrates level.

Mental health diversion and disposal powers are available to the court in E&W and can be used to further inform the legal process, including diversion to the mental health system. The courts have powers to remand defendants to hospital for reports (Section 35 MHA), and assessment (Section 36 MHA – Crown Court only) in order to inform the legal process. These are infrequently used. The law is complex regarding other legal tests which have mental health implications (e.g. fitness to plead, trial of the facts, diminished responsibility and the insanity defence) and is beyond the scope of this chapter. To summarise, in E&W, the Pritchard Criteria (*R* v. Pritchard, 1836) [19] are used to assess whether an individual is fit to plead and the M'Naghten Rules (Daniel M'Naghten's case, 1845) [20] define the

---

Box 17.1 Competencies required of Crown Court Liaison and Diversion Practitioners

- A good working knowledge of the Mental Health Act 1983 (amended 2007) and especially Part III. (Part III of the 1983 Mental Health Act (amended 2007) covers patients concerned with criminal proceedings.) With mental health law arising comparatively rarely in barristers' experience, they may value assistance from the L&Ds navigating mental health pathways.
- A good working knowledge of the Criminal Procedures and Insanity legislation governing unfitness to plead, insanity and alternative disposals.
- A good working knowledge of risk analysis, to advise the court whether pre-sentence psychiatric reports should explicitly address risk.
- Knowledge of potential special experts in forensic psychology and forensic psychiatry, to understand whether experts are available at short notice or have additional areas of expertise (e.g. neuro-psychiatry, neuro-psychology, etc.).
- An understanding of responsibility for assessments and reports on defendants aged below 18. A need to be aware of referral mechanisms, and of who may act as special experts and under what conditions.
- Knowledge of the role and function of court-appointed intermediaries.
- An understanding of referral pathways into local secure units, and relevant high secure services (names, mobile and landline numbers and email addresses). These are to facilitate liaison and develop formal relationships and partnerships. It is important to know how long units take to conduct assessments and achieve transfers from prison.
- A good working knowledge of available general adult mental health services, substance misuse services, learning disability services, CAMHS, transition and old age psychiatry.
- An understanding of the role of the National Offender Management Service Public Protection & Mental Health Group.
- Where the Crown Court has a catchment area wider than that of the provider of the L&D service, the ability to establish formal links with all L&D services whose police stations and magistrates' courts feed into that Crown Court.
- An understanding of what services the prison mental health services and primary care services provide.
- The ability to establish strong working relationships with agencies and services working within Crown Court settings.

(*Source*: NHS England, 2019 [18])

---

criteria to assess whether a defendant is legally 'insane'. If the accused is found to fulfil either of these criteria and have perpetrated the act, they cannot be sent to prison but can receive an absolute discharge, supervision order or hospital order with or without a restriction order.

In terms of 'disposal', the court has powers to 'dispose' of criminal proceedings in a guilty plea/verdict under Section 37 of the MHA (a hospital order), which may include a restriction order under Section 41 of the MHA in cases of the most serious violence sentenced at the Crown Court. The Crown Court also has powers to impose a Section 38 MHA interim hospital order, allowing for a period of assessment of a convicted offender for up to one year in consideration of suitability for a hospital order (with or without restrictions). Finally, for those over 21 years of age, the court may consider a S45A (hybrid order) at the time of sentencing, particularly if the offence is serious and may otherwise attract a hospital order with restrictions or a lengthy custodial sentence; these are controversial and an ongoing source of legal scrutiny. Courts are also able to make community mental health disposals, which will be considered later in the chapter. Table 17.1 shows the changing use of hospital and hybrid orders over time.

Mental Health Factors in Criminal Justice System Sentencing Outcomes

In 2020, the Sentencing Council published new guidelines to take mental health factors into account on sentencing, which came into force on 1 October 2020 [21]. Of particular relevance from the perspective of L&D services, sentencers are advised to take note of the general principles in Box 17.2 pertaining to mental health factors in sentencing.

It is now a requirement that 'where the offender is or appears to be mentally disordered at the date of sentencing, the court must obtain and consider a medical report before passing a custodial sentence other than one fixed by law, unless, in the circumstances of the case, the court is of the opinion that it is unnecessary' [21]. Sentencers are required to assess culpability on the grounds of any mental health condition concomitantly with expert reports (if requested), together with any offence-specific guidelines, and form an overall assessment to support their sentencing decision.

Table 17.1 Use of hospital and hybrid orders on sentencing

	2010	2019
Section 37, hospital order	540	260
Section 37/41, hospital order with restrictions	360	25
Section 45A, hybrid order	5	30

Box 17.2 General principles for mental health factor consideration in sentencing

- Some mental disorders can fluctuate and an offender's state during proceedings may not be representative of their condition at the time the offence was committed.
- Care should be taken to avoid making assumptions. Many mental disorders, neurological impairments or developmental disorders are not easily recognisable.
- No adverse inference should necessarily be drawn if an offender had not previously either been formally diagnosed or willing to disclose an impairment or disorder.
- Offenders may be unaware or unwilling to accept they have an impairment or disorder and may fear stigmatisation if they disclose it.
- It is not uncommon for people to have a number of different impairments and disorders. This is known as 'comorbidity'.
- Drug and/or alcohol dependence can be a factor, and may mask an underlying disorder.
- Difficulties of definition and classification in this field are common. There may be differences of expert opinion and diagnosis in relation to the offender, or it may be that no specific disorder can be identified.
- A formal diagnosis is not always required.
- Where a formal diagnosis is required, a report by a suitably qualified expert will be necessary.

Disposal to the Community

The courts have broad powers to use, with the consent of the offender, various therapeutic community orders in the disposal of MDOs; these rehabilitation activity requirements (RARs) introduced by the Offender Rehabilitation Act 2014 [22] include mental health treatment requirements (MHTRs), drug rehabilitation requirements (DRRs) and alcohol treatment requirements (ATR), as well as potential rehabilitation activities which may be offence-specific (e.g. sexual offence work). These therapeutic orders are regarded as being appropriate for those who do not meet a threshold for MHA detention, but for whom a component of their offending behaviour could be responsive to intervention. In these circumstances, the order could be paired with an element of punishment/supervision. Although, according to the Criminal Justice Statistics Annual Report (2019) [23], the use of community sentences has declined over the last ten years from approximately 35% of all disposals to around 22% in 2019, the new sentencing guidelines may lead to a re-invigoration of courts' willingness to consider treatment-type disposals. However, research has shown that there is little enthusiasm on the part of community mental health services to take up a partnership role with the CJS for supervision and treatment of eligible MDOs [24, 25], at least in part because of concerns about how to progress in the circumstances of a 'breach' [24].

Despite this, there is evidence that including a mental health treatment requirement and alcohol treatment requirement in a community order or suspended sentence order can have a significant and positive impact on reducing reoffending [26]. Specifically, a recent editorial in the British Journal of Psychiatry [27] and a Royal College of Psychiatrists (RCPsych) Position Statement [28] made a strong argument for the evidence, practical use and potential future policy direction of service development to link the criminal justice and mental health components, particularly in less serious offending behaviour to MHTR disposals. Future progress on this is likely, particularly in the light of non-forensic community services that would be likely to receive the majority of such individuals. These services are currently being transformed to achieve closer alignment with primary care networks (PCNs), with caseload durations being reduced to as necessary to provide interventions. Arguably, a MHTR would be one such intervention that would justify longer-term care management on a team, potentially with consultative support from any community forensic team (or similar) operating in the same locality.

Diversion from Prison

Violence and mental disorder within the prison estate amongst remanded and convicted prisoners have been well studied and are discussed elsewhere in this book (Chapter 12). There are now NHS-commissioned mental health in-reach services in all prison establishments in E&W. Such services are required to provide mental health assessment and treatment in line with the Care Programme Approach (CPA) equivalent to services available in the community. However, under certain circumstances it is not safe, feasible or appropriate to provide such care in prison, and transfer under the MHA can take place to a hospital setting at the appropriate level of security, authorised by the Ministry of Justice (MoJ). Section 47 of the MHA is used in the case of a sentenced prisoner and Section 48 of the MHA when the prisoner is unsentenced. The Bradley Report identified unacceptable delays in transfers of prisoners to hospital and mandated a timeframe of 14 days. Despite this, there are still significant delays [29].

Treatment and Risk Management in the Community

MDOs who have been subject to hospital orders and other forms of diversion from custody are likely to be discharged to the care of community mental health services. At present, there exist in E&W several models of community forensic service, having different eligibility criteria, although most commonly they require MDOs to have been in a secure psychiatric setting, and may also be require them to remain under a 'forensic' section of the MHA or under CPA. Another important consideration is whether any risk of violence is associated with mental disorder. Such services are variably called community forensic teams or forensic outreach and liaison services and, as of 2020, include the development of SCFTs. This is an area of ongoing service development, but the thrust of these services is to facilitate the safe discharge of patients from secure services, with knowledge of the legal frameworks surrounding them, and familiarity with specialist risk assessment and management in the community. This includes liaison with other agencies (e.g. MAPPA; see section 'Multi-Agency Public Protection Arrangements') who may also be involved in the care/supervision of such individuals.

An important aspect of community forensic work involves the clinical and social supervision of restricted patients (i.e. those who have been 'conditionally discharged' to the community under Section 42 of the MHA from a Section 37/41 restricted hospital order). In practical terms, the supervision of these patients requires continuing assessment and treatment in conjunction with listed specified conditions agreed at the point of discharge. The presence of restriction means that the MoJ remains involved in the oversight of the individual, and a conditional discharge report (CDR) is sent to them within the first month in the community, and subsequently on a quarterly basis. This report covers multiple areas of the individual's mental health, compliance with conditions and treatment, and other social and risk-related details [30]. Breach of these conditions (e.g. non-compliance with medication, or use of illicit substances, for example) can lead to a recall to hospital, although in practical terms it is also important to consider whether there has been an increase in risk and mental state instability, as well as what additional support structures could be put into place to manage the identified issues.

Community Forensic CAMHS

Community forensic CAMHS (F-CAMHS) services are mentioned elsewhere in this book (Chapter 13). Their role is different from that of forensic community services for adult MDOs. The national service model in England is mainly one of consultation, though assessment and joint intervention can be offered, and the main aim is one of early intervention to avoid placement in a secure setting for the young person.

Community Information-Sharing and Risk Management Structure

The vast majority of offenders in the community are managed by the Probation Service and/or the CJS. However, there are two statutory structures which exist outside the mental health system but which professionals may often be asked to attend and/or contribute to for the purpose of managing individuals with specified risks in the community. This particularly applies when a mental health component has been identified or the individual is known to mental health services; these are the multi-agency public protection arrangements

(MAPPA) and the Channel Panel (counter-terrorism safeguarding strategy). The relationship between such bodies and mental health professionals is not straightforward, since there can be conflicting ethical frameworks between the participants (e.g. CJS and health and social care), for which individuals should seek advice from their employing organisation and professional bodies concerning their obligations to share information.

Information sharing regarding children and young people with risk behaviours is very important as lack of information sharing has been highlighted as contributing to previous serious incidents. It is therefore recommended that there is very close cooperation between all agencies working with young people.

Multi-Agency Public Protection Arrangements

In E&W, the MAPPA were created following the Criminal Justice and Court Services Act 2000 [31], mandating police, prison and probation services to co-operate in the identification and management of offenders whose behaviour is considered to pose significant risk of harm to the public [32]. This development took place against the background of various serious incidents and enquiries before and during the 1990s, where the lack of information sharing about high risk individuals was identified as being a significant contributory factor.

Offenders are 'graded' to determine the level of monitoring and resource allocation provided (see Box 17.3).

At MAPPA meetings, there is always a representative from the relevant mental health organisation, often a forensic psychiatrist or other forensic practitioner. In 2003 the 'duty to co-operate' for health and social care services was introduced by the Criminal Justice Act 2003 [33]. From the perspective of healthcare organisations, professionals and, in particular, psychiatrists, the 'duty to co-operate' and disclosure presents a significant challenge, often hindered by the lack of clear guidelines which take into account the duty of confidentiality clinicians owe to their patients (see Taylor and Yakeley for a comprehensive discussion [34]). Nonetheless, the principle of information sharing on a 'need to know' basis in the public interest for the prevention of serious harm or abuse remains an overarching principle, to be applied on a case-by-case basis, and mental health services benefit from

---

Box 17.3 MAPPA offender management categories and levels

Categories

1. Registered sex offenders
2. Violent and other sex offenders
3. Other offenders considered to pose a risk of serious harm to the public

Levels

1. Ordinary management (low/medium risk being managed by one lead agency)
2. Local inter-agency risk management (active involvement of more than one agency, coordinated at monthly multi-agency meetings)
3. Multi-agency public protection panels [MAPPP] (serious risk and/or requiring complex risk management; monthly level 2 meeting discussion and individual basis at emergency level 3 meetings).

knowledge arising from other organisations in the risk management of high-risk offenders. All healthcare organisations should have clear policies and guidelines that define the relationship with MAPPA.

Prevent and the Channel Process

The Prevent Strategy [35] is a part of the UK government's counter-terrorism strategy, aiming to stop people becoming terrorists or supporting terrorism. In 2007 the Channel process was piloted to provide support to people who were identified as being vulnerable to being drawn into terrorism using a safeguarding framework. The Counter Terrorism and Security Act 2015 [36] places a duty of statutory authorities in health and social care to work as partners to co-operate within a safeguarding framework for vulnerable individuals who may be at risk of radicalisation. The panel is chaired by the local authority and consists of standing representatives of the police counter-terrorism unit for the local area, adult social care, children's services and health.

Channel [37] uses a 'Vulnerability Assessment Framework' consisting of three dimensions: engagement with a group, intent to cause harm and capability to cause harm. When an individual is identified and assessed, Channel is able to approach identified individuals through its partners and seek their consent to engage in the process. Wrap-around interventions can be offered, which may include mentoring support, life-skills development, family support, health awareness contact and substance use interventions. If there is a need for theological or ideological support, Home Office–approved intervention providers are used for the mentoring process, with the aim to increase theological understanding and challenge extremist ideas.

Practitioners may be invited to attend if they have referred, or have a patient under their care, who is known to the process, or a referral from Channel may be received if mental health needs have already been identified. There should be a similar policy from the healthcare organisation defining the relationship with Channel as with MAPPA. Patient consent to share information should be sought in the first instance, but if this is not given it remains the judgement of the individual practitioner as to whether it is appropriate to break medical confidentiality. This decision has to be made in the public interest in the context of preventing serious violence. This is an area of significant controversy with regard to the role of psychiatrists, and the RCPsych has provided a position statement which may be of use in navigating this complex area [38].

National Referral Mechanism

The National Referral Mechanism (NRM) [39] is used when there are concerns about modern human slavery, including criminal and sexual exploitation, for adults and children. Those thought to be at risk of human trafficking and slavery can only be referred into the NRM by social care and the police. If accepted, services are required to offer a multi-agency care plan. For young people, this is often already provided through contextual safeguarding processes; for adults, this places a requirement upon local services.

There has been a change in language about the vulnerability and victimisation of young people in recent years and it is now better understood. Whilst previously those soliciting sexual favours or involved with gangs dealing drugs were criminalised (with the gangs matrix focusing on risk of violence), they are now understood to have been exploited and described as being at risk of (child) sexual exploitation and/or (child) criminal exploitation.

Those at risk of (child) criminal exploitation and on the NRM can still be arrested, charged and convicted of offences, but courts are requested to take these mitigating factors into account.

Conclusion

Over the last decade there have been significant developments in the way in which younger individuals and adults with mental health problems are both regarded by and interact with the CJS, including a dramatic increase in the presence of mental health specialists at the various interfaces with (potential) MDOs, and inter-agency cooperation, sometimes controversially so. Underpinning these developments has been the concept of ensuring that relevant information is available to the CJS about MDOs, in order to ensure their pathway and risks can be identified as early as possible, with a view to improving health outcomes. There remains a need for further development of inter-agency working, particularly in the community with regards to lower-risk offenders, as well as the use of community disposals with mental health and substance use conditions.

References

1. Mullen, P., Burgess, P. Wallace, C., Palmer, S. and Rusctiena, D. Community care and criminal offending in schizophrenia, *The Lancet* 2000; 355:614–17. https://doi.org/10.1016/S0140-6736(05)73088-9

2. Fazel, S. and Grann, M. The population impact of severe mental illness on violent crime. *American Journal of Psychiatry* 2006; 163(8):1397–1403. Available at https://ajp.psychiatryonline.org/doi/full/10.1176/ajp.2006.163.8.1397 [Accessed 28.4.2022].

3. Department of Health. *The Health of the Nation: A Strategy for Health in England.* London: HMSO, 1992.

4. Department of Health and Home Office. *Review of Health and Social Services for Mentally Disordered Offenders and Others Requiring Similar Services.* London: HMSO, 1992.

5. Home Office and Department of Health and Social Care. *Report of the Committee on Mentally Abnormal Offenders* (Butler Report) Cmnd 6244. London: HMSO, 1975.

6. Department of Health. *Best Practice Guidance: Specifications for Adult Medium Secure Services.* London: HMSO, 2007.

7. NHS England. *Developing the 'Forensic Mental Health Community Service' Model.* London: NHS England, 2018.

8. Department of Health. The Bradley Report. London: HMSO, 2009. https://webarchive.nationalarchives.gov.uk/20130105193845/http://www.dh.gov.uk/prod_consum_dh/groups/dh_digitalassets/documents/digitalasset/dh_098698.pdf [Accessed 28.4.2022].

9. NHS England. Webpage: About Liaison and Diversion. 2020. www.england.nhs.uk/commissioning/health-just/liaison-and-diversion/about/ [Accessed 28.4.2022].

10. Department of Health. *The Crisis Care Concordat. Online: The Crisis Care Concordat.* 2014. www.crisiscareconcordat.org.uk/about/#the-concordat [Accessed 28.4.2022].

11. Sainsbury Centre for Mental Health. Briefing 36: The Police and Mental Health. London: The Sainsbury Centre for Mental Health. 2008. www.centreformentalhealth.org.uk/sites/default/files/2018-09/SainsburyCentre_briefing36_police_final_small.pdf [Accessed 28.4.2022].

12. Jones, L. Police dealing with more 'mental health incidents'. London: BBC Online, 2019. www.bbc.co.uk/news/uk-49317060 [Accessed 28.4.2022].

13. HM Government. The Mental Health Act 1983 (as amended 2007). London: TSO. www.legislation.gov.uk/ukpga/1983/20/contents [Accessed 28.4.2022]

14. Keown, P., French, J., Gibson, G. et al (2016). Too much detention? Street triage and detentions under Section 136 Mental Health Act in the north-east of England: A descriptive study of the effects of a street triage intervention. *BMJ Open*, 2016; 6: e011837. https://doi.org/10.1136/bmjo pen-2016-011837. https://bmjopen .bmj.com/content/bmjopen/6/11/e011837 .full.pdf [Accessed 28.4.2022].

15. HM Government. The Police and Criminal Evidence Act 1984. London: TSO. www .legislation.gov.uk/ukpga/1984/60/con tents [Accessed 28.4.2022].

16. McKinnon, I., Srivastava, S., Kaler, G. and Grubin, D. Screening for psychiatric morbidity in police custody: Results from the HELP-PC project. *The Psychiatrist* 2013 37(12):389–94. https://doi.org/10.1192/pb .bp.112.041608 [Accessed 28.4.2022].

17. National Appropriate Adult Network. *There to Help 3*. Online: NAAN 2020. https://appr opriateadult.org.uk/policy/research/thereto help3 [Accessed 28.4.2022].

18. NHS England. Liaison and Diversion Standard Service Specifications. London: NHS England. 2019. www.england.nhs.uk/ wp-content/uploads/2019/12/national- liaison-and-diversion-service-specification- 2019.pdf [Accessed 28.4.2022].

19. *R v. Pritchard* (1836) 7 Car & P 303, 7 Car and P 304, 173 ER 135, [1836] EWHC KB 1, 7 Car & P 303. www.bailii.org/ew/cases/E WHC/KB/1836/1.html [Accessed 28.4.2022].

20. Daniel M'Naghten's Case [1843] UKHL J16, 8 ER 718. www.bailii.org/uk/cases/UK HL/1843/J16.html [Accessed 28.4.2022].

21. Sentencing Council. *Sentencing offenders with mental disorders, developmental disorders, or neurological impairments*. London: Sentencing Council 2020. www .sentencingcouncil.org.uk/overarching- guides/magistrates-court/item/sentencing- offenders-with-mental-disorders- developmental-disorders-or-neurological- impairments/ [Accessed 28.4.2022].

22. HM Government. The Offender Rehabilitation Act 2014. London: TSO. www.legislation.gov.uk/ukpga/2014/11/co ntents [Accessed 28.4.2022].

23. Ministry of Justice. Criminal Justice Statistics Annual Report December 2019. London: Ministry of Justice. 2020. https:// assets.publishing.service.gov.uk/govern ment/uploads/system/uploads/attach ment_data/file/888301/criminal-justice- statistics-quarterly-december-2019.pdf [Accessed 28.4.2022].

24. Khanom, H., Samele, C. and Rutherford, M. *A Missed Opportunity? Community Sentences and the Mental Health Treatment Requirement*. London: Sainsbury Centre for Mental Health, 2009.

25. National Offender Management Service. Mental Health Treatment Requirement; A Guide to Integrated Delivery. London: NOMS. 2014. https://assets .publishing.service.gov.uk/government/up loads/system/uploads/attachment_data/fil e/391162/Mental_Health_Treatment_Req uirement_-_A_Guide_to_Integrated_Deli very.pdf [Accessed 28.4.2022].

26. Ministry of Justice. Do offender characteristics affect the impact of short custodial sentences and court orders on reoffending? London: Ministry of Justice. 2018. www.gov.uk/government/publica tions/do-offender-characteristics-affect- the-impact-of-short-custodial-sentences- and-court-orders-on-reoffending [Accessed 28.4.2022].

27. Taylor, P., Eastman, N., Latham, R., and Holloway, J. Sentencing offenders with mental disorders, developmental disorders or neurological impairments: What does the new Sentencing Council Guideline mean for psychiatrists? *The British Journal of Psychiatry* 2021; 218(6):299–301. https:// doi.org/10.1192/bjp.2021.21.

28. Royal College of Psychiatrists. Position Statement PS04/21: Mental Health Treatment Requirements (MHTRs). London: RCPsych. 2021. www .rcpsych.ac.uk/docs/default-source/improv ing-care/better-mh-policy/position- statements/ps04_21--mental-health- treatment-requirements.pdf?sfvrsn=b0e2 e006_8 [Accessed 28.4.2022].

29. Woods, L., Craster, L., and Forrester, A. Mental Health Act transfers from prison to psychiatric hospital over a six-year period in a region of England. *Journal of Criminal Psychology* 2020; 10(3):219–31. https://doi.org/10.1108/JCP-03-2020-0013.

30. Ministry of Justice. Guidance for clinical supervisors. London: Ministry of Justice. 2009. https://assets.publishing.service.gov.uk/government/uploads/system/uploads/attachment_data/file/631272/guidance-for-clinical-supervisors-0909.pdf [Accessed 28.4.2022].

31. HM Government. The Criminal Justice and Court Services Act 2000. London: TSO. www.legislation.gov.uk/ukpga/2000/43/contents [Accessed 28.4.2022].

32. HM Prison and Probation Service. MAPPA Guidance 2012 v 4.5 (updated July 2019). London: HMPPS.2019. https://assets.publishing.service.gov.uk/government/uploads/system/uploads/attachment_data/file/819400/MAPPA_Guidance.odt [Accessed 28.4.2022].

33. HM Government. The Criminal Justice Act 2003. London: TSO. www.legislation.gov.uk/ukpga/2003/44/contents [Accessed 28.4.2022].

34. Taylor, R. and Yakeley, J. Working with MAPPA: Ethics and pragmatics. *BJPsych Advances*, 2019; 24(3); 157–65. https://doi.org/10.1192/bja.2018.5.

35. HM Government. The Prevent Strategy. London: TSO. 2011. https://assets.publishing.service.gov.uk/government/uploads/system/uploads/attachment_data/file/97976/prevent-strategy-review.pdf [Accessed 28.4.2022].

36. HM Government. The Counter-terrorism and Security Act 2015. London: TSO. www.legislation.gov.uk/ukpga/2015/6/contents [Accessed 28.4.2022].

37. HM Government. Channel Duty Guidance: Protecting vulnerable people from being drawn into terrorism. London: TSO. 2015. https://assets.publishing.service.gov.uk/government/uploads/system/uploads/attachment_data/file/964567/6.6271_HO_HMG_Channel_Duty_Guidance_v14_Web.pdf [Accessed 28.4.2022].

38. Royal College of Psychiatrists. Counterterrorism and Psychiatry Position Statement PS-04/16. London: RCPsych. 2016. www.rcpsych.ac.uk/pdf/PS04_16.pdf [Accessed 28.4.2022].

39. HM Government. National Referral Mechanism Online Guidance. 2020. www.gov.uk/government/publications/human-trafficking-victims-referral-and-assessment-forms/guidance-on-the-national-referral-mechanism-for-potential-adult-victims-of-modern-slavery-england-and-wales [Accessed 28.4.2022].

Information-Sharing, Including With Victims of Crime Committed by Persons With Mental Disorders

Masum Khwaja, Miriam Barrett and David Cochrane

Introduction

The use and disclosure of information is governed primarily by legislation such as the Data Protection Act 2018 and the Human Rights Act 1998. There is also guidance on confidentiality provided in the Code of Practice for the Mental Health Act (MHA) and by professional bodies such as the General Medical Council (GMC) and the Royal College of Psychiatrists (RCPsych).

In general, a patient's treatment and progress in hospital is confidential and, unless the patient has given consent, the information that can be disclosed is limited.

However, information about a patient can be disclosed to a third party (e.g. a victim) if other statutes, such as the Domestic Violence, Crime and Victims Act 2004, and the MHA 1983 (amended 2007) permit this. Information can also be disclosed in the public interest or if another person is at risk of harm if the information is not disclosed. Furthermore, the victims of specific violent and sexual offences have certain rights to information about the offender. This includes offenders who are subject to the MHA and are detained in hospital or subject to compulsion in the community.

Patients can both be the victims as well as the perpetrators of crime, and professionals working in health, social care and the justice system require a robust understanding of when to share confidential information.

The first half of this chapter provides information on legislation and guidance to be considered when sharing information about patients. The second half is focused on legislation and guidance on information-sharing by organisations supporting victims of crimes (also referred to as offences) committed by mentally disordered offenders and includes discussion of liaison with victims. Inevitably, there is overlap between the two halves of the chapter.

Useful references are provided for readers who wish to expand on the subject matter discussed.

Legislation and Guidance to Be Considered When Sharing Information About Patients, Including Those Who Are Victims of Crime

The Common Law Duty of Confidence

The general position is that if information is given in circumstances where it is expected that a duty of confidence applies, then that information cannot normally be disclosed without the information provider's consent [1].

If the patient has not consented, confidential information may still be released but only if disclosure is necessary to safeguard the individual or others, is in the public interest or there is a legal duty to do so (e.g. a court order).

Disclosure in the public interest requires solid justification and a clear explanation of why the individual's rights to confidentiality are being waived, and it is advisable to seek specialist or legal advice if disclosure is being considered. Any decision to disclose should be fully documented.

The General Data Protection Regulation and the Data Protection Act 2018

The Data Protection Act 2018 is the UK's implementation of the General Data Protection Regulation (GDPR) [2, 3]. The act controls how your personal information is used by organisations, businesses or the government. Everyone responsible for using personal data has to follow strict rules called data protection principles. They must make sure, for example, that the information is used fairly, lawfully and transparently and for specified, explicit purposes. There are separate safeguards for personal data relating to criminal convictions and offences [4].

The Human Rights Act 1998

The Human Rights Act became part of UK law on 2 October 2000. It incorporates the European Convention on Human Rights into UK law, allowing an individual to assert their convention rights in UK courts and tribunals, rather than at the European Court in Strasbourg [5].

The Human Rights Act can only be used against a public body, therefore health and social care organisations, as public bodies, are subject to the Act. Article 8 of the Convention, the right to respect for private and family life, is the most relevant to the health and social care setting and contains four rights: (i) the right of respect for private life, (ii) the right of respect for family life, (iii) the right of respect for one's home and (iv) the right of respect for correspondence.

Article 8 impacts on subject access requests, consent, confidentiality and disclosure issues. Article 8 rights are qualified rights; this means that in certain circumstances they can be interfered with by the state. However, this interference must be lawful, for a legitimate social aim, necessary to achieve that aim, and proportionate to the objective to be achieved. Legitimate social aims include national security, protection of public safety, protection of health or morals, prevention of crime or disorder, protection of the economic well-being of the country and protection of the rights and freedoms of others.

The Crime and Disorder Act 1998

Any person may disclose information to a relevant authority or to a person acting on behalf of such an authority under Section 115 of the Crime and Disorder Act 1998, 'where disclosure is necessary or expedient for the purposes of the Act (reduction and prevention of crime and disorder)' [6].

The 'relevant authority' includes a chief officer of police in England, Wales or Scotland, a local policing board, a local authority, a health authority, a social landlord, a probation board, an NHS commissioning board or a fire and rescue authority in England and Wales.

Safeguarding Aspects of the Care Act 2014 and the Mental Capacity Act

The local authority has the lead responsibility for safeguarding adults with care and support needs, and the police and the NHS also have clear safeguarding duties under the Care Act 2014. Sharing the right information, at the right time, with the right people, is fundamental to good practice in safeguarding adults. However, sharing information is a difficult area of practice and organisations should ensure that policies and training are in place to support staff in feeling confident about raising concerns and sharing information appropriately.

A Social Care Institute for Excellence (SCIE) guide summarises key aspects of relevant legislation regarding information-sharing and discusses basic principles in relation to safeguarding practice and the sharing of safeguarding information [7].

In practice, if a person refuses support with a safeguarding concern, or requests that information about them is not shared with other safeguarding partners, their wishes should be respected. The exceptions are:

- The person lacks the mental capacity to make that decision – this must be properly explored and recorded in line with the Mental Capacity Act (MCA)
- Other people are, or may be, at risk, including children
- The alleged abuser has care and support needs and may also be at risk
- A serious crime has been committed
- Staff are implicated
- The person has the mental capacity to make that decision but they may be under duress or being coerced
- Sharing the information could prevent a crime
- The risk is unreasonably high and meets the criteria for a Multi-Agency Risk Assessment Conference referral
- A court order or other legal authority has requested the information.

Sharing information between organisations about known or suspected risks may help to prevent abuse taking place, but it may also increase risk to the patient and others. For this reason, information-sharing decisions should always be based on considerations of the safety and well-being of the person and others who may be affected by their actions.

MHA Code of Practice

Chapter 10 of the MHA Code of Practice discusses confidentiality and information-sharing arising in connection with the MHA [8]. The code states that the law on confidentiality is the same for those patients subject to the MHA as it is for any other patients, except where the Act says otherwise.

Under the MHA, there are some situations where confidential information about a patient is legally authorised to be disclosed, even if the patient does not consent. Guidance is given on the sharing of information by professionals and agencies to manage serious risks which certain patients pose to others.

Part 3 of the MHA, known as the 'Forensic Sections', deals with mentally disordered offenders. Chapter 40 of the MHA Code of Practice provides information about the rights of victims of serious violent and sexual offences with regard to a Part 3 patient's treatment and discharge.

General Medical Council

Professional independent regulators, such as the GMC, provide useful advice on confidentiality, including when to break confidentiality in the public interest [9, 10].

Royal College of Psychiatrists

The RCPsych have produced a college report: 'Good Psychiatric Practice Confidentiality and information sharing' (CR209) [11].

Codes of Practice for Handling Information in Health and Care

There are various codes of practice for handling information in health and social care [12]. These include the Health and Social Care Information Centre (HSCIC) Guide to Confidentiality (2013), which advises health and care workers on what they should do and why, to share information safely while following rules on confidentiality, and the Confidentiality: NHS Code of Practice (2003), which sets out what health and care organisations have to do to meet their responsibilities around confidentiality and patients' consent to use their health records.

Legislation and Guiding Principles for Sharing Information with Victims of Crimes Committed by Mentally Disordered Offenders

Domestic Violence, Crime and Victims Act 2004 (DVCA 2004)

The Domestic Violence, Crime and Victims Act 2004 (DVCA 2004) is concerned with criminal justice and concentrates on legal protection and assistance to victims of crime, particularly domestic violence. Its purpose is to ensure that victims of particular crimes are able to express their views about both the sentencing and the release of the offender concerned.

Chapter 2 of Part 3 of the DVCA 2004 is concerned with victims' rights to representation and information about patients who have committed a crime that places them under Chapter 2 of Part 3 of the DVCA (often referred to as 'Chapter 2 patients') [13].

The offences covered in the DVCA 2004 which apply to those convicted or to those dealt with using a hospital order or restriction order include:

- Murder or an offence specified in Schedule 18 of the Sentencing Act 2020;
- An offence in respect of which the patient or offender is subject to the notification requirements of Part 2 of the Sexual Offences Act 2003;
- An offence against a child within the meaning of Part 2 of the Criminal Justice and Court Services Act 2000.

A comprehensive list of offences is available in a government guide on the extension of victims' rights under the DVCA 2004 [14].

The DVCA 2004, from July 2005, gave, for the first time, the victims of certain mentally disordered offenders, detained in hospital under Part 3 of the MHA as restricted patients or in the community subject to a conditional discharge, rights to receive information and to make representations about conditions to which the offender may be subject on discharge from hospital. This could include letting the victim know how and when the offender will be released. It also allows victims to express their views about licence conditions the offender must follow if they are to serve the remainder of their sentence in the community (e.g. not to contact the victim or the victim's family members).

In November 2008, provisions in Schedule 6 of the MHA 2007 amended the DVCA 2004 to extend these rights to the victims of unrestricted patients: those detained in hospital under Part III of the 1983 MHA following conviction for a specified sexual or violent offence, who are not subject to special restrictions, including those who are later discharged from hospital on a community treatment order (CTO) [15].

Specifically, the DVCA 2004 provisions apply if:

- The offender is convicted on or after 1 July 2005, and
- The offence is a listed sexual or violent offence (see earlier) and, in the case of a sentenced prisoner, the sentence was 12 months or more.
- For restricted patients, the patient became subject to one of the following sections after 1 July 2005: a hospital order with a restriction order (s37[1]) and s41 MHA 1983), a hospital and limitation direction (s45 MHA 1983), or a transfer direction with a restriction direction (s47 and s49 MHA 1983).
- For unrestricted patients, the patient became subject to one of the following sections after 3 November 2008: s37 MHA (hospital order including an unrestricted order under the Criminal Procedure and Investigations Act [CPIA]), s47 MHA (transfer direction), notional s37 MHA (notional hospital order – starts when prison sentence ends), and s17A MHA (CTO – following a s37 or notional s37 if the aforementioned criteria apply).

Code of Practice for Victims of Crime

The Code of Practice for Victims of Crime (Victims' Code) is a statutory government document. The original Victim Code came into effect in 2006, having become necessary through the Domestic Violence, Crime and Victims Act 2004. It built on the support for victims within the Victim Charter, which was introduced in 1990 and which set out for the first time the levels of service victims of crime should expect. The Code has been updated several times, and the most recent revision, the Code of Practice for Victims of Crime 2020, came into force on 1st April 2021 [16].

The new code brings together 12 overarching rights that outline the minimum level of information, support and services victims can expect at each stage of the justice process. It also explains what information victims are entitled to under the Victim Contact Scheme, as set out in the DVCA 2004.

In contrast to the previous Victims' Code, the new code applies equally to victims in respect of restricted and unrestricted Part 3 MHA patients.

Hence, under the Code, victims of all such patients where the conviction relates to a specified sexual or violent offence for which the offender receives a sentence of 12 months or more or has been detained in a hospital for treatment under the MHA 1983, are now entitled to receive certain information about the mentally disordered offender via a probation service (PS) victim liaison officer (VLO) under the Victim Contact Scheme (VCS).

The new code has also made referral to the VCS automatic as opposed to 'opt in'. The victim may opt out following referral, and may opt in again at a later date if they choose to do so. More detail on the VCS is given later in the chapter.

. Other rights, pertinent to information-sharing, include:

– the right to be informed of the reasons why a suspect will not be prosecuted. If unhappy, victims will also be able to ask the police or Crown Prosecution Service (CPS) to review this decision.

– for the first time, the rights of victims of foreign national offenders to be updated on when an offender's deportation may occur.

Should Information Be Shared With Victims of Mentally Disordered Offenders Who Do Not Have a Statutory Right to Receive Information?

Section 40 of the MHA 1983 Code of Practice states that it is good practice for the PS to consider providing support to any victim of a restricted patient, even those who do not fall within the scope of the DVCA 2004, for statutory contact under the VCS. Such non-statutory victims of Part 3 MHA restricted patients include, for example, those where the conviction occurred prior to the DVCA 2004 but the victim has now made contact, the victim of a non-qualifying offence or sentence length (s47/49) where the victim has expressed concerns about their safety and the victims of co-defendants convicted in connection with the same incident.

Similarly, it is good practice to 'offer a service' on a discretionary basis to 'non-statutory' victims of unrestricted mentally disordered offenders. This includes those wishing to make representations about an unrestricted patient who is the subject of an order or direction made before the November 2008 (schedule 6 MHA 2007) amendments to the DVCA 2004 came into force. In addition, it is good practice to offer contact to victims where the patient was transferred from prison under s47 of the MHA 1983 but the prison sentence ended prior to the legislation coming in.

Victim Liaison Protocol

The Victim Liaison Protocol (VLP) was developed jointly by the PS and the Ministry of Justice (MoJ). It provides information on procedures for information-sharing, joint working and the forwarding of victims' written representations about discharge conditions to Mental Health Tribunals (MHT) and other decision-makers, as well as guidance on non-statutory good practice. The protocol at the time of writing has been widely circulated but has yet to be formally published, but we have permission to copy parts of the protocol to inform this chapter.

Liaison with Victim
Referral to the Victim Contact Scheme

Referral is automatic in this scheme and the witness care unit has a statutory requirement to pass on the details of any statutory victim to the PS's VCS within ten working days of the date of sentence of an offender who has received a hospital order, with or without restrictions. This includes those who have been found unfit to plead or found not guilty by reason of insanity, or who are the subject of a hospital direction and limitation direction.

The catchment areas for mental health services are not aligned with the areas covered by the PS. Work with the victim is undertaken by the local victim liaison unit (VLU) covering the victim's current address, irrespective of where the patient originated from or is currently placed. Referrals are made to the VLU local to the sentencing court and, where the victim lives in a different area, the referral is then passed to that area's VLU.

Victim Opt-in to Victim Contact Scheme

A named VLO will write to the victim and offer contact to the victim(s) or to the victim's family. If the victim chooses to opt into the VCS, the VLO will offer them a home visit. In some cases, joint visits with the responsible clinician, forensic social workers or other appropriate professionals may be appropriate. The initial letter should include an offer of an interpreter if one is needed, and a clear statement to the effect that refusing contact now does not debar contact in the future.

At the meeting, the VLO will explain what the sentence of the court means in terms of the offender's detention in prison or hospital, and the victim's entitlement to certain information, but should not divulge details of the patient's treatment or location to the victim(s), although this may already be known to them (in many cases, victims are family members of the patient).

The VLO will also explain that they will provide updates on offenders at key stages (see later in the chapter) of their sentence and over the course of their treatment. Victims may opt in to or out of the VCS at any time during the life of the hospital order/direction.

Liaison with Key Professionals

With restricted cases, the VLU is tasked to inform the mental health casework section (MHCS) which VLOs have been assigned to a case. Multiple victims of the same offender may be located in different geographical areas, which will require different VLOs.

The VLO is responsible for identifying and contacting key professionals involved in the case and for gathering the necessary information. The VLO will seek contact details for the nominated single point of contact (SPOC), clinical team and/or the responsible clinician (RC) responsible for the patient's care from the MHCS and/or the hospital. The SPOC is usually an MHA administrator, care co-ordinator, social worker or the RC.

With unrestricted cases, the MHCS is not involved and the VLO contacts the hospital directly via the SPOC to identify themselves and the fact they have victim contact, giving office details and requesting similar contact details for the SPOC and involved professionals as for restricted patients. For both restricted and unrestricted cases, the hospital manager, usually via the SPOC, should record the involvement of the VLO and ensure that the RC and care team are aware that the victim has requested to receive information under the VCS.

Passing on Information to the Victim

For the victims of unrestricted mentally disordered offenders, prior to the Victims' Code 2020, statutory duty for contact was held by the hospital managers and the VLO would seek the victim's consent to pass the victim's details to hospital managers (via the MHA office).

However, as now directed by the new Victims' Code 2020, victims of unrestricted patients, as for victims of restricted mentally disordered offenders, should receive information via a probation service VLU or VLO.

Hospital managers, SPOCS and RCs should maintain links with designated VLOs, share appropriate information in a timely fashion and also continue, as they did before the new Victims' Code, to maintain records of which patients are 'Chapter 2 patients' and hence eligible to receive information and to make representations.

Confidentiality of Patient Information

The DVCV Act 2004 does not place any statutory requirements on the RC to disclose any personal information about the patient. The information which is required to be disclosed under the DVCV Act relates to discharge and conditions of discharge.

Under the Act, the VLO or hospital managers may also provide 'such other information to the victim as the VLO or hospital managers consider appropriate in all the circumstances of the case'. This is intended to allow the VLO or hospital managers the discretion to give information which will reassure the victims, such as the actual date of discharge (usual practice under the VCS is to provide the week of discharge before it takes place, and then confirm the actual date after the fact). It is not intended to lead to the disclosure of information that is covered by patient confidentiality. In some cases, it may be appropriate to seek the patient's permission to disclose anything regarded as personal information.

In other circumstances, professionals should encourage (but may not require) mentally disordered offender patients to agree to share information that will enable victims and victims' families to be informed about their progress. Amongst other benefits, disclosure of such information can sometimes serve to reduce the danger of harmful confrontations after a discharge of which victims were unaware. Professionals should be ready to discuss with patients the benefits of enabling some information to be given by professionals to victims, within the spirit of the Code of Practice for Victims of Crime 2020.

Key Stages in Restricted Patients

For restricted patients only, the MHCS must, as the decision maker, contact VLOs in order to pass on information about the key stages in the offender's sentence, including:

- To request victim representation when considering a proposal for discharge.
- Details of any agreed conditions of discharge relating to the victim or their family.
- Consideration being given to varying victim-related conditions of discharge.
- Decision made to discharge patient, regardless of whether the patient will be subject to conditions (i.e. absolute or conditional discharge).
- If a patient previously found unfit to plead is remitted back to court.
- If a patient is remitted to prison.
- Hospital transfer.
- Escorted/unescorted leave (see section 'Leave from Hospital').
- When restrictions cease.
- Recall for treatment under the MHA 1983.

The MHCS expects the RC to liaise with the VLO prior to making any application for leave, transfer or discharge, and its application forms include a section for the clinician to complete, setting out the VLOs details and any representations the victim wishes to make about conditions.

Key Stages in Unrestricted Patients

The MHCS is not involved in cases where there is no restriction. Information pertaining to key stages will be provided to the VLO at the discretion of the RC.

The statutory minimum information which should be communicated to victims includes:

- The date a patient is to be discharged
- Whether a CTO is to be made, including allowing the victim to make representations about conditions
- The date on which the authority to detain the patient expires
- The conditions of the CTO relevant to the victim
- The details of any variation to the CTO which relates to contact with the victim or his family.

The provision of information about a key stage of a patient's sentence may be limited if this stage is considered to be medical treatment, as this would mean that as the information was medical it would be confidential.

Following Admission/Transfer to Hospital

Once it has been established that there is victim contact, the clinical team should decide with the VLO the level of contact between them. This may include, for example, whether or not the VLO should attend any meetings with the team about the case.

The clinical team should identify in the clinical record the 'key stages' (as detailed earlier) in a patient's sentence and/or rehabilitation, and communicate these to the VLU so that the VLO is prepared to consult with victims as and when the need arises.

Information about any identified victims is confidential and must not be disclosed to the patient. Any reports sent to the hospital by the VLU are also strictly confidential (unless otherwise advised) and should be kept in the third-party section of the clinical file with the victim's consent.

Essential victim information should, however, be readily available to senior nursing staff and other disciplines if the patient absconds. In the event of a patient absconding, staff at the hospital should notify the police, the VLU (where there is victim contact) and, in restricted cases, the MHCS. Should the clinical team wish to have discussions with victims in order to gather information relating to risk assessment formulation, then it is most appropriate for members of the care team to meet the victim jointly with the VLO. Due consideration should be given to the language and diversity needs of victims in order to ensure effective two-way communication.

When carrying out risk assessments for the purpose of making applications for leave (in the case of restricted patients to the MHCS), members of the clinical team will consider, with the victim's consent, information given by the VLO about the victim's circumstances. In cases of intra-familial violence, the clinical team should consider the professional conflicts of interest that may arise and, in the circumstances, how best to support the victim(s). In cases where the victim has continued contact with the patient, further discussions should take place as to the appropriateness or need for victim contact via the VLO.

In appropriate cases, the clinical team will liaise with the VLO to request facilitation of any work under restorative justice, which is provided through contracts by the relevant Police and Crime Commissioner (PCC).

Leave from Hospital

Informing victims of leave is not a statutory requirement. However, following a ministerial commitment in April 2014, victims of restricted patients, who have opted into the VCS, should be told if permission for community leave is granted by the Secretary of State unless there are exceptional reasons why they should not be told. Exceptional reasons include risk to the patient.

In practice, the MHCS ascertains whether the victim wishes to make any representations about conditions to be attached to consent to community leave in advance of making the decision. The RC should contact the VLO in advance of the application and provide details of any request when completing the application form to be sent to MHCS. Any concerns about this must be flagged up to the MHCS in the application for community leave. When the MHCS gives permission to the RC for a restricted patient to take escorted or unescorted leave, they will inform the VLO and tell them if any conditions relating to the victim were attached to that permission. The MHCS will also inform the VLO if permission for leave is refused, or granted but later rescinded, although reasons for that would not be provided unless they are already in the public domain (e.g. if the offender has been charged with a further offence and appeared in court).

Although, in contrast to victims of restricted mentally disordered offenders, the victims of unrestricted mentally disordered offenders do not have to be informed about escorted or unescorted leave, the VLP strongly recommends that a similar procedure as is used for restricted patients should be followed when considering community leave for unrestricted patients. The protocol states that 'As well as upholding the spirit of the Code of Practice for Victims of Crime, it will help prevent possible harmful situations or issues around potential exclusion zones that victims may request on the patient's eventual discharge.'

Conditions of Discharge

General rules:

a. The clinical team are asked to consider conditions of discharge relevant to the victim on receipt of their representations, such as 'no contact' conditions or exclusion zones, in liaison with the VLO; in making recommendations through the RC in their reports to the MHT or the MHCS, it will be down to either the MHT or MHCS to decide what conditions should be included.

b. Such conditions must be proportionate and necessary, although 'necessary' can mean that they are required for the reassurance and mental well-being of the victim.

c. The clinical team should not ordinarily divulge the proposed discharge address of the patient to the VLO.

d. The clinical team should, as a matter of courtesy, inform the VLO as quickly as possible of any discharge conditions that relate to the victim following a MHT hearing.

e. In cases where the decision was taken by the Secretary of State, the MHCS will inform the VLO.

f. Care plan meeting documentation prepared by the clinical team should include information on victim issues, details of any conditions and exclusion zones relating to the victim that have been imposed and the action required if the patient breaches those conditions.

g. The clinical team must maintain established links with the VLO so that the latter can report promptly any concerns about the patient breaching the conditions attached to their discharge. The VLO, in consultation with the MHCS (if involved), RC and clinical team will agree what information can be reported back to the victim about the action that has been taken. In line with standard practice, victims should be advised to contact the police if they fear they are in immediate danger from any individual.

Recall to Hospital of Conditionally Discharged Patients or Those on a Community Treatment Order

Restricted Patients

Breach of the conditions imposed on a discharged patient may not in itself lead to recall to hospital. In order to manage victims' expectations, it is important that this is made clear from the outset. A restricted patient may not be recalled to hospital, except in an emergency, unless there is medical evidence that the patient's mental health has deteriorated. However, information about breaches of any conditions may also lead to recall. The same conditions also apply to conditionally charged patients whom, if arrested for any reason, can still be prosecuted through the criminal justice system.

Victims should be informed when a patient is recalled to hospital. In restricted cases, the MHCS will inform the VLO.

Unrestricted Patients

Similarly, an unrestricted patient subject to a CTO may be recalled to hospital by the RC and, if recall is needed, victims should be informed by the VLO.

Hospital-to-Hospital Transfer

The MHCS will also consider where the victim is living when considering a request to transfer to a different hospital. The victim is not entitled to make representations about where the patient is detained, but the MHCS will consider whether a move to a particular hospital puts the patient inside, or very close to, a requested exclusion zone, which could make progression to leave and discharge in that area very difficult. In such cases, the MHCS will raise concerns with the RC and discuss whether an alternative placement could be identified and considered. The MHCS will not inform the victim where a patient is detained or where he or she is being transferred to but, where the victim has asked to be informed of key decisions, will inform them that a patient has been moved up or down in security.

As with applications for discharge, the MHCS expects the hospital to have liaised with the VLO prior to any application for leave or transfer, so that there is no delay in considering the application on receipt.

Transfers Between Prison and Hospital

For transferred prisoners, it is the responsibility of the MHCS to notify the patient's Probation Practitioner (PP) or Prison Offender Manager (POM) of a transfer from prison to hospital. The PP/POM must then notify the VLO. However, it is good practice for the relevant mental health assessor of the prisoner to contact the VLU before admission if it is known that victim contact is statutory in the case. This would ensure there are no problems associated with the location of the victims to the nominated hospital. Where a patient is remitted to prison to continue their sentence, the MHCS will inform the VLO.

Mental Health Tribunals: Restricted Patients

When the Secretary of State refers a patient to the Mental Health Tribunal or receives notification from the MHT that a patient has applied, the MHCS will forward the details of the relevant VLO to the MHT office. The MHT Secretariat will then inform the VLO of the tribunal date once it has been set, as well as the date by which a victim's representations must be received so that they can be considered at the hearing.

Victims can apply to the tribunal to direct that their representations be withheld from the patient, but no guarantees can be given that such an application will be granted. The expectation is that all documents are disclosed to the patient; the circumstances in which documents can be withheld are very limited, but would be based on concerns that disclosure would adversely affect the health or welfare of the patient or others.

The MHT will inform the VLO if it refuses a request to withhold victim representations from the patient. The clinical team will also advise the VLU, as soon as practicable, of a decision by the MHT to disclose to the patient information provided by the victim for which confidentiality had been requested.

Mental Health Tribunals: Unrestricted Patients

When an unrestricted patient applies for a review by the MHT, or a referral is made on their behalf, the MHT must inform the managers or SPOC of the relevant hospital. The hospital manager or SPOC must then pass the VLO contact details to the MHT and inform the VLO(s) of the victim or victims who have opted to receive information of the application and invite them to make written representations about conditions that they would wish attached to any discharge (in practice, this would be a no contact condition and/or exclusion zones where the victim or victim's family live, work and frequent).

Any written representations made by the victim must be forwarded to the MHT.

Under the DVCV Act, the MHT must inform the managers or SPOC of the relevant hospital of the need to:

a. Inform the victim whether the patient is to be discharged;
b. Inform that person whether a CTO is to be made in respect of the patient;
c. State that if a CTO is to be made in respect of the patient it should specify the conditions which relate to contact with the victim or his family, and to provide that person with details of those conditions;
d. State that if a CTO is in force in respect of the patient and the conditions specified in the order are to be varied, then provide that person with details of any variation relating to contact with the victim or his family;
e. State that if a CTO in respect of the patient is no longer in force, to inform that person of the date on which it is to cease to be in force;
f. Clarify, if following the examination of the patient under section 20 of the MHA 1983, the authority for the patient's detention is not to be renewed, to inform that person of the date on which the authority is to expire;
g. Provide that person with such other information as the managers of the relevant hospital consider appropriate in all the circumstances of the case.

Victim Application to Attend MHT Hearing

Any application by a victim to attend the MHT hearing and give oral evidence must be considered by the MHT. There is no obligation to accede to this request, with respect to either attendance at the MHTs or oral evidence heard by the MHTs. Representations made by a victim can cover only a limited range of issues and the victim is not a party to the proceedings. In most cases, therefore, a written statement is the most satisfactory way for the victim to express their views. Amongst other matters, direct involvement by the victim in mental health proceedings, or a procedure that brings the victim into direct conflict with the patient, is unlikely to be helpful to the victim, to the patient or to the tribunal. If the victim believes that their attendance at the hearing is necessary, he or she will have to demonstrate that the opportunity to make written representations is insufficient for the tribunal to deal with the case fairly and justly, and that there is a need for the victim to be heard in person in relation to the relevant matters.

Conclusion

Patients can be both the victims as well as perpetrators of crime.

Professionals working in health, social care and the justice system require a robust understanding of when to share confidential information, and organisations should ensure that policies and training are in place to support staff in feeling confident about sharing information appropriately.

In practice, when considering sharing information, the patient should first be asked whether they consent to information being disclosed, with an explanation given as to why the information should be shared and who the information will be shared with. If the patient refuses then information may still be shared if it is necessary to safeguard the individual or others, it is in the public interest or there is a legal duty to do so.

The most recent version of the Code of Practice for Victims of Crime, also known as the 'Victims' Code', applies equally to victims in respect of restricted and unrestricted Part 3 MHA patients and provides details of what information victims are entitled to receive under the VCS.

References

1. NHS. Consent and Confidential patient information, 16 Mar. 2022. [Online]. https://transform.england.nhs.uk/information-governance/guidance/consent-and-confidential-patient-information/ [Accessed 16.04.2022].

2. UK Government. The Data Protection Act 2018. [Online] www.gov.uk/data-protection [Accessed 16.04.2022].

3. UK Government. Guide to the General Data Protection Regulation. 5 May 2018. [Online] https://ico.org.uk/for-organisations/guide-to-data-protection/guide-to-the-general-data-protection-regulation-gdpr/. [Accessed 16 April 2022].

4. Information Commissioners Office. Criminal Offence Data. [Online] https://ico.org.uk/for-organisations/guide-to-data-protection/guide-to-the-general-data-protection-regulation-gdpr/lawful-basis-for-processing/criminal-offence-data [Accessed 16.04.2022].

5. Department of Health Northern Ireland. The Human Rights Act 1998. [Online]. www.health-ni.gov.uk/articles/human-rights-act-1998 [Accessed 16.04.2022].

6. UK Government. Crime and Disorder Act 1998 [Online] www.legislation.gov.uk/ukpga/1998/37/section/115/2018-11-02 [Accessed 16.04.2022].

7. Social Care Institute for Excellence. Safeguarding Adults: sharing information. Last updated January 2019. [Online] www.scie.org.uk/safeguarding/adults/practice/sharing-information [Accessed 16.04.2022].

8. UK Government. Code of Practice: Mental Health Act 1983. Last updated 31 October 2017. [Online] www.gov.uk/government/publications/code-of-practice-mental-health-act-1983 [Accessed 16.04.2022].

9. General Medical Council. Confidentiality: good practice in handling patient information. [Online] www.gmc-uk.org/ethical-guidance/ethical-guidance-for-doctors/confidentiality [Accessed 16.04.2022].

10. General Medical Council. Disclosures for the protection of patients and others. [Online] www.gmc-uk.org/ethical-guidance/ethical-guidance-for-doctors/confidentiality/disclosures-for-the-protection-of-patients-and-others [Accessed 16.04.2022].

11. Royal College of Psychiatrists. Third Edition of the College Report CR209. Good Psychiatric Practice: Confidentiality and information sharing. [Online] www.rcpsych.ac.uk/docs/default-source/improving-care/better-mh-policy/college-reports/college-report-cr209.pdf?sfvrsn=23858153_2 [Accessed 16.04.2022].

12. NHS Digital. Codes of practice for handling information in health and care. [Online] https://digital.nhs.uk/data-and-information/looking-after-information/data-security-and-information-governance/codes-of-practice-for-handling-information-in-health-and-care [Accessed 16.04.2022].

13. UK Government. Domestic Violence, Crime and Victims Act 2004. [Online] www.legislation.gov.uk/ukpga/2004/28/part/3/chapter/2/2020-12-01 [Accessed 16.04.2022].

14. Department of Health; Ministry of Justice; National Offender Management Service. Mental Health Act 2007: Guidance on the Extension of Victims' Rights under the Domestic Violence, Crime and Victims Act 2004. Published 2008. [Online] https://webarchive.nationalarchives.gov.uk/20130104164723/http://www.dh.gov.uk/en/Publicationsandstatistics/Publications/PublicationsPolicyAndGuidance/DH_089408 [Accessed 16.04.2022].

15. UK Government. Schedule 6 Mental Health Act 2007. [Online] www.legislation.gov.uk/ukpga/2007/12/schedule/6 [Accessed 16.04.2022].

16. Ministry of Justice. Code of Practice for Victims of Crime in England and Wales. November 2020. [Online]. https://assets.publishing.service.gov.uk/government/uploads/system/uploads/attachment_data/file/974376/victims-code-2020.pdf [Accessed 16.04.2022].

Chapter 19

Victims of Violence

Alexis Theodorou, Saima Ali and Masum Khwaja

Introduction

This chapter provides an overview of the impact of violence and victimisation on the people who suffer from it, and, to a lesser extent, on the perpetrators of violence. The chapter concludes with a list of contact details of organisations that provide information and support for victims and perpetrators of violence.

The following topics are discussed:

- The relationship between mental health and violence.
- The association between COVID-19, lockdown and domestic violence.
- A public health approach to violence prevention.
- The history and development of legal protection and statutory services for victims in the United Kingdom, including information on the 2021 Victims' Code.
- Current support for victims and perpetrators of violence.
- Potential for future development within this field.

Mental Health, Violence and Violent Victimisation

Violence often devastates the lives of affected individuals and their families, leaving a lasting impact on both perpetrators and their victims. Research interests have traditionally focused on the relationship between mental illness and the risk of perpetrating violence. This is likely to have contributed to a negative public perception of, and stigma against, psychiatric patients [1]. Certain psychiatric disorders, such as schizophrenia, are allegedly associated in the public mind with an increased risk of violence. However, this is not true for schizophrenia itself, but only relevant when schizophrenia is associated with comorbid substance misuse and personality disorder [2, 3].

There is a growing body of evidence that illustrates the elevated risk of victimisation and the high violence burden experienced by those with mental health problems. Contrary to general societal belief, psychiatric patients are more likely to be victims of violent crime than they are perpetrators [4]. They are also more likely to be victims when compared to the general population. It is estimated that those suffering from mental illness are five times more likely than the general public to have experienced assault, and this risk rises to up to ten times for women [4].

Violent victimisation is associated with a number of negative consequences for psychiatric patients. Such experiences may impact on existing psychopathology as symptoms are exacerbated, and also increases the likelihood of contact with services and dissatisfaction with that received [4, 5]. In addition, victimisation has been linked to greater substance misuse problems [6], an increased risk of re-victimisation [7] and a poorer quality of life [5].

The relationship between mental illness and violent victimisation is nuanced and complex. Bi-directional relationships have been documented in intimate partner violence and depression: violence impacts upon depressive symptoms, and depression increases the risk of violence [8]. There is also significant overlap between the risk of becoming a perpetrator and that of being a victim [9], and this is observed across clinical practice. The reality is that victimisation encompasses a number of individual, socio-cultural and environmental factors [10].

This is illustrated in the current difficulties associated with the coronavirus pandemic. A global increase in domestic violence figures has been reported. Enforced isolation, possible increases in substance misuse and financial uncertainty have all been postulated as potential reasons for this [11, 12]. Limitations of travel, alongside a reduction in access to usual resources, may have contributed to increased difficulty in escaping abusive households [13].

A Public Health Approach to Violence Prevention

A public health perspective is helpful in conceptualising and addressing the pressing issue of violence and violent victimisation. Violence disproportionately impacts the most deprived communities, contributes substantially to worldwide mortality and morbidity rates and is a financial burden to the health service, costing the NHS in England and Wales £2.5 billion a year [14]. This is likely to be an underestimation, as exposure to violence as a child can also increase the risk of obesity, heart disease, substance misuse and other mental illness in later life [15].

In 1996, the 49th World Health Assembly passed Resolution WHA49.25 declaring that violence 'is a leading worldwide public health problem' [16]. This has helped develop a clearer recognition of this significant problem, alongside enabling further research regarding identification of the complex underlying causes. These are illustrated in Figure 19.1.

This has enabled the development of clear violence prevention strategies. These are divided into categories according to the level of intervention, as shown in Table 19.1

Overview of the History and Development of Legal Protection and Statutory Services for Victims in the UK

The Domestic Violence, Crime and Victims Act (2004) [18] led to significant changes in the representation and support victims of crime receive. The position of Victims' Commissioner was created, and the first commissioner was appointed in 2010. This role is a ministerial appointment, tasked with maintaining independence from governmental agencies in order to promote the interests of victims and liaise with all criminal justice agencies to promote good practice [19]. Alongside this, the Code of Practice for Victims of Crime (the Victim's Code) was established in 2006 and most recently revised in 2021 [20]. This is a statutory code that delineates the level of support victims must receive from all criminal justice agencies, from the moment they report a crime to the sentencing of an offender. The revised code is discussed later in the chapter.

The Police Reform and Social Responsibility Act 2011 led to the creation of Police and Crime Commissioners (PCCs) to replace the existing police authorities. These are elected officials, serving fixed terms of representation. They are responsible for the creation of local

Table 19.1 Violence prevention strategies: Levels of intervention

Level of Intervention	Aim
Primary	Preventing incidents of violence before they occur
Secondary	Risk reduction following an incident of violence
Tertiary	Longer-term interventions aimed at risk minimisation

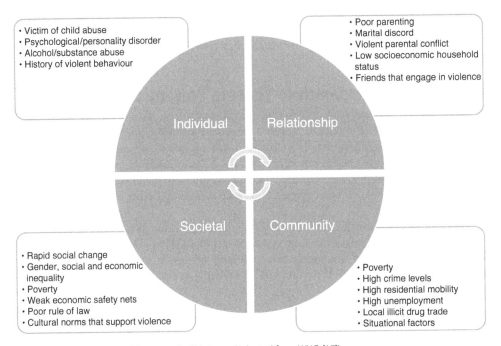

Figure 19.1 The Ecological Framework of Violence (Adapted from WHO [17])

police crime plans, the appointment and scrutiny of chief constables and the resource allocation of police forces and constabularies across England and Wales [21]. They are also allocated funding for the development of victim support services locally [22].

In 2018, HM Government published the 'Victims Strategy' policy paper [23]. This details the strengthening of the Victims' Code, with an increase in spending on support services, and introduces changes in police and court approach in relation to victims and modifications to the Victim Contact Scheme.

The same year, HM Government published its Serious Violence Strategy [24]. Although this initially did not adopt a clear public health approach, subsequent consultations resulted in an announcement in July 2019 of a 'new legal duty to underpin a 'public health' approach to tackling serious violence' [25]. This was developed into the Serious Violence Bill 2019/20, which was announced in the Queen's Speech on 19 December 2019 [26]. At the time of writing, it has not been scheduled for a second reading in Parliament.

Current Support for Victims of Violence

The development of identification strategies and provision of effective care and support for victims of violence is key to their health and well-being and to break the cycle of violence [15]. As discussed earlier, violent victimisation is a risk factor for re-victimisation and can also increase the likelihood of perpetrating violence in future [27].

Enshrining victim support in legislation has enabled the development of services. Tailored criminal justice measures, such as protection orders, can help mitigate the risk of further violence [28]. Specialist domestic violence courts (SDVC) have been helpful in enabling successful prosecutions, and witness care units have been shown to improve court attendance, trial outcomes and victim satisfaction [29, 30].

The recognition that NHS staff were at increased risk of aggression and violence led to the development of the NHS violence reduction strategy in 2018. The aim is to protect NHS workers from violence, with a zero-tolerance approach, by creating more robust links between the NHS, the Crown Prosecution Service (CPS) and the police [31]. Unfortunately, it is clear that a lot of work remains to be done, as the 2019 NHS Staff Survey showed that 17% of staff had experienced violence at work in the preceding 12 months [32].

Screening programmes are implemented with the aim of detecting victims of violence and providing appropriate support. Currently, most available tools are focused on intimate partner violence and child maltreatment. Although use of screening tools is widely advocated, there is a paucity of evidence supporting long-term sustainability or effectiveness in violence reduction [33].

There has been an expansion of specialist training provision for professionals, aimed at raising awareness of signs and symptoms of abuse, as well as improving knowledge about local protocols for reporting and referrals. Evidence shows that training can improve clinician knowledge, attitudes and confidence in relation to supporting victims of interpersonal violence and child maltreatment. In England, the Identification and Referral to Improve Safety (IRIS) programme trains primary healthcare staff to recognise and refer cases of domestic violence. It was found to improve identification of victims three-fold, and also yielded a six-fold increase in referral of victims to advocacy services [34]. There is no current equivalent programme for mental health clinicians, but the BRAVE (Better Reduction through Assessment of Violence and Evaluation) study is an ongoing trial that aims to improve detection of and response to domestic violence in both male and female psychiatric patients [35].

Advocacy programmes range from providing counselling to victims and families to job support and substance abuse treatment referrals and assistance with social and legal services. Although advocacy services have been shown to reduce physical abuse in some incidents of intimate partner violence, in extreme cases some interventions may increase the risk of abuse [36]. A broad range of psychological interventions have been used to support victims of violence. The evidence base for efficacy, however, remains limited, and two recent systematic reviews of psychological interventions for the victims of intimate partner violence have suggested that it is not possible to draw meaningful conclusions at present [37, 38].

Creating and maintaining coordinated multi-agency efforts can result in effective victim support. The Multi-Agency Risk Assessment Conference (MARAC) was originally set up in Cardiff in 2003, involving various parties from mental health staff to the police and social services. This operates on a tertiary prevention level. After a period of one year following MARAC intervention, around four in ten women did not report further violence [39]. In England, people over 14 who have been raped or sexually assaulted can attend a national network of Sexual Assault Referral Centres (SARCs), which also provide multidisciplinary support including physical examination, psychological support and follow-up care, regardless of whether victims choose to report an incident [40].

The Victims' Code

In April 2021, a new Victims' Code also came into force in England and Wales, aiming to give victims of crime better support from the police and improve public confidence in the criminal justice system [20].

The Victims' Code applies to all criminal justice agencies, including the police, the CPS, the Courts Service and the Probation Service.

The code focuses on 12 overarching rights for victims:

1. To be able to understand and to be understood.
2. To have the details of the crime recorded without unjustified delay.
3. To be provided with information when reporting the crime.
4. To be referred to victim support services and have services and support tailored to their needs.
5. To be provided with information about compensation.
6. To be provided with information about the investigation and prosecution.
7. To be able to make a Victim Personal Statement.
8. To be given information about any trial, trial process and their role as a witness.
9. To be given information about the outcome of the case and any appeals.
10. To be paid expenses and have property returned.
11. To be given information about the offender following a conviction.
12. To make a complaint about rights not being met.

Which rights apply will depend on individual circumstances, including whether there has been a police report, if the case goes to trial and whether a conviction has been made.

The Code acknowledges that victims who are considered vulnerable or intimidated, are a victim of the most serious crime (including a bereaved close relative) or have been persistently targeted are more likely to require specialised assistance (some victims may fall into one or more of these categories). Such support may include being offered a referral to a specialist support service, being contacted sooner after key decisions and having access to special measures (see Right 4). Within each individual Right this Code highlights 'where such (enhanced) rights apply'. [20]

In cases where the offender has been convicted of a serious violent or sexual offence (or cases where death or serious injury has been caused by dangerous driving, or instances of coercive or controlling behaviour in an intimate relationship), victims or bereaved relatives will now be automatically referred to the probation service Victim Contact Scheme and be assigned a victim liaison officer (VLO). This includes cases where the sentence is one of detention in hospital for treatment under the Mental Health Act 1983 (2007). This is irrespective of whether a restriction order has been requested. VLOs are able to offer information support to victims around issues such as sentencing, offender movement to open conditions and parole board hearings.

Notably, victims will now be automatically informed when a perpetrator is due to leave prison. Victims of sexual violence will be able to choose the sex of their police officer, be informed when foreign national offenders are deported and be given clearer advice on when evidence can be pre-recorded ahead of trials.

Suggestions for Future Development

The future of support for victims of violence appears directly linked to the implementation of a public health approach and the proposed new legal duty on agencies. This raises the possibility of the development of a broad range of primary, secondary and tertiary interventions.

Taken holistically, these interventions could be aimed at both the individual and the societal levels. At the individual level, outreach work aimed at engaging and supporting vulnerable households, alongside comprehensive education packages, should aim at reducing the frequency of adverse childhood events. The Early Start Project, a home-based family support programme in New Zealand, was shown to be associated with reduced rates of violence towards children [41].

Societally, the role of poverty, inequity and low socio-economic status in the development of violence is clear. This calls for significant investment in these communities and the creation of good-quality employment opportunities. There is a clear need for re-establishment and expansion of substance misuse services and development of improved education out of school services. In planning interventions at this level, the impact of austerity policies should be kept in mind in order to account for the years of disproportionate impact borne by these communities [42].

Secondary-level interventions can aim to build on the existing legal framework and statutory duties developed over the past 16 years. This relies on the effective and timely intervention by authorities trained in supporting victims of crime and their particular psychological needs, such as the expansion of sensitive and focused screening for victims of domestic violence and coercive control.

Tertiary-level interventions can be structured along a two-pronged approach: support for the victims of violence and effective interventions for the perpetrators. As can be seen in the list of resources, there are a number of governmental and third-sector organisations in place to support victims. The vast majority are aimed at women, with only three services dedicated to male victims. This is likely due to men being disproportionally convicted of being the perpetrators of violent offences. Further research is needed, however, to explore what impact this resource disparity may have on male victims seeking help, alongside possible internalised sexist biases. As well as male victims of violence, elderly abuse victims, victims of abuse by caregivers, human trafficking victims and victims of honour-based violence are examples of groups that are at risk of being missed by the healthcare system. Further efforts are required to learn how to best support these victims [43].

It is also notable that there is a paucity of available resources providing specialist interventions to the perpetrators of violence; it is estimated that only 1% of perpetrators will have access to such support. The Drive Project is a new multi-agency intervention targeted at domestic violence perpetrators that has recently completed a three-year pilot. Preliminary findings have been encouraging, demonstrating a reduction in physical and sexual abuse alongside harassment and coercive control [44]. The further development of such interventions at this level would form part of the tertiary strategy against violence and in turn aid in supporting risk minimisation measures for the victims of these offences. There is evidence to support interventions provided by specialist units such as Grendon therapeutic community prison [45], the Millfields Unit [46] and the Portman clinic [47, 48]. This is an area that remains underdeveloped.

In considering the above, a common thread is apparent: without significant and sustained financial investment, these interventions are unlikely to achieve the outcomes that are hoped.

Conclusion

In contrast to public perception, people with severe mental illness (SMI) are more likely to be victims of violent and non-violent crime than they are perpetrators. They are also at a higher risk of violence than the general population, with women with SMI being particularly vulnerable.

Violence often devastates the lives of affected individuals, families and communities and may leave a lasting impact on both perpetrators and their victims. Identification and early intervention strategies and the provision of effective care and support for victims of violence are essential if the risk of re-victimisation and, in some cases, perpetration of violence are to be reduced.

Violence disproportionately impacts the most deprived communities. Public health principles provide a useful framework to understand the causes and impact of violence and a public health approach is required to tackle violent crime.

The most recent version of the Victims' Code acknowledges that those who are the victims of the most serious crimes are more likely to require specialised assistance.

List of Resources

Below is a list of organisations that victims of crime can contact for advice and support.

General: Governmental and Devolved Nations

Name	Contact Details	Information
Community Safety Partnerships (CSPs)	www.gov.uk/govern ment/publications/com munity-safety-partnerships-contact-details	CSPs are made up of five responsible authorities: police, local authority, fire and rescue authority, probation provider and clinical commissioning groups. This website provides more information and advises on how to get in touch with your local community safety unit.
Directory and Book Services (DABS)	www.dabs.uk.com/the-directory-2	DABS is a not-for-profit organisation that

(cont.)

Name	Contact Details	Information
		produces a national resource directory of charities and organisations throughout the UK and Ireland working to support victims of abuse and sexual violence.
Foreign and Commonwealth Office	www.gov.uk/victim-crime-abroad Telephone: 020 7008 1500	Support for British victims of crime perpetrated outside the UK.
Home Office	www.gov.uk/get-support-as-a-victim-of-crime	This is the website for the UK government. Provides links to victim information, Victim Contact Scheme and restorative justice for victims of crime in England and Wales.
Ministry of Justice	www.victimandwitnessinformation.org.uk/ Telephone: 0808 168 9293	Information for victims and witnesses of crime in England and Wales.
Mygov.scot	www.mygov.scot/victim-witness-support/	Online resource for people in Scotland to access public services. Provides links to support services after a crime, support through court proceedings and practical information for victims of crime in Scotland.
NIdirect	www.nidirect.gov.uk/articles/support-services-victims	The official government website for Northern Ireland citizens Provides a range of support services for victims of crime in Northern Ireland.

HM Prison Service

Name	Contact Details	Information
HM Prison and Probation Service (HMPPS)	victim.helpline@justice.gov.uk Telephone: 0300 060 6699	Contact the Victims Helpline for any unwanted contact from a prisoner

Third-Sector Organisations: National Resources for Victims of Crime

Name	Contact Details	Information
Catch-22	www.catch-22.org.uk/victims/	This is a national not-for-profit business with a broad range of work. They provide services for victims, including emotional and practical support.
Victim Support	www.victimsupport.org.uk Telephone: 08 08 16 89 111 Available 24 hours a day throughout the year	This is an independent charity providing free advice and support for people affected by crime. They also advocate victims' rights by conducting research, creating reports and advocating changes to national policy.

Mediation, Conflict Resolution and Restorative Justice

Name	Contact Details	Information
Crime Concern UK	www.crimeconcernuk.net Telephone: 01206 868359	A national crime reduction charity which provides mediation, restorative justice and professional witness services.
The Restorative Justice Council (RJC)	https://restorativejustice.org.uk/do-you-need-restorative-justice	The RJC is the membership body for restorative practice. The group aims to empower victims by giving them an opportunity to communicate the impact of crime to the perpetrators. This website provides more information and links to local groups.

Linking Abuse and Recovery Through Advocacy for Victims and Perpetrators (LARA-VP)

LARA-VP is an excellent online guide to help mental health professionals identify and respond to domestic violence and abuse (DVA) [49].

LARA-VP	www.kcl.ac.uk/mental-health-and-psychological-sciences/assets/lara-vp-online-resource.pdf
Appendix 5	Provides details of services for women experiencing DVA.
Appendix 6	Details of services for men experiencing DVA.
Appendix 7	Details of services for Lesbian Gay Bisexual, Transgender and related communities (LGBTQ+) people who are experiencing DVA.
Appendix 8	Details of services for Black and Minority Ethnic (BAME) people experiencing DVA.
Appendix 9	Details of services for children and young people experiencing DVA.

Women's Services: Sexual Violence or Domestic Abuse

Name	Contact Details	Information
Black Association of Women Step Out (BAWSO)	https://bawso.org.uk/en/ Telephone: 0800 731 8147 Website at time of writing under maintenance. Helpline functioning.	BAWSO is a Welsh organisation providing support and temporary accommodation for those affected by domestic abuse, female genital mutilation, forced marriage, honour-based violence, human trafficking and modern slavery.
Jewish Women's Aid (JWA)	www.jwa.org.uk Telephone: 0808 801 0500	JWA is an organisation that supports Jewish women and children affected by domestic abuse and sexual violence across the UK.
Live Fear Free	https://gov.wales/live-fear-free/contact-live-fear-free Telephone: 0808 80 10 800	This is a service provided by the Welsh government for women experiencing domestic abuse.
Rape Crisis Federation	www.rapecrisis.org.uk Telephone: 0808 802 9999	National voice for female survivors of sexual violence and abuse in England and Wales. It provides specialist advice and support.
	www.rapecrisisscotland.org.uk/ Telephone: 08088 01 03 02	As above, for Scotland.

(cont.)

Name	Contact Details	Information
	www.rcni.ie/ Telephone: 1800 778888	As above, for Northern Ireland and the Republic of Ireland.
	https://jaar.je/ Telephone: 01534 482800	As above, for Jersey.
Refuge	www.refuge.org.uk National Domestic Abuse Help Line: 0808 2000 247	Refuge is a charity aimed at supporting women and children victimised by domestic violence. They provide a range of services, including emergency accommodation, community outreach support and advocacy. They also lobby government and advocate for change in policies and legislations.
Rights of Women	www.rightsofwomen.org.uk	Charity that provides free legal advice for women on a broad range of areas, including family, criminal, immigration and asylum law as well as advice on sexual harassment at work. For England and Wales.
Southall Black Sisters	www.southallblacksisters.org.uk Telephone: 020 8571 9595	This is an organisation in West London that provides for women in London who have experienced gender-based violence.
The Kiran Project	http://kiranss.org.uk/ Telephone: 020 8558 1986	The Kiran Project provides support and temporary accommodation to Asian women and children who have experienced domestic violence and abuse.
Women's Aid	www.womensaid.org.uk/	National charity working to end domestic violence against women and children. They provide a broad range of resources for victims in England.
	https://womensaid.scot/ Scotland's Domestic Abuse and Forced Marriage Help line: 0800 027 1234	As above, for Scotland.
	www.welshwomensaid.org.uk/	As above, for Wales.
	www.womensaidni.org/	As above, for Northern Ireland.

Men's Services: Sexual Violence or Domestic Abuse

Name	Contact Details	Information
ManKind	www.mankind.org.uk/ Telephone: 01823 334244	Provides a helpline, support services and information to male victims of domestic abuse and domestic violence.
Men's Advice Line	https://mensadviceline.org.uk/ Telephone: 0808 8010327	A confidential helpline for male victims of domestic abuse and those supporting them.
Survivors UK	www.survivorsuk.org Telephone: 02035983898	Supports and provides resources for men who have experienced any form of sexual violence. They are an inclusive service and provide support for anyone who identifies as male.

Children and Child Abuse

Name	Contact Details	Information
Children Experiencing Domestic Abuse Recovery (CEDAR)	www .cedarnetwork.org.uk/ho w-to-access-cedar/	This is a Scottish organisation supporting the recovery of children who experienced domestic abuse.
Childline	www.childline.org.uk/ge t-support/	Childline is a service provided by the NSPCC. It provides a phone line, online messaging and email platform for anyone under the age of 19 in the UK.
The National Association for People Abused in Childhood (NAPAC)	https://napac.org.uk/oth er-support/ Telephone: 0808 801 0331	NAPAC offers support to adult survivors of childhood abuse.
The National Society for the Prevention of Cruelty to Children (NSPCC)	www.nspcc.org.uk/what-you-can-do/get-advice-and-support/ Telephone: 0808 800 500	The NSPCC can be contacted for help or advice if you are worried about a child.

Lesbian, Gay, Bisexual, Transgender, Queer or Questioning and Other Identities (LGBTQ+): Specific Support

Name	Contact Details	Information
Stonewall	www.stonewall.org.uk/help-and-advice Telephone: 0800 0502020 www.stonewall.org.uk/domestic-violence-and-abuse-resources-lgbt-people	Information and support for LGBTQ+ community. Domestic violence and abuse – resources for LGBTQ+ people.
Galop (previously known as Broken Rainbow)	www.galop.org.uk/ Telephone: 0800 999 5428	This is a national LGBTQ+ charity that provides advice and support for victims of domestic violence.

Refugees and Asylum Seekers: Specific Support

Name	Contact Details	Information
Freedom from Torture	www.freedomfromtorture.org Telephone: 0207 697 7777	A charity providing therapy and support to torture survivors.
Helen Bamber Foundation	www.helenbamber.org Telephone: 0203 058 2020	Human rights charity providing support to asylum-seekers and refugees who are survivors of extreme human cruelty.

Disability Support Services: Specific Support

Name	Contact Details	Information
Respond	www.respond.org.uk Telephone: 0207 383 0700	A charity for children and adults with learning disabilities who have experienced abuse or trauma.
Apna Ghar Housing Association	www.agha.org.uk Telephone: 020 8795 5405	Housing association for people with disabilities.
Stay Safe East	www.staysafe-east.org.uk Telephone: 0208 519 7241	Charity operating in East London supporting adults and families with disabilities who experience hate crime, domestic or sexual abuse.

Support for Perpetrators of Violence

Name	Contact Details	Information
Respect	https://respectphoneline.org.uk Telephone: 0808 802 40 40	This is charity funded by the Home Office, Government of Scotland and Northern Ireland's Department of Justice. It runs a confidential helpline for domestic abuse perpetrators. Respect provide training and accreditation to smaller, regional charities. The complete list is available on their website.
Selected Respect Accredited Services		
Ahimsa	www.ahimsa.org.uk Telephone: 01752 213535	Run specialist intervention programmes for perpetrators of domestic violence and abuse in the Devon & Cornwall area.
The Change Project	www.thechange-project.org Telephone: 01245 258680	Offer group interventions for domestic abuse perpetrators in Essex, Hertfordshire and Norfolk.
The Evolve Programme (run by Eve)	https://eveda.org.uk Telephone: 01604 230 577	The Evolve programme is run by Eve, a domestic violence support and prevention charity. Evolve is a behavioural change programme for perpetrators of domestic violence.
Harbour	www.myharbour.org.uk Telephone: 03000 20 25 25 25	A charity providing support to perpetrators of domestic violence and abuse in the North of England.
Relate Cymru	www.relate.org.uk/cymru/ help-domestic-violence Telephone: 0300 003 2340	Relate is a charity offering the Choose2Change Programme for perpetrators living in Wales.
Rise	www.risemutual.org Telephone: 07495 099694	Rise offer a Ministry of Justice accredited intervention for perpetrators of violence. The programme, called Building Better Relationships, is delivered in London.
Talk, Listen, Change	www.talklistenchange.org.uk Telephone: 0161 872 1100	Offers a range of violence prevention programmes for men and women living in Manchester, Stockport and Salford.

References

1. Corrigan, P. How stigma interferes with mental health care. *American Psychologist* 2004; 59(7):614–25.

2. Fazel, S., Gulati, G., Linsell, L., Geddes, J.R., Grann, M. Schizophrenia and violence: Systematic review and meta-analysis. *PLOS Med* 2009; 6(8): e1000120.

3. Putkonen, A., Kotilainen, I., Joyal, C. C. and Tiihonen, J. Comorbid personality disorders and substance use disorders of mentally ill homicide offenders: a structured clinical study on dual and triple diagnoses. *Schizophrenia Bulletin* 2004; 30:59–72.

4. Pettitt, B., Greenhead, S., Khalifeh, H. et al. At risk, yet dismissed: The criminal victimisation of people with mental health problems. [online]: www.mind.org.uk/me dia-a/4121/at-risk-yet-dismissed-report.pdf [Accessed 12.5.2022].

5. Hind, K., Oram, S., Osborn, D., Howard, L. M. and Johnson, S. Recent physical and sexual violence against adults with severe mental illness: A systematic review and meta-analysis. *International Review of Psychiatry* 2016; 28(5):433–51.

6. Bhavsar, V., Dean, K., Hatch, S. L., MacCabe, J. H. and Hotopf, M. Psychiatric symptoms and risk of victimisation: a population-based study from Southeast London. *Epidemiology and Psychiatric Sciences* 2019; 28(2):168–78.

7. Lam, J. A., Rosenheck, R. The effect of victimization on clinical outcomes of homeless persons with serious mental illness. *Psychiatric Services* 1998; 49(5):678–83.

8. Devries, K. M., Mak, J. Y., Bacchus, L. J. et al. Intimate partner violence and incident depressive symptoms and suicide attempts: A systematic review of longitudinal studies. *PLOS Med* 2013;10(5):e1001439.

9. Choe, J. Y., Teplin, L. A., Abram, K. M. Perpetration of violence, violent victimization, and severe mental illness: Balancing public health concerns. *Psychiatric Services* 2008;59(2):153–64.

10. Bhavsar, V. and Ventriglio, A. Violence, victimisation and mental health.

11. Yahya, A. S., Khawaja, S. and Chukwuma, J. Association of COVID-19 with intimate partner violence. *Primary Care Companion for CNS Disorders* 2020;22 (3):20com02634.

12. Bradley, N. L., DiPasquale, A. M., Dillabough, K. and Schneider, P. S. Healthcare practitioners' responsibility to address intimate partner violence related to the COVID-19 pandemic. *Canadian Medical Association Journal* 2020;192(22): E609–E610.

13. Gulati, G. and Kelly, B. D. Domestic violence against women and the COVID-19 pandemic: What is the role of psychiatry? *International Journal of Law Psychiatry* 2020;71:101594. https://doi.org/10.1016/j.ijlp.2020.101594.

14. Senior, M., Fazel, S. and Tsiachristas, A. The economic impact of violence perpetration in severe mental illness: a retrospective, prevalence-based analysis in England and Wales. *Lancet Public Health* 2020;5(2):e99–106.

15. Department of Health, NHS (UK). Protecting people Promoting health: A public health approach to violence prevention for England. [online]: https://assets.publishing.service.gov.uk/government/uploads/system/uploads/attachment_data/file/216977/Violence-prevention.pdf [Accessed 12.5.2022].

16. World Health Organisation. Forty-ninth WHO Assembly Resolutions and decisions annexes. 2016. [online]. https://apps.who.int/iris/bitstream/handle/10665/178941/WHA49_1996-REC-1_eng.pdf [Accessed 12.5.2022].

17. World Health Organization. The Violence Prevention Alliance (VPA) approach. [online]. www.who.int/groups/violence-prevention-alliance/approach [Accessed 12.5.2022].

18. Home Office. The Domestic Violence, Crime and Victims Act 2004. March 2005. [online]. www.gov.uk/government/publica

International Journal of Social Psychiatry 2017;63(6):475–9.

tions/the-domestic-violence-crime-and-victims-act-2004 [Accessed 12.5.2022].

19. Victims Commissioner. Role of the Victims' Commissioner. [online]. https://victimscommissioner.org.uk/victims-commissioner [Accessed 12.5.2022].

20. Ministry of Justice. Statutory guidance. The Code of Practice for Victims of Crime in England and Wales and supporting public information materials. [online]. www.cps.gov.uk/sites/default/files/documents/legal_guidance/OD_000049.pdf [Accessed 12.5.2022].

21. Association of Police and Crime Commissioners. The role of the Police and Crime Commissioner. [online]. www.apccs.police.uk/role-of-the-pcc/ [Accessed 12.5.2022].

22. Home Office. Local forums and the role of Police and Crime Commissioners. 30 May 2019. [online]. www.gov.uk/government/publications/police-and-crime-commissioners-engagement-protocols/local-forums-and-the-role-of-police-and-crime-commissioners [Accessed 12.5.2022].

23. Ministry of Justice. 'Victims Strategy'. 10 September 2018. [online]. www.gov.uk/government/publications/victims-strategy [Accessed 12.5.2022].

24. HM Government. Serious Violence Strategy. April 2018. [online]. https://assets.publishing.service.gov.uk/government/uploads/system/uploads/attachment_data/file/698009/serious-violence-strategy.pdf [Accessed 12.5.2022].

25. House of Commons Library. How is the Government implementing a 'public health approach' to serious violence? July 2019. [online]. https://commonslibrary.parliament.uk/home-affairs/crime/how-is-the-government-implementing-a-public-health-approach-to-serious-violence [Accessed 12.5.2022].

26. Prime Minister's Office, 10 Downing Street. December 2019. Her Majesty's most gracious speech to both Houses of Parliament. [online]. www.gov.uk/government/speeches/queens-speech-december-2019 [Accessed 12.5.2022].

27. Krug, E. G., Dahlberg, L. L., Mercy, J. A., Zwi, A. B. and Lozano, R. World report on violence and health. Geneva, World Health Organization (2002) [online]. https://apps.who.int/iris/bitstream/handle/10665/42495/9241545615_eng.pdf,jsessionid=F6FA31118E2A84B9560E381C24F5C0F6?sequence=1 [Accessed 12.5.2022].

28. Holt, V. L., Kernic, M. A., Wolf, M. E. et al. Do protection orders affect the likelihood of future partner violence and injury? *American Journal of Preventive Medicine* 2003;24(1):16–21.

29. Crown Prosecution Service (UK). Specialist domestic violence courts review 2007–08. [online]. www.cps.gov.uk/sites/default/files/documents/publications/sdvc_review_2007-08_justice_and_safety.pdf [Accessed 12.5.2022].

30. Avail Consulting. No Witness, No Justice (NWNJ) pilot evaluation. Executive summary. Avail Consulting, London. 2004. [online]. www.yumpu.com/en/document/view/37527934/no-witness-no-justice-nwnj-pilot-evaluation-executive-summary [Accessed 12.5.2022].

31. Department of Health & Social Care. Stronger Protection from Violence for NHS staff, gov.uk. [online] www.gov.uk/government/news/stronger-protection-from-violence-for-nhs-staff [Accessed 12.5.2022]

32. NHS Staff Survey 2019: National Results Briefing (Survey Coordination Centre). [online] www.nhsstaffsurveys.com/Caches/Files/ST19_National%20briefing_FINAL%20V2.pdf [Accessed 12.5.2022].

33. Centre for Public Health, Liverpool JMU & World Health Organisation (WHO). Violence Prevention: The Evidence. reducing violence through victim identification, care and support programmes. [online]: https://apps.who.int/iris/handle/10665/44176 [Accessed 12.5.2022].

34. Feder, G., Davies, R.A., Baird, K. et al. Identification and Referral to Improve Safety (IRIS) of women experiencing domestic violence with a primary care training and support programme: a cluster

randomised controlled trial. *The Lancet* 2011;378(9805):1788–95.

35. Rujine, R. E., Howard, L. M., Trevillion, K. et al. Detection of domestic violence by community mental health teams: A multi-centre, cluster randomised controlled trial. *BMC Psychiatry* 2017;17(1):288.

36. Oram, S., Khalifeh, H., Howard, L. M. Violence against women and mental health. *Lancet Psychiatry* 2017;4(2):159–70.

37. Hameed, M., O'Doherty, L., Gilchrist, G. et al. Psychological therapies for women who experience intimate partner violence. *Cochrane Database of Systematic Reviews* 2020, Issue 7. Art. No.: CD013017. https://doi.org/10.1002/14651858.CD013017.pub2.

38. Keynejad, R. C., Hanlon, C. and Howard, L. M. Psychological interventions for common mental disorders in women experiencing intimate partner violence in low-income and middle-income countries: A systematic review and meta-analysis. *The Lancet Psychiatry* 7(2)2020:173–90. https://doi.org/10.1016/S2215-0366(19)30510-3.

39. Robinson, A. L. and Tregidga, J. The perceptions of high-risk victims of domestic violence to a coordinated community response in Cardiff, Wales. *Violence Against Women* 2007;13 (11):1130–48.

40. Eogan, M., McHugh, A. and Holohan, M. The role of the sexual assault centre. *Best Practice & Research Clinical Obstetrics & Gynaecology* 2013;27(1):47–58.

41. Fergusson, D. M., Grant, H., Horwood, L. J. and Ridder, E. M. Randomised trial of the early state program of home visitation. *Paediatrics* 2005;116(6): e803–e809.

42. Carastathis, A. The politics of austerity and the affective economy of hostility: racialised gendered violence and crises of belonging in Greece. *Feminist Review* 2015;109(1), 73–95. https://doi.org/10.1057/fr.2014.50

43. Viergever, R. F., Thorogood, N., Wolf, J. R. L. M. and Durand, M. A. Supporting ALL victims of violence, abuse, neglect of exploitation: Guidance for health providers. *BMC International Health and Human Rights* (2018;18:39.

44. Marianne Hester, M., Eisenstadt, N., Ortega-Avila, A. et al. Evaluation of the Drive Project. A three-year pilot to address high-risk, high-harm perpetrators of domestic abuse. 2020. University of Bristol. [online]. http://driveproject.org.uk/wp-content/uploads/2020/02/Executive-Summary_Final2020.pdf [Accessed 12.5.2022].

45. Bennett, J. and Shuker, R. The potential of prison-based democratic therapeutic communities. *International Journal of Prison Health* 2017,13(1):19–24. https://doi.org/10.1108/IJPH-08-2016-0036.

46. Freestone, M., Taylor, C., Milsom, S. et al. Assessments and admissions during the first 6 years of a UK medium secure DSPD service. *Criminal Behavior and Mental Health* 2012;22(2):91–107. https://doi.org/10.1002/cbm.1823.

47. Adshead, G., Moore, E., Humphrey, M., Wilson, C. and Tapp, J. The role of mentalising in the management of violence. *Advances in Psychiatric Treatment* 2013;Jan. 19(1):67–76.

48. Yakeley, J. (2014) Mentalization-based group treatment for antisocial personality disorder. In *Forensic Group Psychotherapy. The Portman Papers*. London: Karnac, pp. 151–82. ISBN 9781780490496.

49. Yapp, E. J., Oram, S., Lempp, H. K. et al. LARA-VP: A resource to help mental health professionals identify and respond to domestic violence and abuse (DVA). King's College London. [online]. 2018. www.kcl.ac.uk/mental-health-and-psychological-sciences/assets/lara-vp-online-resource.pdf [Accessed 12.5.2022].

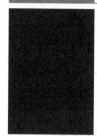

Introduction to Section 6

Section 6: Opinions, Attitudes, Support and Engagement

The final two chapters add a more personal touch to the book. When there are so many directives, requirements, management advice and instructions around the subject of violence we must not forget that each episode represents a common universal experience, one in which many feelings are engendered, from deep hurt to anger. The staff exposed to violence need emotional and practical support too, and the initiatives in these concluding chapters show that these can be provided by many who are conventionally 'outside the system'. Looking at a problem with completely fresh eyes can often be an enormous help. It offers a new sense of direction, better understanding and a more specifically personal impact that can help resolution. Together, these accounts end the book on a note of quiet optimism. Oh brave new world, that has such people in it – long may they thrive.

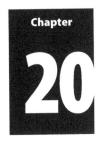

Chapter

20

An Account of Service Users' Involvement in Training Delivery on the Prevention and Management of Violence and Aggression: The Impact on Practice

Jane Obi-Udeaja, Kate Crosby and Garry Ryan

Introduction

This chapter is divided into two parts. The first part discusses service user (SU) involvement in training and describes the involvement of mental health service users (SUs) in the development and delivery of a short training course on the prevention and management of violence and aggression (PMVA) at Middlesex University. It considers the impact of training with SUs who themselves have experienced being restrained in acute mental health settings from the perspectives of course participants and the SU trainers. The account given by the SU trainers is supported by a description of the outcome of a research study (discussed in the second part of the chapter) carried out by a member of the PMVA training team. The aim of the research study was to trace the outcome of the SU contribution to the training onto the hospital wards in order to determine what influence (if any) it had on staff practice.

It is acknowledged that the accounts of the SUs are anecdotal; they are their individual and subjective experiences. In the setting, however, the training participants are the providers of care for the SU trainers. Amongst them, therefore, could be the staff members who participated in the restraint scenarios being described by the SU trainers. In that situation, one would assume it would be unlikely that the SU trainers would deliberately distort facts. Additionally, the narration is specifically about the PMVA training as provided at Middlesex University. It makes no claim whatsoever as regards any other training provision or setting. The reader is invited to read, compare and make their own judgement with regard to similarities and therefore lessons, if any, to take away.

Background

There is a growing understanding of the important contribution that SUs can make to the development of the mental health practitioners that care for them [1–4]. The expanding body of literature [5–8] exploring the subject area is an indication of the current interest on

The authors of this chapter are members of the prevention and management of violence and aggression (PMVA) training team at Middlesex University London. The team comprises staff members of the university and mental health service users.

user and carer involvement in the education and training of health and social care professionals. In the United Kingdom, Higher education institutions are mandated by policies and guidelines to involve users of services in the education and training of the health and social care professionals [9–11]. For example, the Nursing and Midwifery Council's new standards for nurse education require providers to demonstrate user involvement activities and student nurses to show user-involvement skills in practice [11]. Indeed, significant literature and reviews [5, 12, 13] have emerged confirming that SU involvement has become the norm in mental health education and training.

The involvement of users of services and carers in the training of social and healthcare practitioners in normal teaching and learning settings has become a common practice and a mandatory requirement. However, their involvement in PMVA training, a unique subject area, is a new phenomenon.

The General Services Association (GSA) [14] model is recognised as one of the leading models in PMVA training, and this is the model that we provide to mental health inpatient staff of the local NHS hospital trusts and to the university's final year mental health nursing students. The model is guided by recommendations made in the National Institute for Health and Care Excellence (NICE) guidance (NG10) [9] for dealing with violent situations before, during and after they occur. NG10 offers specific guidance on prevention and de-escalation through to safe interventions and post-incident debrief. The theoretical component of the GSA model lays emphasis on prevention and de-escalation, achieved mainly through assessment and effective communication. The physical component describes a hierarchy of holds that runs from low level to high level. This enables staff to choose the holds most appropriate to the patient's level of agitation. Efforts to de-escalate the situation should continue throughout the process.

PMVA training at Middlesex University is delivered in a non-operational setting away from the ward environment. As trainers, the team recognise the potential rift between the theoretical principles emphasised in training and the staff practice on the ward. An example of this theory–practice gap is the varying practices of 'field modification' of restraint techniques which can occur for various reasons, including fear, as noted by Terkelsen and Larsen [15] and by Paterson [16]. One of the ways that the team try to bridge the rift is by inviting mental health SUs living in the community, who have experienced being restrained during a hospital admission, to join them in delivering the training. The SU element of the training enables the course participants to have a face-to-face discussion with the service users. Repper and Breeze [17] offer 'tentative evidence' (p. 1) that involving SUs in the education of mental health practitioners is important for providing students with the opportunity to develop greater awareness and understanding through the unique insights of people's lived experience of mental health conditions. The SU session is developed on the principle of active interaction with the course participants. It uses their lived experience of physical restraint to inform course participants to adopt a patient and caring approach, especially when managing patients' anger and aggression on the ward. Their contribution to the training since they joined the PMVA team in 2008 has consistently earned positive feedback from course participants.

Service User Involvement: Is It All Tokenistic?

The value of SU involvement, either in service development and delivery or in the education and training of health and social care professionals, continues to be questioned [2, 18, 19]. There is even a lack of consensus about what constitutes meaningful

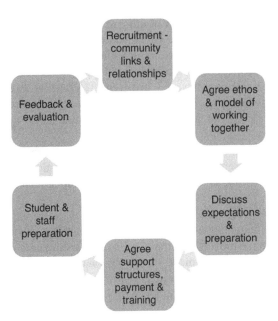

Figure 20.1 Essential processes in the cycle of user and carer involvement. Modified from Terry [19] (p. 203)

involvement [20]. There is also a concern that such involvement, particularly in the education and training of the professionals who care for them, is nought but rhetoric. In other words, there is suspicion about the genuineness of such involvement and how balanced the powers of the parties are in those situations. To mitigate such concern, Gilburt et al. [21] used emancipatory/user-led research to ensure a balance of power between the SU researchers and the SU research participants in their study. The point here is to emphasise that the onus is on the training providers to prove that their SU involvement is genuine. Authors including Terry [19] and Tew et al. [4] recommend criteria for achieving genuine and productive user involvement. Our team's SU involvement activities are mapped against what the staff and service users in Terry's study [19] consider as the prerequisite processes and good practice for effective involvement. This is intended to enable readers to judge for themselves whether the SUs' involvement in our training delivery is genuine or not. Figure 20.1 shows the criteria, as explained in Terry [19].

PMVA Service User Involvement in PMVA Training – How We Did It

Initial Recruitment of a Service User

The Middlesex University PMVA team's co-training with SUs started in 2008 when members of the team decided to find out whether any of the SUs already engaged in the mental health department's teaching and learning activities had experienced being physically restrained. Would such individuals want to join the PMVA team in order to share their experiences with course participants? One of the SUs had been physically restrained and was keen to work with the PMVA team.

Recruitment: Community Links and Relationships

As explained earlier, the first SU trainer was subsequently recruited through the existing SU educators on the mental health nurse training programmes at Middlesex University. The second SU trainer was recruited when the PMVA team co-ordinator visited a local community centre for African-Caribbean mental health SUs to specifically seek representation from this group. Studies including that carried out by Browne [22] for the Campaign for Racial Equality and the Mental Health Act Commission found that 75% of all professionals interviewed thought that Black clients were more likely to be seen as dangerous. By purposely recruiting from this ethnic group, the intention was to better reflect the perceptions and experiences of staff and SUs on the inpatient units.

Agreed Ethos and Model of Working Together

Prior to the first SU joining the team, a meeting was arranged between her and two staff members of PMVA team. Some of the staff members on the team had been concerned that the SUs might use the training opportunity to only express their anger about physical restraint. On the contrary: this particular SU had a very balanced view. In the meeting, she talked about her positive and negative experiences of being restrained. The tutors were impressed and were convinced that such a balanced and touching perspective would support the philosophy that lay behind the GSA model of training. Initially, a slot of one hour for each SU session was proposed, but to allow flexibility more or less time was allowed – the longer period being chosen when two users facilitated together. The hope was that participants on the course would benefit most from any flexibility they had introduced.

Expectations and Preparations

The first SU was very experienced and an active member of the local community user groups. Because she was already involved in teaching and learning activities in the university, she needed minimal induction. Our proposed training and team function were explained to her. Potential challenges and difficulties were discussed and considered. For example, we were concerned that sharing and discussing her restraint experiences with practitioners on the course might leave her feeling vulnerable, especially as some of the practitioners on the course worked within the trust where she received her care and treatment. However, she was satisfied with the questions and gave positive answers.

Support Structure, Payment and Training

The first SU's strong educational background, her positive experiences of involvement in other aspects of teaching and learning at the university, especially teaching pre-registration nurses, and the support and reflective feedback after these sessions boosted her confidence about the PMVA training role. Subsequently, she volunteered to mentor the second SU trainer when he joined the team. The second SU trainer, although very keen to share his experiences of being physically restrained, was initially anxious about the prospect as he had not been previously involved in a similar role in a higher institution. Interestingly, the support and reassurances from the staff members of the team did little to soothe his anxiety. But the moment the first SU took him under her wings, he became a different person. The two have worked consistently together ever since. They regularly update and modify their delivery approach for greater impact. When they first started on the training, they used to go straight into sharing their experiences of being restrained on the wards. Led by the more experienced colleague, they continue to modify, tweak, update and enrich both the content and their style of delivery to suit the audience. They appear driven by their sole motivation for joining the PMVA training team which, according to them, is to help in bringing about positive changes in the use of physical restraint.

Student and Staff Preparation

The PMVA training is a short course that runs consecutively from Monday to Friday. The SU session is on the final day of the course. Students on the course are informed about the session during their introduction to the course on the first day. This information is also contained in the course programme. In the early days of the SUs' involvement, the PMVA staff trainers used to sit in the session as a gesture of support. Now, the SU trainers prefer the staff not to sit in. They seem convinced that the course participants will talk with less inhibition if the staff trainers are not in the room. In effect, our SU colleagues have control over both the content and the style of delivery of their session. An example of their demonstration of this control was when, at an international conference in Dublin, we had a well-prepared and well-rehearsed PowerPoint presentation. Just before we went in, one of the SU trainers suggested that we should go in and assess our audience first, adding that if we could stimulate them for a lively interactive session then we would use the power point selectively to support the discussion. That was exactly what we did and the delegates, in the words of the conference chairman, 'were blown away'.

Challenges Encountered

Delivering the training with SUs comes with occasional challenges. For example, the SU trainers are occasionally unavailable for training. Flexibility in such situations enables alteration of the time and/or the day of their session to suit them. Our two colleagues may also decide that one instead of both come in to run the session. Because the two SUs that started this training complement each other very well and are totally committed to the course, the team is yet to make a concerted effort to recruit more SUs. Other challenges are discussed later in the chapter.

Service Users' Description of Their Experience of Participating in the Delivery of the PMVA Training

Box 20.1 contains the SUs' moving description of their experience of participating in the delivery of the PMVA training.

Food for Thought

The SUs' account raised questions for us. Do the staff take seriously the lessons from their session? Do they make the effort to implement them? Does the contribution of the SUs actually make a difference to staff practice on the ward? In the search for answers to these questions, a member of the PMVA team decided to research the phenomenon. The final section presents a brief account of the research project which she carried out for the partial fulfilment of her doctoral degree. The account offers insight into the value of SU involvement in PMVA training.

Box 20.1 Service Users' Account of Being Involved in the PMVA Training

Introduction

I am writing this with some trepidation. I know that there are many within my community who disagree and feel very strongly about restraint and control. I too have issues around this. I firmly believe that 99.9999% of all restraints that happen on a mental health ward should not have occurred. Which is why I got involved in the PMVA training delivered to qualified and soon-to-be qualified staff.

I am a woman who uses and at times has been forced to use mental health services. I have had a long career both as a service user of mental health services and as an advocate and service user trainer. There have been many changes – good and bad – within the services, but restraint and control are still very much in use and although I have no concrete evidence, I feel they can be and are often used as a means to subdue individuals/to punish us.

I strongly believe that if the use of restraint is to be drastically reduced then mental health service users who have been on the receiving end need to tell their stories.

How I Became Involved With the PMVA Training

For many years now, I have been involved with Middlesex University, helping to train student nurses. In 2008, a member of the Middlesex University PMVA training team approached the service users involved at Middlesex University and asked if anyone was interested in meeting with her to discuss having some form of service user input into the 5-day PMVA training.

I have experienced restraint; one was very humiliating and definitely was a means to punish and control me. However, on another occasion I have been restrained and I am convinced that had that not been the case I would no longer be on this earth. Having experienced what I would term 'good' and 'bad' restraints is why I feel it is so important to be part of a team who delivers the PMVA to mental health staff. So, I put myself forward.

Shortly after I started, another colleague joined me: a young African-Caribbean man who also has been restrained by mental health staff.

Implications of Being Part of the PMVA Team

It was not an easy decision to make. Talking about ones' experience of being restrained and the effect this can have might be damaging and possibly dangerous to us service user trainers. The training is sometimes delivered to trust staff where we both receive care. Would that have a negative impact for us? What support would be available for us if we felt threatened, worried or if a session went badly? These and other issues have raised their ugly heads. Fortunately, this has been on very rare occasions, and we have had the full support of our colleagues within the team.

Most of our sessions have been very productive, and the participants taking part have been very appreciative.

How We Facilitate Our Sessions

We facilitate an hour-long session on the last day of the training. This hour is ours and it is up to us what we include and how we run it.

We like the session to be interactive and at times we have to agree to disagree. However, that is quite rare.

The participants can be qualified nursing staff or student nurses about to qualify. We start with first having a session exploring what makes the participants happy, sad, angry and frightened. We all experience these emotions. Most of us have similar examples of what makes us have these emotions. Interestingly when we give an example of what makes us angry – for example, someone invading our personal space in a queue to use the cash machine – all the participants can relate to that feeling of someone being too close and how irritating it can be.

Box 20.1 (cont.)

My service user colleague and I then give an example each of what we (and we do stress that this is our and only our experience) feel was a 'bad' and what was a 'good' restraint that was done to us. We ask the participants to identify why we felt that the 'bad' restraint was bad and vice versa for the 'good' restraint. Interestingly, the participants usually identify the same factors as to why we feel the restraint was 'good' or 'bad'.

We want staff to realise that the ward environment can influence how we can feel. No milk for a cup of tea but the staff in the office have tea! Would that not make you angry? Also, we want staff to realise that the way and reason for restraining us can influence how we as service users of mental health services view staff and how it can affect our very own recovery. The example I give of a particularly bad experience is one which to this day has affected me. I cannot go into that hospital where I was humiliated, punished and treated in an undignified way without feeling physically sick. Lucky, then, that I am no longer treated by that hospital!

What We Hope That Our Involvement Achieves

We both hope that by being involved in the training, staff seeing mental health service users well and delivering the training with the power reversed, those who make decisions around control and restraint will stop and think, 'oh that person has feelings and emotions and is a person who is frightened, scared, angry, etc.' And instead of resorting to physical restraint, greater effort is made to resolve problems by talking with patients.

Our Response on Tokenism

The reason I have stayed and been part of the PMVA training for so long is because of the support the other team members give us. I feel, and am made to feel, that my involvement is as important as theirs. If an issue were to occur during the session which affected us, we know that the team members are there, and we can approach them at any time if need be for support. The PMVA team have been invited to various conferences here and abroad to talk about service users being involved in the PMVA training and we have always been asked if we wish to be part of these. I have never been made to feel tokenistic.

WITHOUT SERVICE
USERS BEING INVOLVED
AND TELLING THEIR
STORIES THINGS MAY
NEVER CHANGE.

Research Project

The research project sought to find out whether the SUs' contribution to PMVA training delivery actually influenced staff management of patients' anger and aggression on the wards.

The researcher studied staff members' accounts of the impact on their practice when SUs are involved in staff training on PMVA in local NHS mental health inpatient wards. The contribution of SUs to the PMVA team's training had not previously been evaluated and the hope was that the findings might provide a further evidence base to support SU involvement in PMVA training delivery.

The research question was 'Do SUs make a sustainable contribution to mental health staff practice in the PMVA through active participation in training and development?'

The objectives were:

- To find out the training participants' perspectives on PMVA before the SU session.
- To identify changes in perspectives (if any) as a result of the training.
- To determine the implementation and sustainability of changed perspectives in practice.
- To identify from previous SU training evaluation records participants' intents to apply learning into practice.

A qualitative descriptive research design [23, 24] was adopted for the study. Purposive sampling was employed in selecting data sources (see Figure 20.2) who participated in the PMVA SU session and could talk about the experience [25]. Two focus group interviews of ten new mental health inpatient ward staff and ten mental health final year students were conducted. Semi-structured interviews of ten experienced mental health inpatient ward staff were carried out. A review of a sample from 111 records of feedback from previous PMVA training participants was carried out.

Tape-recorded responses from the participants were cross-checked with their signed written responses. The thematic analytical method [26–28] was used for the analysis. Collaboration, criticality and reflexivity were employed to enhance rigour [29]. Themes and categories were cross-checked against colleague's independently identified ones. Core themes and sub-themes were used to present the findings and to guide the discussion. Table 20.1 presents the analytical structure used in presenting the findings.

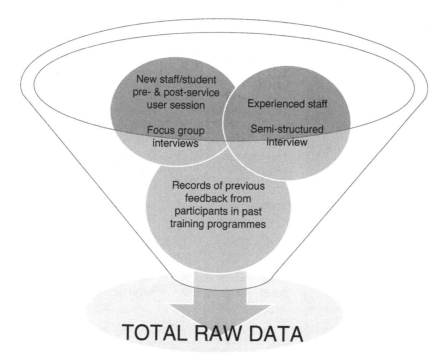

Figure 20.2 An illustration of the sources of data

The themes, sub-themes and candidate themes in Table 20.1 were derived from a combination of all the data sets. The contents of the table were followed in presenting the abundant materials from the findings [30, 31], of which the samples that follow are a very small fraction.

Sample of findings: The SU element of the PMVA training is a driven search for effective ways to prevent or at least reduce untoward incidents on mental health wards and, in so doing, avoid the need for physical restraint (PR). If PR has to happen, their involvement is also a search for ways to minimise the negative effects of PR on those involved (patients, staff and observers).

The SU contribution to the training is discussed across the themes (Table 20.1). The participants thought that their involvement was important because it enabled the practitioners to gain knowledge and insight into the views and feelings of the recipients of physical restraint (PR). The importance of getting alternative views of physical restraint, particularly from the recipients of PR themselves, was emphasised.

> I think it (SU contribution) gives a different perspective of what PMVA is about from the person who has actually being restrained. Because, in that situation emotions are heightened and people can be quite aroused and quite emotional and we are looking at it from our point of view as nurses ... But to actually hear it from their point of view ...
>
> (Roger, experienced staff, semi-structured interview)

Table 20.1 Themes, sub-themes and candidate themes

Themes	Sub-themes	Candidate themes
Mental health SUs contribution to PMVA training	An essential element of PMVA training	SUs contribution draws attention to patients' perspectives
		Their contribution is invaluable
	Translating learning into practice	SUs contribution affects people differently
		Their contribution is useful for practice
Working with patients	Engage with patient	Planning care with patients
		Effective communication
		Therapeutic relationship
	Preventing physical restraint (PR)	Minimising incidents
		Is PR inevitable?
		Debriefing
Challenges to implementation of SU contribution	Staffing issues	Staff issues
		Emergency Response Team
		Breakdown in Relationship
		Raising issues
	Policies	Policies
	Environmental issues	Environmental issues
	Additional relevant issues	Allied professionals

Source: Adapted from [26]

The SU contribution triggered thoughts about de-escalation and using PR as a last resort only. Expressing her thoughts, a new staff member responded:

Fabulous! Their experience really helped me to understand the effect restraints have on service users. But also helped me to acknowledge the importance of de-escalation and definitely using restraint as a last resort.   (Vicky, trust staff, focus group interview).

Some of the other issues that were emphasised by the SU trainers (such as debriefing after incidents) were practices that appeared uncommon in inpatient wards. Commenting on her new awareness, a participant said:

Yes, it has made me try to avoid using restraint. I always try to minimise, like if someone's not taking their medication, maybe give them a bit more time to think about it. Talk to them a bit more rather than just saying, 'Okay we need to give this medication now' and then call the team. It's also the de-brief as well. I've started doing that. I've started talking to patients after the restraint.   (Helen, experienced staff, semi-structured interview)

Helen went further to give an example of her debriefing practice which, according to her, was useful in retaining patient's trust:

Yeah, I've had to restrain someone and then I spoke to them afterwards and the trust wasn't broken ... They still respected me as a professional. I think because they understood why I had to do it. Instead of them thinking that I just did it because I could. There's a difference.
(Helen, experienced staff, semi-structured interview)

Overall, the study found that the participants were highly impressed by the confidence with which the SUs delivered their session, the rich and balanced content, as well as the interactive nature of the session. Each group of study participants expressed a resolve to implement the lessons from the session in their ward practice.

The new staff and students were determined to reflect lessons from the SU session in their practice:

It [the SU contribution] helps us to keep them in mind when we're restraining them because usually, when we do a restraint, it's more like about the safety of us and keeping the patient in control and in the ward. But now, when you go in, you think, 'Are they alright?' or 'How are they going to experience this?'   (Ada, trust staff, focus group interview)

Adding her voice, a student participant said:

And also, in the service user session we were talking about if the restraint is done in a communal area so all the other patients are watching. It's just about going to the patient who hasn't been restrained and saying 'are you okay'? They might feel scared of the nurses like 'oh it might happen to me if I don't do something' ... to reassure them.   (Lisa, student, focus group interview)

The experienced staff were reflecting lessons from the SU session in ward practices. A participant shared what the SU suggested could lessen the trauma of the experience and his adoption of the suggestion in his practice:

And he mentioned how to make it a better experience by letting him, if you're having to restrain a person or a service user, just letting him know what the process is, who you are and who the team is, and that has been what I have done throughout my practice. (Andy, experienced staff, semi-structured interview)

Asked whether the lesson from the SU session changed the way he treated all his patients on the ward, Sam said:

It does quite a lot. Because I try as much as possible to make it final, final, last resort before we get to the point of restraining ... I try and talk to them. I try and give them option of calming down. I tell them whatever I can to calm down the situation. It works out well as well. . . . at least they see you've tried and the next time it builds up rapport and forms that kind of therapeutic relationship ... (Sam, experienced staff, semi-structured interview)

The previous evaluation records held expressed intentions by the participants to reflect in practice lessons learnt from the SU session. A course participant said:

The service user session was the most interesting and helpful part of the whole training. Hearing a real-life experience who had one bad experience and one good experience of being restrained really ingrained the whole process of how to treat a patient with respect and dignity whilst keeping them safe, as well as the importance of attitude and communication especially after restraint. It is a thought I'll remember when working and I will encourage my colleagues to do the same. The service user said it took one person to talk to her and treat her well for her life to change. For that reason, I will always take on board what she said in the session.
(Angela, Record of Feedback)

Echoing this, another course participant said:

The SU session was excellent as I really like his presentation about lack of debriefing and how staff lack relationship with patients. The presentation has broadened my knowledge and I hope to go and practice what I have learnt from the session in the ward.
(Tasia, Record of Feedback)

There were challenges to the implementation of the SU contribution, such as staffing issues, environmental problems and policies.

Participants believed that problems directly linked to staffing at the work places tended to undermine their effort to practice as discussed in the training. They explained that their inability to give their best to patients was sometimes a direct result of staff shortage:

It's just to understand ... I know you cannot get it 100%, like getting to know a patient 100%. But I think we need to learn how to communicate more and shortage of staff does not help it. That's a big issue. (Susan, experienced staff, semi-structured interview)

Reiterating, another participant said:

I definitely agree with the communication part because I feel like the level of contact with the patient itself would have made a difference for the SU trainer when he said that he had been on the ward for two and a half days and nobody had spoken to him.
(Jill, student, focus group interview)

The research concluded that SU trainers sought to motivate the participants to avoid PR or to use it compassionately if it became necessary. Their session enabled the training participants to hear and discuss service users' views on PR – an exercise that could promote a reflection on practice and hopefully enhance practice. The diverse subjective perspectives from the research participants portrayed how relaxed the atmosphere was during the interviews. With confidentiality guaranteed, they uninhibitedly shared their experiences, their practices and their intentions for future practice with regard to PR. In the theme 'Their contribution is useful for practice' (see Table 20.1), the resolve to reflect lessons from the SU session in practice was clearly expressed in the records of feedback and by the focus group participants. Meanwhile, the practitioner participants convincingly articulated how the lessons were being reflected in their practices. The study confirms findings from previous studies on SU involvement which claim that their involvement in the education and training of professionals has the potential to positively influence practice [32, 33].

The research has made a difference. When it was presented in Dublin in 2014 at the European Network for Training in the Management of Aggression Conference (ENTMA08) it triggered the development of guidelines on SU involvement in PMVA training delivery. To quote the chairman of the organisation in response to the team's presentation, 'You have convinced me that developing guidelines on best practice in service user involvement in training should be on our next work plan' [34]. In 2019, the Restraint Reduction Network (RRN) training standards recommended the involvement of service users in the development and delivery of any training which involves the use of restrictive interventions [35]. The findings from this study justify these developments.

Conclusion

In the United Kingdom, higher education institutions are mandated by policies and guidelines to involve users of services in the education and training of the health and social care professionals. There is a potential rift between theoretical principles and practice in PMVA, and it is practicable and beneficial to involve service users with lived experience of PR in training in order to motivate practitioners to translate theory into practice. Our experience and the research we carried out suggest that using trainers with lived experience of being restrained is effective in helping staff to better understand the impact of restrictive practices on patients. The training reinforced best practice, was appreciated by staff and showed potential to positively influence practice post-training. Future researchers on the phenomenon should also work with service users/patients in order to gain their perspectives on the subject.

References

1. Nash, M. *A Mixed Methods Approach to Exploring Mental Health Nurses Diabetes Education and Skills Needs*. London: Middlesex University's Research Repository, 2014.

2. McCusker, P., MacIntyre, G., Stewart, A. and Jackson, J. Evaluating the effectiveness of service user and carer involvement in post qualifying mental health social work education in Scotland: Challenges and opportunities. *Journal of Mental Health Training, Education and Practice* 2012; 7 (3):143–53. https://doi.org/10.1108/17556221211269956.

3. Obi-Udeaja, J., Crosby, K., Ryan, G., Sukhram, D. and Holmshaw, J. Service user involvement in training for the therapeutic management of violence and aggression. *Mental Health and Learning Disabilities Research and Practice* 2010; 7(2),185–94.

4. Tew, J., Gell, C. and Forster, S. *Learning from Experience: Involving Service Users and Carers in Mental Health Education and Training*. West Midlands: National institute for mental health in England (NIMHE); 2004.

5. McIntosh, G. L. Exploration of the perceived impact of carer involvement in mental health nurse education: Values, attitudes

and making a difference. *Nurse Education in Practice* 2018, 29:172–8. https://doi.org/10.1016/j.nepr.2018.01.009 [Accessed 30.4.2022].

6. Poreddi, V., Gandhi, S., Thimmaiah, R. and Suresh, B. M. Attitudes toward consumer involvement in mental health services: A cross-sectional survey of Indian medical and nursing undergraduates. *Investigación y Educación en Enfermería* 2016; 34 (2):243–51.

7. Happell, B., Byrne, L., McAllister, M. et al. Consumer involvement in the tertiary-level education of mental health professionals: A systematic review. *International Journal of Mental Health Nursing* 2014; 23:3–16.

8. Rush, B. Mental health service user involvement in England: Lessons from history. *Journal of Psychiatric and Mental Health Nursing* 2004; 11:313–18.

9. NICE. Violence and aggression: Short-term management in mental health, health and community settings: NICE guideline. National Institute for Health and Care Excellence 2015; www.nice.org.uk/guidance/NG10 [Accessed 29.4.2022].

10. Department of Health. A positive and proactive workforce: a guide to workforce development for commissioners and employers seeking to minimise the use of restrictive practices in social care and health. 2014. www.skillsforhealth.org.uk [Accessed 24.4.2022].

11. NMC. Standards for pre-registration nursing education, 2010. http://standards.nmc-uk.org/PublishedDocuments/Standards%20for%20pre-registration%20nursing%20education%2016082010.pdf [Accessed 22.4.2022].

12. Russell, S. Engaging undergraduate mental health nursing students in recovery orientated practice through service user involvement: A mixed methods study. 2014; http://doras.dcu.ie/20195/1/Submitted_PhD_thesis_September_2014.pdf [Accessed 30.4.2022].

13. Perry, J., Watkins, M., Gilbert, A. and Rawlinson, J. A systematic review of the evidence on service user involvement in interpersonal skills training of mental health students. *Journal of Psychiatric and Mental Health Nursing* 2013; 20:525–40.

14. GSA. *Physical skills core curriculum.* General Services Association 2015; www.thegsa.co.uk [Accessed 30.4.2022].

15. Terkelsen, T. B. and Larsen, I. B. Fear, danger and aggression in a Norwegian locked psychiatric ward: dialogue and ethics of care as contributions to combating difficult situations. *Nursing Ethics* 2016:1–10.

16. Paterson, B. Millfields Charter: Drawing the wrong conclusions. *Learning Disability Practice* 2007; vol 10 (no3).

17. Repper, J. and Breeze, J. User and carer involvement in the training and education of health professionals: A review of the literature. *International Journal of Nursing Studies* 2007; 44:511–19. www.qub.ac.uk/sites/PatientandCarerEducationPartnership/Filestore/Filetoupload,822710,en.pdf.

18. Hatton, K. A critical examination of the knowledge contribution service user and carer involvement brings to social work education. *Social Work Education* 2017; 36 (2):154–71. https://doi.org/10.1080/02615479.2016.1254769.

19. Terry, J. M. The pursuit of excellence and innovation in service user involvement in nurse education programmes: Report from a travel scholarship. *Nurse Education in Practice* 2013; 13:202–6.

20. Webber, M. and Robinson, K. The meaningful involvement of service users and carers in Advanced-Level Post-Qualifying Social Work Education: A qualitative study. *British Journal of Social Work* 2011; 42:1256–74.

21. Gilburt, H., Rose, D. and Slade, M. The importance of relationships in mental health care: A qualitative study of service users' experiences of psychiatric hospital admission in the UK. *BMC Health Services Research* 2008; 8:92.

22. Browne, D. *Black People and Sectioning.* Arkansas: Little Rock Publishing; 1997.

23. Bradshaw, C., Atkinson, S. and Doody, O. Employing a qualitative

description approach in health care research. *Global Qualitative Nursing Research* 2017;4:1–8.

24. Sandelowski, M. Focus on research methods: Whatever happened to qualitative description? *Research in Nursing & Health* 2000; 23:334–40.

25. Polit, D. F. and Beck, C. T. *Essentials of Nursing Research*, 9th ed. *Appraising Evidence for Nursing Practice*. New Delhi: Wolters Kluwer (India) Pvt Ltd, 2017.

26. Braun, V., Clarke, V., Hayfield, N. and Terry, G. Thematic analysis. In P. Liamputtong (ed.) *Handbook of Research Methods in Health Social Sciences*. Singapore: Springer; 2018, pp.1–18. https://doi.org/10.1007/978-98 1-10-2779-6_103-1.

27. Braun, V. and Clarke, V. *Successful Qualitative Research: A Practical Guide for Beginners* (1st ed.) 2013. London: Sage Publications Limited.

28. Braun, V. and Clarke, V. Using thematic analysis in psychology. *Qualitative Research in Psychology* 2006; 3(2):77–101. ISSN1478-0887.

29. Ravitch, S. M. and Carl, N. M. *Qualitative Research: Bridging the Conceptual, Theoretical, and Methodological* (2nd ed.). Los Angeles: Sage Publications Inc., 2021.

30. Obi-Udeaja, J. *Exploring the Impact on Practice when Service Users are Involved in Staff Training on the Prevention and Management of Violence and Aggression in Local NHS Mental Health Inpatient Wards.* London: Middlesex University's Research Repository, 2021.

31. Obi-Udeaja, J., Kerr, C. and Weller, G. Impacts of service user involvement in mental health nurse training on management of aggression: a qualitative description research. *Work Based Learning e-Journal* 2020; 9(2.b). https://files .eric.ed.gov/fulltext/EJ1280816.pdf [Accessed 30.4.2022].

32. Spencer, J., Godolphin, W., Karpenko, N. and Towle, A. *Can Patients be Teachers? Involving Patients and Service Users in Healthcare Professionals' Education.* London: The Health Foundation, 2011.

33. Turnbull, P. and Weeley, F. M. Service user involvement: inspiring student nurses to make a difference to patient care. *Nurse Education in Practice* 2013; 13:454–8.

34. Paterson, B. Email communication, Jan. 2015.

35. Ridley, J. and Leitch, S. *Restraint Reduction Network (RRN)Training Standards*, 1st ed. Birmingham: BILD Publications, 2019.

Chapter

21

Engagement With Patients and Carers to Address and Reduce the Risk of Violence and Aggression

Mary Moss (final draft completed by Masum Khwaja)

Introduction

The aim of the chapter is to stimulate and encourage readers to consider how best to involve and engage patients and carers in their own place of work. The chapter is opinion as well as evidence-based and has been developed in collaboration with local carers, patients and patient leaders. Those who agreed to be mentioned by name include Raf Hamaiza, Vanessa Lee, Alex Garner and David Gilbert. Professional colleagues also made suggestions, and encouragingly, there were major overlaps regarding the suggestions and aspirations of each group.

Those patients and carers I met raised broadly similar concerns about offering insight to support the writing of this chapter, including:

- That their narrative would be responded to only emotionally, as an anecdote, rather than as a meaningful source of information to develop change or to influence service delivery.
- Attempts to systematically use feedback data is seen by some user groups as patient leaders and carers 'selling out' and becoming part of the 'system'.
- Carers and people with lived experience are expected to contribute time and effort without being adequately remunerated, thereby working for free to support services. This confirmed the sense of being used rather than valued and respected.

Despite such concerns, I am deeply grateful that so many agreed to be involved in informing this chapter.

Working with patients and carers in a collaborative way is beset with challenges including the terminology. This chapter adopts the terms used in David Gilbert's *The Patient Revolution*[1], in which those who receive services are described as 'patients' and those who have lived experience and are contributing to influence and change services are 'patient leaders', whilst carers are carers throughout, in line with the Care Act (2014) rather than the earlier, more restrictive definition of the Carers Act (2004). The 2014 act defines a carer as an adult who provides or intends to provide care for another adult (an 'adult needing care') [2]. It should be noted that 'care' can mean practical help or emotional support.

This chapter is dedicated to Fenella Lemonsky, who had lived experience of multiple conditions and sadly died during preparation of the initial draft: she was a generous and forthright person who tirelessly campaigned to improve quality of care using her intuition and sense of fun to help people of all backgrounds make meaningful connections. She challenged the exclusion of service-user-led experience and made sure that use of language was appropriate and respectful.

The United Nations (UN) have adopted the widely used phrase 'nothing about us without us' to emphasise the important principle of equal participation of persons with disabilities in society including in the development of services and policy. The United Nations Convention on the Rights of Persons with Disabilities, was ratified by the UK in 2009 but is yet to be fully implemented [3].

Health service provision is undergoing a period of change wherein the principles of co-production and co-design should be embedded in service models, but this radical egalitarian approach is often substituted by 'inclusion' or 'participation' – terms which do not permit the same level of influence and respect for diverse experience [4]. Education and training of mental health professionals is also lagging, and research often does not include studies or data from the perspective of carers and patients.

Initiatives in trauma-informed care are a good start in reframing the basis for distress and behaviour, but these have not replaced the terminology of personality disorder which is distressing and unacceptable to many [5].

Engaging with patients and carers is an essential part of understanding and developing therapeutic approaches to reduce the risk of aggression and violence, for example, by identifying early warning signs, triggers and minimisation strategies.

Definitions of patient engagement share an underlying theme: 'the facilitation and strengthening of the role of those using services as co-producers of health, and health care policy and practice' [6].

My own journey with this topic began with a relocation to working in a psychiatric intensive care (PICU) setting and my request to spend time in seclusion: this involved me being forcibly taken by the team and laid prone before they exited and locked the door. The whole experience was frightening (even as an experienced consultant who gave capacitous consent to the process), and I encourage colleagues to expose themselves to similar experience and reflect on the impact restrictive practices have on patients who are usually acutely unwell, frightened and have little ability to influence their situation.

Community Engagement

The World Health Organisation (WHO) defines community engagement as 'a process of developing relationships that enable stakeholders to work together to address health-related issues and promote well-being to achieve positive health impact and outcomes' [7, p. vii].

To plan services that effectively serve a population, it is necessary to quantify the demographics and needs of a population and to identify *barriers to engagement*. Raising awareness of mental illness, challenging stigma and improving the acceptability of services are necessary considerations if barriers to engagement are to be overcome and equity of mental health care achieved for all members of a community.

The empowering principles of social inclusion, citizenship and recovery have influenced mental health policy in several English-speaking countries, including the United Kingdom, Ireland, the USA, Canada Australia and New Zealand, and are concepts mental health staff are increasingly familiar with and supportive of [8].

In a recently published paper, Khan and Tracy [9] discuss the difficulties in embedding 'recovery concepts into professionally directed treatment of disease' (p. 1) without moving away from ('distortion') of what matters most to service users. The Sainsburys centre has described a practical methodology to help mental health services and their local partners become more 'recovery-oriented' in their organisation and practices [10].

The value of citizenship in promoting mental health is explained in a paper by Macintyre and colleagues [11]. The promotion of the voting rights of mental health patients by Central and North West London Foundation Trust (CNWL FT) is a good example of an initiative that acknowledges the importance of citizenship and social inclusion in facilitating recovery from mental illness. CNWL FT actively support patients to register to vote and to cast their vote, should they wish to, prior to local and national elections. Interested readers should access the information and resources available on the CNWL website and consider co-producing a similar initiative in their own Trusts [12].

Service Engagement

The principles of co-production and co-design are central here, with patient leaders helping determine the shape of services and individual patients making a meaningful contribution to and having influence over their care plan. Patient leaders should have a clear role in the organisation, with access to senior staff, to ensure that their views are incorporated into service developments. There should be open and honest dialogue about the reality of funding and changes to services that are being considered.

There should be clear governance arrangements to ensure that patients and carers are represented at all levels of the organisation. In Sussex Partnership NHS Foundation Trust, those in senior patient leader and carer roles have mentors drawn from director- and board-level staff so that they are engaged at the highest levels of the service and their development and influence is embedded within the organisational structure. Engagement with patients extends from the ward in which day-to-day frustrations are raised and addressed using a 'you said we did' model with a poster confirming concerns of patients ('you said') and actions in response by staff ('we did') to more formal structures of feedback and engagement. Ideally, each department or ward feeds back to a locality service management meeting, which should include service users, carers, clinicians and managers and, if necessary, progress to directorate and board level if the issue of concern is not resolved.

This model of collating, sharing and addressing issues is common to many parts of the NHS (and to some private sector providers). For example, Leicestershire Partnership NHS Trust (LPT) have established a 'Peoples Council' whose purpose is 'to help shape the Trusts approach to engagement and to improving patient experience by advising on the best ways to reach out to communities and individuals and to feedback and review the experience of those who use or who are impacted by the service delivered by LPT' [13].

For governance structures to have an impact on reducing the risk of violence, there must be a clear pathway for addressing concerns and assurance that they will be acted upon. This will help reduce some of the frustration felt by those with lived experience who are asked to present their narratives to senior staff only to feel re-traumatised by experiencing the events again without any discernible gain for themselves or peers.

Building a culture of gathering and responding to feedback from those using the service is likely to improve patient satisfaction, quality of care and safety. An example of a small local change actioned following patient feedback was a proposal to change the layout of the intercom for the seclusion room as the relative position of the speakers meant that people could not make eye contact, which was frightening and caused unnecessary additional distress. Patients were happy that staff had responded to their concerns and staff were pleased that a potential trigger for behavioural disturbance had been identified and removed.

Following the use of restrictive interventions, post-incident debriefs are useful to identify and address factors that led to an incident. Debriefs use a framework for anticipating and reducing violence and aggression and aim to reduce the likelihood of the incident happening again. The principle that patients and carers, as well as staff who were directly involved or witnessed the incident, are involved in debriefs is endorsed by the National Collaborating Centre for Mental Health programme to reduce restrictive practices [14]. The National Institute for Health and Care Excellence (NICE) emphasises the importance of ensuring patients have an opportunity 'to talk about what happened, why the restraint was used and how they feel about it' [15, p. 23].

Mental health services should consider involvement in the RCPsych accreditation programmes and quality care networks which seek to improve the quality of care provided for patients and their carers. The quality networks use a process of regular peer review and self-review against service standards to promote high-quality care. Service standards include standards for engagement. Patient and carer involvement in all stages of the development programme is emphasised [16].

Engagement With Staff

A major concern raised by patients and carers is the lack of continuity of care. This is inherent in the functional model of care, wherein people fall under multiple teams even during a single episode of ill health, and is exacerbated by recruitment and retention issues in mental health staffing. Repeating a history to multiple staff across many teams is invalidating, frustrating and traumatic, often representing an early trigger for distress and outbursts.

Furthermore, the previous view of severe and enduring mental illness (SMI) requiring long-term support from specialist mental health services has been replaced by a recovery-based approach with the aim of discharge back to primary care and peer-led services.

The switch from the combined community and inpatient care (sectorised) model to the functional inpatient one aimed to improve 'patient flow' and provide consistency for the ward multidisciplinary team, but it broke an important link at a time when patients are most vulnerable. In a large European study, the move to functional inpatient care has been shown to lead to much greater patient dissatisfaction than with the sectorised system [17].

Continuity of care is as important to address in primary care as it is in secondary care, as highlighted by a recent observational cohort study in primary care which showed that, for those with SMI, seeing the same primary care professional ('higher relational continuity') and having a care plan were both associated with a significantly lower risk of unplanned hospital use for physical and mental health problems [18].

It is noteworthy that the early studies of continuity of care were written from the clinician's point of view [19], whilst more recent ones use patient and carer appraisal to assess continuity of care [20] and give more emphasis to the patient experience and value.

Boredom on the wards is strongly associated with poor outcomes, particularly self-harming behaviours and aggression. Initiatives such as Star Wards found that 60% of participating wards reported a reduction in aggression with implementation of their activity and well-being-based programme [21]. Activities should be routinely available on each ward, with an emphasis on the preferences and needs of each patient with regard to the duration and intensity they can tolerate: for some it may be an activity to make a connection with staff, such as a board game or sporting activity, whilst others may wish for a more therapeutic and exploratory session, such as psychology or art therapy.

I was originally approached to write this chapter because of my work with Mutley, my therapy dog, who regularly visits the ward, and his impact on the engagement with staff and patients [22]. He is a model for positive engagement and is very enthusiastic about coming to work; during each visit, he usually interacts with 80% of the patients, and he respects the space of those who are not interested in him. During his visits I noticed a marked increase in positive interactions between patients and increased interaction with staff. Repeatedly, patients de-escalated themselves and each other because 'we mustn't worry Mutley'. I noticed I was being approached regularly by patients for one-to-one time and realised it was because they wanted to spend time with the dog. Mutley's presence reduced the sense of hierarchy and enabled us to talk more freely. Mutley's positive impact is replicated by Buddy, the therapy dog affiliated to the Safe Wards [23] model, whose owner is a service user and who developed Safe Wards. Readers interested in animal-assisted therapy (AAT) are directed to an interesting narrative expert review with a systematic literature search which 'highlights the promising potential of AAT to relieve symptoms leading to aggressive behavior' [24].

Changing the model of staff deployment is also important in reducing the risk of incidents. Shoreditch Ward, a fourteen-bedded medium-secure service for men with intellectual disabilities in East London, identified that most of the staff time was spent on responding to incidents rather than providing care which might have reduced the risk of incidents. This observation was formulated into the 'Flip the Triangle' model, which aims to redirect the bulk of staff time taken up by dealing with crisis situations to increasing focus on positive and proactive interventions, with the intention of maintaining the ward as a settled therapeutic environment [25].

Staff Training

Various initiatives to manage violence have been developed over the years, and increasingly staff training involves those with lived experience.

For those with intellectual disabilities, initiatives such as Positive Behaviour Support and Calm Cards are useful to help staff understand and de-escalate potentially volatile situations without resort to restrictive practice or medication [26].

The Safe Wards Programme works alongside the Star Wards initiative and focuses on changing the interactions on the ward between staff and patients. Staff are taught about conflict-originating factors and flashpoints, and they learn how to identify and reduce the potential for conflict [21, 23].

Prevention Management of Violence and Aggression (PMVA) and de-escalation training is a requirement when working in a mental health environment; service-user involvement in PMVA is discussed in Chapter 20.

Many of the perceived benefits, fallacies and obstacles to involving service users in the design and delivery of education and training are discussed in a useful document produced by the Health Professionals Council [27].

Involvement of those with lived experience should be an essential part of staff training; however, it is often overlooked and undervalued. For example, the statutory training courses for Section 12 doctors and approved clinicians under the Mental Health Act 1983 require input by service-user representatives; yet in many instances this is covered by a video or a service user attending for a brief presentation. There is a powerful difference if the service user is present and remains throughout the day as attendees switch their focus from the arcana of the Mental Health Act to the implications of depriving someone of their liberty.

Simulation training is a burgeoning part of health education and offers an opportunity to enact clinical scenarios in controlled conditions with professional actors. This gives staff the chance to reflect on their own, and other participants', interaction style(s) with patients. As well as actors, it is useful to employ those with lived experience, who may be helpfully engaged in scenarios or providing feedback.

Videos featuring people with lived experience are also useful educational tools. To aid staff in collaborative and supportive working for autistic individuals, Sussex Partnership Trust produced a patient-led video that demonstrated the agitation and overwhelming distress experienced by those with fixed routines and sensory processing problems when they are rushed into a noisy and crowded environment. The video offered valuable insight and was considered particularly effective because it was patient led.

Engaging With Family and Carers

Carers I spoke to raised concerns regarding lack of information-sharing and a misunderstanding about listening to family experiences versus confidential information-sharing. Carers were also concerned about the impact on relationships if they were seen to work with staff in a collaborative way, and of the potential to themselves become victims of aggression and violence due to the closeness of their relationship with the person they were caring for.

A family member's inability to articulate the wish for and/or a lack of capacity to agree to family involvement in care was also a concern and parents of those with neurodevelopmental disorders and learning disabilities explained how they may find themselves excluded from information-sharing and decision-making when their family member reaches adulthood. An inability to articulate the wish for and/or a lack of capacity to agree to family involvement in care was also a concern.

In many incidents and inquiries, lack of engagement with carers is identified as an area of concern. Initiatives such as the Triangle of Care emphasise that the provision of safe, good-quality care requires a three-way relationship between carers, patients and staff [28]. The key standards identified for this are:

1. Carers and the essential role they play are identified at the first contact or as soon as possible thereafter.
2. Staff are 'carer aware' and trained in carer-engagement strategies.
3. Policy and practice protocols with regard to confidentiality and sharing information are in place.
4. Defined post(s) responsible for carers are in place.
5. A carer introduction to the service and staff is available, with a relevant range of information across the care pathway.
6. A range of carer support services is available.

The carers involved in providing information for this chapter all wished for direct contact and support, whether it be from staff or peers. They said that finding oneself 'dismissed' with a pile of leaflets felt disrespectful and disempowering, and it did not give them the opportunity they wanted to share or receive information about the person they were caring for.

Carers usually have a unique knowledge of patients and involving carers, especially at a time when a patient may be too unwell to make their own choices regarding care, may help to ensure patient preferences for treatment are taken into consideration when establishing a care plan. Carers may also pass on useful information, such as support strategies to help calm a patient, preferred interests and sources of reassurance (plus things to avoid) that can help staff to build a therapeutic relationship with a patient and thereby reduce the risk of aggression.

Discharge planning should be co-produced with patients and their support networks, and involving carers is likely to ensure better outcomes.

One of the frustrations voiced by carers and those with lived experience who contributed to this chapter, and shared by me both as a recipient of services and as a practitioner, is the repeated cycle of 'rediscovery' of effective models of care, with initiatives being dismantled only to reappear in slightly different guises. Family-work initiatives were identified as highly beneficial from the 1970s, with Vaughan and Leff's [29] studies on expressed emotion, the specialist Thorn training schemes for community nurses in the 1990s, inpatient Star Ward training in the early 2000s, and the family intervention models for early intervention for psychosis with open dialogue being implemented most recently [30]. One way to reduce some of this frustration is to ensure that patients and carers are fully informed of the drivers behind change and are meaningfully involved in the decision-making process when changes to service provision are proposed.

Engaging With the Patients

The flashpoints identified by service users I spoke to were very much in line with the framework used in the Safe Wards model, with boundaries, delays and restrictions, combined with a feeling of being disrespected by staff, all being potent triggers.

There is an inherent power differential for patients who face the reality of imposed treatment and admission under the Mental Health Act due to the undermining of choice and personal autonomy. This can lead to frustration and an escalation in volatility as a response to the coercive nature of treatment. Attempts to redress this power differential by changing terminology (e.g. using the term 'service leaders') is seen by many as patronising and disingenuous. The change in terminology, they would argue, represents superficial change only, and one that attempts to mask the reality of the power differential.

Care planning, whether for admission or discharge, offers staff an opportunity to listen and respond to patient and carer concerns by meaningfully involving them in the care-planning process. Section 10 of the Care Act 2014 states that patients and carers should be in control of their care, actively involved in care planning and have an opportunity to lead or strongly influence the planning and subsequent content of their care plan [31]. Co-producing comprehensive care plans that meet people's changing needs and that are patient-centred is a key message of NICE guideline NG53 [32].

It must be remembered that patients in an acute setting will also be feeling vulnerable and unfamiliar with their surroundings and care team. Good provision of information and clear signage can help to reduce anxiety by ensuring information is given in a direct and unambiguous manner to reduce uncertainty. Documenting times of meetings or leave and adhering to this both shows respect and gives reassurance.

The concept of relational security ('See Think Act') gives the staff the opportunity to consider not only the individual patient but also the patient mix on the ward as well as ensuring that boundaries are implemented in a consistent fashion for individual patients and by the team as a whole [32]. This can reduce the sense of favouritism that may be a trigger for alienation and retaliation.

The Other Victims of Violence

The original brief of this chapter was about engagement of users and carers in strategies for the prevention and management of aggression. Implicit in this was the notion that service users were the perpetrators of the violence. However, many narratives from service users and carers, particularly with regard to experiences in assessment and treatment units, or when subject to restraint and forced medication, identified the service users as victims of violence at the hands of staff. This is endorsed by the recent inquiries into the care provided in settings such as Whorlton Hall [34], St Andrews [35] and Winterbourne View [36], and there is an increasing sense of frustration that, despite regular inspection regimes, these matters are not identified and managed in a timely way. Too often the responsibility is passed on to the most junior and unqualified members of the staff team. Concerns were also raised about the utility of the Care Quality Commission (CQC) Inspection process. This is highly significant as patients are often marginalised and unheard; the duty of professionals is not merely to manage them into safe conformity, but to ensure they have access to all safeguards. Each professional must remember their duty of care, duty of candour and the access to a Freedom to Speak Up Guardian. Each unit should also clearly display information on how to register a complaint and how to contact the patient advice and liaison service (PALS) and the CQC.

Conclusion

There is no doubt that patients want to be involved in decisions about their treatment and that carers want to be listened to and supported in their role as carers. Acknowledging that people who use mental health services have invaluable knowledge and expertise that can be harnessed for the benefit of research, policy and practice in mental health is the fundamental principle behind co-production. Patients and carers should be meaningfully involved in education, research and policy development, and at all levels of a service, from the frontline ward or community team to the executive-board level.

References

1. Gilbert, D. *The Patient Revolution: How We Can Heal the Healthcare System*. Illustrated ed. London: Jessica Kingsley Publishers. 2019.

2. GOV.UK. Care Act 2014. [online]. www.legislation.gov.uk/ukpga/2014/23/section/10 [Accessed 14.4.2022].

3. United Nations. Convention on the Rights of Persons with Disabilities. www.un.org/development/desa/disabilities/convention-on-the-rights-of-persons-with-disabilities.html [Accessed 31.12.22].

4. Writer, A., Coproduction – Radical Roots, Radical Results. [Blog] Fragments from a half-life Ally Writes. [Online]. 2019. https://allywritesblog.wordpress.com/2019/11/10/ [Accessed 14.4.2022].

5. Sweeney, A., Filson, B., Kennedy, A., Collinson, L. and Gillard, S. A paradigm shift: Relationships in trauma-informed mental health services. *BJPsych Advances* 2018 Sep;24(5):319–33. https://doi.org/10.1192/bja.2018.29. PMID: 30174829; PMCID: PMC6088388.

6. Carman, K. L., Dardess, P., Maurer, M. et al. Patient and family engagement: A framework for understanding the elements and developing interventions and policies. *Health Affairs (Millwood)* 2013 Feb;32(2):223–31. https://doi.org/10.1377/hlthaff.2012.1133. PMID: 23381514.

7. World Health Organization. Community engagement: A health promotion guide for universal health coverage in the hands of the people. October 2020. Community engagement: a health promotion guide for universal health coverage in the hands of the people. www.who.int/publications/i/item/9789240010529 [Accessed 10.4.2022].

8. Boardman, J. and Shepherd, G. RECOVERY: Implementing recovery in mental health services. *International Psychiatry* 2012 Feb 1;9(1):6–8. PMID: 31508109; PMCID: PMC6735049.

9. Khan, N. and Tracy, D. K. The challenges and necessity of situating 'illness narratives' in recovery and mental health treatment. *BJPsych Bulletin.* 2022 Apr;46 (2):77–82. https://doi.org/10.1192/bjb.2021.4. PMID: 33597058.

10. Shepherd, G., Boardman, J. and Burns, M. *Implementing Recovery: A Methodology for Organisation Change.* London: Sainsbury Centre for Mental Health. 2010.

11. MacIntyre, G., Cogan, N. A., Stewart, A. E. et al. 'What's citizenship got to do with mental health? Rationale for inclusion of citizenship as part of a mental health strategy', *Journal of Public Mental Health* 2019. 18(3):157–61. https://doi.org/10.1108/JPMH-04-2019-0040.

12. CNWL NHS FT. Voting Rights of Patients with Mental illness or intellectual disability. [online], 2022. www.cnwl.nhs.uk/patients-and-carers/voting-rights [Accessed 21.4.2022].

13. Leicestershire Partnership NHS Trust. The Peoples council. www.leicspart.nhs.uk/involving-you/the-peoples-council/ [Accessed 1.4.2022].

14. National Collaborating Centre for Mental Health. [online]. 2018. www.rcpsych.ac.uk/improving-care/nccmh/reducing-restrictive-practice [Accessed 14.4.2022].

15. NICE. Violent and aggressive behaviours in people with mental health problems. Quality standard [QS154]; Quality statement 5: Immediate post-incident debrief. [online], June 2017. www.nice.org.uk/guidance/qs154/chapter/quality-statement-5-immediate-post-incident-debrief [Accessed 21.4.2022].

16. Royal College of Psychiatrists. Quality networks and accreditation. www.rcpsych.ac.uk/improving-care/ccqi/quality-networks-accreditation [Accessed 10.4.2022].

17. Bird, V. J., Giacco, D., Nicaise, P. et al. In-patient treatment in functional and sectorised care: patient satisfaction and length of stay. *British Journal of Psychiatry* 2018;212(2):81–7.

18. Ride, J., Kasteridis, P., Gutacker, N. et al. Impact of family practice continuity of care on unplanned hospital use for people with serious mental illness. *Health Services Research* 2019 Dec;54(6):1316–25. https://doi.org/10.1111/1475-6773.13211. Epub 2019 Oct 9. PMID: 31598965; PMCID: PMC6863233.

19. Bindman, J., Johnson, S., Szmukler, G. et al. Continuity of care and clinical outcome: A prospective cohort study. *Social Psychiatry and Psychiatric Epidemiology* 2000 Jun;35(6):242–7. https://doi.org/10.1007/s001270050234. PMID: 10939422.

20. Burns, T., Catty, J., Harvey, K. et al. Continuity of care for carers of people with severe mental illness: results of a longitudinal study. *International Journal of Social Psychiatry* 2013 Nov;59(7):663–70. https://doi.org/10.1177/0020764012450996. Epub 2012 Aug 17. PMID: 22904167.

21. Star Wards. [online]. 2004. www.starwards.org.uk/ [Accessed 14.4.2022].

22. Sussex Partnerships NHS Foundation Trust. Mutley Moss, the therapy dog. [online]. www.sussexpartnership.nhs.uk/positive-practice-awards/mutley-moss-therapy-dog [Accessed 14.4.2022].

23. Safe wards. [online]. www.safewards.net/ [Accessed 14.4.2022].

24. Widmayer, S., Borgwardt, S., Lang, U. E. and Huber, C. G. Could animal-assisted

therapy help to reduce coercive treatment in psychiatry? *Frontiers in Psychiatry* 2019 Nov 14;10:794. https://doi.org/10 .3389/fpsyt.2019.00794. PMID: 31798469; PMCID: PMC6867966.

25. Whittle, C., Chingosho, G., Parker, K. et al. Flip the triangle: Using quality improvement methods to embed a positive behaviour support approach on a medium secure forensic ward for men with intellectual disabilities. *BMJ Open Quality* 2021 Oct;10(4): e001514. https://doi.org/10 .1136/bmjoq-2021-001514. PMID: 34667033; PMCID: PMC8527158.

26. The Challenging Behaviour Foundation. Positive behaviour support. www .challengingbehaviour.org.uk/information-and-guidance/positive-behaviour-support/p bs-your-questions/ [Accessed 10.4.2022].

27. Faculty of Health & Social Care Sciences, Kingston University and St George's, University of London. Professor Mary Chambers & Dr Gary Hickey. Service user involvement in the design and delivery of education and training programmes leading to registration with the Health Professions Council. www.hcpc-uk.org/glo balassets/resources/reports/service-user-involvement-in-the-design-and-delivery-of-education-and-training-programmes.pdf [Accessed 10.4.2022].

28. Carerstrust. The Triangle of Care. Carers Included: A Guide to Best Practice in Mental Health Care. [online]. 2013. https:// carers.org/downloads/resources-pdfs/tri angle-of-care-england/the-triangle-of-care -carers-included-second-edition.pdf [Accessed 14.4.2022].

29. Vaughn, C. E. and Leff, J. P. The influence of family and social factors on the course of psychiatric illness: A comparison of schizophrenic and depressed neurotic patients. *British Journal of Psychiatry* 1976 Aug;129:125–37. https://doi.org/10.1192/b jp.129.2.125. PMID: 963348.

30. North East London NHS Foundation Trust. The NHS Open Dialogue Project. [online].

www.nelft.nhs.uk/aboutus-initiatives-opendialogue [Accessed 14.4.2022].

31. Department of Health. Care and Support Statutory Guidance Issued under the Care Act 2014. 2014 [online]. https://assets.publishing.service.gov.uk/ government/uploads/system/uploads/att achment_data/file/506202/23902777_ Care_Act_Book.pdf [Accessed 22.4.2022].

32. NICE. Transition between inpatient mental health settings and community or care home settings. NICE guideline [NG53] Key message 3: Co-producing comprehensive care plans that meet people's changing needs [online 2016] www.nice.org.uk/guidance/ng53/resource s/tailored-resources-4429245855/chapter/ 3-co-producing-comprehensive-care-plans-that-meet-peoples-changing-needs#the-guideline-and-legislation-3 [Accessed 22.4.2022].

33. Royal College of Psychiatrists. See Think Act. 2nd ed. [online]. 2015. www .rcpsych.ac.uk/docs/default-source/improv ing-care/ccqi/quality-networks/secure-forensic/forensic-see-think-act-qnfmhs/st a_hndbk_2nded_web.pdf?sfvrsn=90e1f c26_4 [Accessed 14.4.2022].

34. Triggle, N. Whorlton Hall: Hospital 'abused' vulnerable adults. BBC, May 2019 [online]. www.bbc.co.uk/news/health-483 67071 [Accessed 14.4.2022].

35. Bowden, G., The Huffington Post. Dispatches Investigation Finds Shocking Treatment Of Child Mental Health Patients [online]. March 2017. www .huffingtonpost.co.uk/entry/dispatches-channel-4-investigation-finds-shocking-treatment-of-child-mental-health-patients_uk_58b6d894e4b0a8a9b787c89d [Accessed 14.4.2022].

36. BBC. Undercover reporter 'haunted' by abuse of patients. Panorama. [online]. 2011. www.bbc.co.uk/panorama/hi/front_ page/newsid_9501000/9501531.stm [Accessed 14.4.2022].

Index

Printed in the United States
by Baker & Taylor Publisher Services